重庆市高等教育医学专业英语精品规划教材

A Coursebook for Writing English Biomedical Journal Paper

生物医学期刊英文论文写作教程

主 编 王 燕 刘 艳

副主编 田俊英 谭阳阳

编 者（按姓氏笔画顺序排列）

王 燕 田俊英 牟 君

刘 艳 张志全 谭阳阳

重庆大学出版社

内容提要

本教程贯穿专业、规范、实用的编写思想,选用英美著名医学期刊论文为素材,从介绍英文论文的选词、造句和成段特点入手,深入讲解论文各部分的内容、结构、语言特点与写作要点。既可以供医学专业高年级本科生和研究生作为教科书使用,也可以供医学工作者、双语教师或医学英语教师作为参考书使用。

图书在版编目(CIP)数据

生物医学期刊英文论文写作教程／王燕,刘艳主编. --重庆:重庆大学出版社,2020.8(2022.7 重印)
ISBN 978-7-5689-2191-6

Ⅰ.①生… Ⅱ.①王… ②刘… Ⅲ.①生物医学工程—论文—英语—写作—教材 Ⅳ.①R318

中国版本图书馆 CIP 数据核字(2020)第 093478 号

生物医学期刊英文论文写作教程
主 编 王 燕 刘 艳
责任编辑:高小平 版式设计:高小平
责任校对:夏 宇 责任印制:赵 晟

＊

重庆大学出版社出版发行
出版人:饶帮华
社址:重庆市沙坪坝区大学城西路 21 号
邮编:401331
电话:(023)88617190 88617185(中小学)
传真:(023)88617186 88617166
网址:http://www.cqup.com.cn
邮箱:fxk@cqup.com.cn(营销中心)
全国新华书店经销
重庆升光电力印务有限公司印刷

＊

开本:787mm×1092mm 1/16 印张:17.5 字数:479 千
2020 年 8 月第 1 版 2022 年 7 月第 3 次印刷
ISBN 978-7-5689-2191-6 定价:55.00 元

前　言

1. 编写说明

当今社会,国际交流日趋频繁和专业,高校英语教学迎来了重要的转向,即由通用英语向专门用途英语的范式转移。在医科院校的英语教学中,将通用英语向医学专业英语扩展,实施专门化教学,既符合英语与专业知识相长的教学规律,也有助于学生掌握学科特定的语言交流方式,为融入学科的话语团体,实现准确、有效的国际交流打下基础。为此,重庆医科大学的外语教学进行了课程改革以及配套的教材建设。

《生物医学期刊英文论文写作教程》的编写主要针对医学研究生。高校研究生阶段培养的是高层次的专业人才,对应的英语教学应同时体现专业性、学术性和实用性,学术论文写作能力的培养则是其中重要的一环。教育部办公厅《关于进一步规范和加强研究生培养管理的通知》(教研厅〔2019〕1号)就明确要求"把论文写作指导课程作为必修课纳入研究生培养环节"。我校早在2005年就开设了针对研究生层次的"医学英语写作"课程,于2008年编写出版了《医学英语翻译与写作教程》并沿用至今。经过多年的建设发展,该课程于2019年获批重庆市研究生教育优质课程建设项目,并更名为"SCI论文阅读与写作",教授内容更具针对性和学术性。本教程受该项目经费资助,基于课程团队多年的理论研究和教学实践,对现用教材进行优化编写而成。

2. 编写原则

课程团队在教学中采用了基于语篇体裁的专门用途英语教学法。本教程的编写沿用此思路,重点选择研究论文、文献综述和病例报告三种论文体裁,以研究论文为主,其他类型为辅;同时,对论文内容化整为零,分层介绍,涉及字词、语句、段落和篇章四个层次。遵循真实性、代表性、时效性原则,本教程优选了英美著名医学期刊上发表的论文,向学习者展示论文的体裁结构和语言样式,并针对重要语言现象进行专题讲解以帮助学习者掌握论文写作的基本语言知识,培养其运用体裁进行知识阅读和论文写作的能力。本教程贯彻专业、规范、实用的编写思想,既可以供医学专业高年级本科生和研究生作为教科书使用,也可以供医学工作者、双语教师或医学英语教师作为参考书使用。

3. 编写特色

(1)医学英语的词汇特征

生物医学期刊英文论文写作的质量很大程度上依赖于学习者对医学英语文体特点的熟

悉和掌握程度。医学英语文体特点中最突出的是医学英语词汇。掌握医学英语词汇的构词特点及使用原则对医学英语文献的阅读、理解和写作至关重要。本教程全面介绍了医学英语的词汇类型及其特征,包括来源于希腊和拉丁语的医学术语,以人名、地名等冠名的冠名术语,以及从普通英语中借用的两栖医学词汇、医学形象性描述语等,学习者学习之后对纷繁复杂的医学英语词汇一定会有豁然开朗的感觉。

(2)英文医学论文的写作规范

不积跬步,无以至千里。论文写作的基础是单个的语句,医学英语的语句与普通英语的语句有显著不同,着力于准确、简练、规范。本教程以编辑纠错的视角对论文语句写作中的常犯错误进行了举例和分析说明,旨在帮助学习者掌握正确的语句写作知识。在熟悉语句写作规范的基础上,本教程还对段落内以及段落间的逻辑架构进行了介绍和说明,配以详实的例子,让学习者对论文写作的认识自然过渡到篇章,也希望借此让学习者触类旁通,了解并掌握医学论文的谋篇布局。

(3)生物医学期刊英文论文的写作指要

生物医学期刊英文论文是一种具有特定内容、风格及受众的固定体裁,遵循研究性论文的传统结构,包括引言、方法、结果和讨论。本教程根据国际医学期刊编辑委员会公布的国际标准《学术研究实施与报告和医学期刊编辑与发表的推荐规范》,简称"ICMJE 推荐规范",运用专门用途英语研究中的文本学(Text Typology)理论,对论文各部分的体裁结构和语言表现样式作了详实的讲解。该教程注重专业性和实用性,所选论文素材涵盖基础和临床类生物医学论文,既呈现论文的统一写作标准,又反映目标杂志的特殊要求,为学习者提供可效仿的内容结构和语言形式,同时借助翻译实践活动帮助学习者强化体裁意识和运用体裁知识的能力。

《生物医学期刊英文论文写作教程》由重庆医科大学和新乡医学院长期从事本科生和研究生医学英语教学和研究的骨干教师及重庆医科大学附属第一医院的医生编写。在编写过程中,编者优选了《柳叶刀》《新英格兰医学杂志》《英国医学会杂志》《美国医学会杂志》《细胞》和其他国外医学杂志期刊及医学信息检索网站 PubMed 上刊登的许多宝贵资料,我们向这些期刊的编辑部和论文作者表示诚挚的谢意!除此之外,我们还使用了在平时的医学论文英文摘要编辑和医学英语教学工作中收集到的第一手资料,目的是反映国内医学工作者在撰写英文摘要和论文时存在的问题,以便进行针对性的讲解。重庆医科大学翻译专业的硕士研究生也参与了资料的收集工作,在此我们对这些作者和学生表示感谢!最后,向支持本教程出版的重庆大学出版社表示感谢!

编　者

2020 年 7 月

目　录

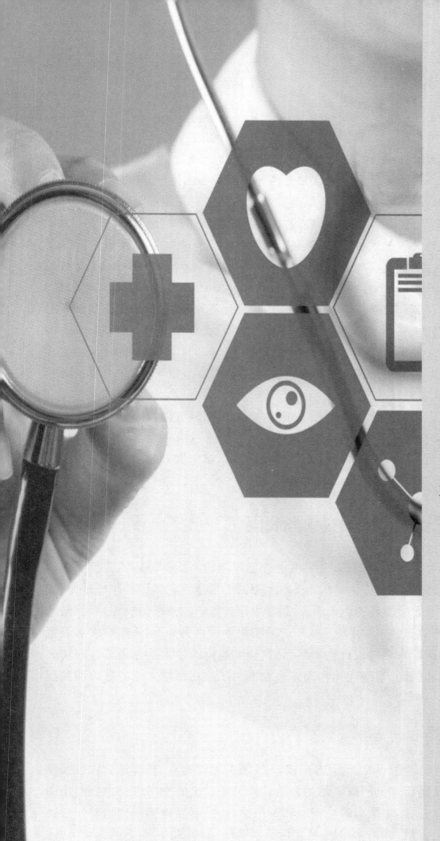

第

1

章

生物医学英文
文献的语言特
征

生物医学文献是经过人类组织、加工,可以存取并能够满足人类需求的各种医学文献的集合。生物医学文献按照不同的划分方法可以划分为不同的类型。第一,按载体类型可分为书写型、印刷型、缩微型、视听型和电子型文献。其中印刷型文献是图书馆收藏文献的主要类型。第二,按出版类型可分为图书、期刊、会议文献、科技报告、政府出版物、专利文献、技术标准、产品资料、学位论文和技术档案。其中的图书基本上分两大类:一类是供读者阅读的图书,如专著、教科书,著名的医学教科书有:《格氏解剖学》(Gray's Anatomy)、《希式内科学》(Cecil Textbook of Medicine)、《克氏外科学》(Sabiston Textbook of Surgery)等;一类是供读者查阅的图书,如字典、百科全书等。其中的期刊,又称杂志,是一种连续出版发行的文献,著名的医学期刊有:《新英格兰医学杂志》(The New England Journal of Medicine)、《柳叶刀》(The Lancet)等。自然科学期刊有:《科学》(Science)、《自然》(Nature)、《细胞》(Cell)等。第三,按文献内容的加工深度和内容性质可分为一次文献(即原始文献)、二次文献、三次文献和零次文献。①

生物医学英文文献具有严谨的写作原则和固定的内容结构,撰写生物医学期刊英文论文,首先要熟悉生物医学英文文献的语言特征。下面将从医学术语的基础知识(构词成分、构成形式、拼读和复数规则)、医学专业特异性词汇和生物医学英文文献的文体特点三个方面进行详细阐述。

1.1　源于希腊语和拉丁语的医学术语

医学术语是一类具有专门用途的词汇,主要供医务工作者使用或在特定的医疗卫生语境中使用。作为英语词汇的一个分支,医学术语基本上遵循了普通英语单词的构成规律、拼写原则和读音规则。但由于医学发展的历史渊源,医学术语大量吸收外来语词汇,特别是希腊语和拉丁语成分,这就使得部分医学术语不同于普通英语单词。另外,由于医学发展源远流长,学科分支细密,大量医学术语得以产生。然而,这些大量的医学术语在形成过程中大体上都遵循着一定的规律和原则,这些规律和原则也就成为了学习医学术语的基础和前提条件。

1.1.1　医学术语的构词成分

医学英语词汇来源广泛,数量巨大,构词方法多异,主要包括派生法、转类法、合成法、缩略法和逆生法,其中派生法是最常见和最常用的方法。本节所讨论的医学术语主要是指由派生法构成的一系列词汇。派生法是指派生词缀和词根结合,或者黏着词根和黏着词根结合构成单词的方法。因而,医学术语的构词成分包括医学词根、医学词缀(包括前缀和后缀)

---

① 本段对生物医学文献的论述主要参阅郭继军,《医学文献检索与论文写作》,第 5 版,北京:人民卫生出版社,2018 年,第 13-17 页。

和连接元音。

1.1.1.1　医学词根

　　医学词根是医学术语的核心成分,既承载着单词的核心意义,也是单词构成最基本的单位。在意义表达上,医学词根意义单一,无论与单词的其他成分以何种方式搭配,意义均保持不变。如 cardiopathy(心脏病)、myocarditis(心肌炎) 和 electrocardiogram(心电图) 中,共同的词根 cardi-,意义均为"心脏(的)"。在单词形态学意义上,医学词根是将医学单词附加成分全部去掉后,剩下的不可再分的最基本的单位。如 gastritis(胃炎)、transgastric(经胃的) 和 epigastric(上腹部的) 中的 gastr-,以及前例中的 cardi-。

　　医学词根包括两大类:自由词根和黏着词根。自由词根可独立存在,并具有实在的意义,同时也可与其他构词成分连接形成新词。例如 gene(基因),可独立成词,也可参与构成其他词汇,如 oncogene(致癌基因)、genotype(基因型)、genealogy(家族,家谱;家系)、homogeneity(同质)。与自由词根不同,黏着词根虽然具有实在意义,但是不能独立成词,必须与其他构词成分结合才能构成单词。医学词根主要是黏着词根,它们大都来源于希腊语和拉丁语语素,构词能力强大,极大地适应了医学发展对医学新词的需要。

　　按身体各器官系统分,常用词根主要如下:

1. 皮肤系统(integumentary system)

例1

adip(o)-, lip(o)- 脂、脂肪	coll(o)-, coll(a)- 胶
derm(o)-, dermat(o)- 皮肤	epitheli(o)- 上皮
kerat(o)- 角质,角膜	seb(o)-, seb(i)- 皮脂
sudor(o)-, diaphor(o)-, hidr(o)- 汗	therm(o)- 热,温度
trich(o)-, pil(o)- 毛发	ungu(o), onych(o)- 指甲、趾甲

2. 肌肉骨骼系统(musculoskeletal system)

例2

arthr(o)-, articul(o)- 关节	brachi(o)- 臂
carp(o)- 手腕	cervic(o)- 颈
chir(o)- 手	chondri(o)-, chondr(o)- 软骨
clavicul(o)- 锁骨	cost(o)- 肋骨
crani(o)- 颅骨	dors(o)- 背
fibr(o)-, in(o)- 纤维	ligament(o)-, syndesm(o)- 韧带
lumb(o)- 腰	maxill(o)- 上颌
my(o)-, muscul(o)- 肌肉	oste(o)-, osse(o)- 骨
pelv(o)-, pelvi(o)- 骨盆	pod(o)- 足,脚
rachi(o)- 脊柱	radi(o)- 桡骨
sacr(o)- 骶骨	sarc(o)- 肌,肉
thorac(o)- 胸	vertebr(o)-, spondyl(o)- 脊椎

3. 神经系统(nervous system)

例3

aesthesi(o)- 感觉	cerebell(o)- 小脑
cerebr(o)- 大脑	crani(o)- 颅骨
encephal(o)- 脑	gangli(o)- 神经节
medull(o)- 髓	mening(o)- 脑膜
myel(o)- 脊髓	neur(o)- 神经
pont(o)- 脑桥	thalam(o)- 丘脑
vag(o)- 迷走神经	ventricul(o)- 室(心室,脑室)
sympath(o)-, sympathic(o)-, sympathetic(o)- 交感神经	

4. 感觉系统(sensory system)

例4

ambly(o)- 模糊	audi(o)-, aur(i)- 听
aur(o)-, ot(o)- 耳	blephar(o)-, palpebr(o)- 眼睑
cochle(o)- 耳蜗	conjunctiv(o)- 结膜
corne(o)-, kerat(o)-, cerat(o)- 角膜	cycl(o)- 睫状体
dacry(o)-, lacrim(o)- 泪	ir(o)-, irid(o)- 虹膜
myring(o)- 鼓膜	nas(o)-, rhin(o)- 鼻
ocul(o)-, ophthalm(o)- 眼睛	optic(o)-, opt(o)- 视力
phac(o)-, phak(o)- 晶状体	pupill(o)-, cor(o)- 瞳孔
retin(o)- 视网膜	scler(o)- 巩膜
sin(o)- 窦	tonsill(o)- 扁桃体

5. 心血管系统(cardiovascular system)

例5

agglutin(o)- 凝集	angi(o)-, vas(o)- 血管
arteri(o)- 动脉	ather(o)- 粥样的
atri(o)- 心房	capill(o)-, capillari(o)- 毛细血管
cardi(o)- 心脏	circul(o)- 循环
coron(o)- 冠状	electr(o)- 电
erythr(o)- 红,红细胞	hem(o)-, hemat(o)- 血
leuc(o)-, leuk(o)- 白细胞	pericardi(o)- 心包膜
plasm(o)- 血浆	rrhythm(o)- 节律
ser(o)- 血清	sphygm(o)- 脉搏
thromb(o)- 血栓	valv(o)- 瓣膜
ven(o)-, phleb(o)- 静脉	ventricul(o)- 心室

6. 呼吸系统 (respiratory system)

例6

alveol (o) - 肺泡

bronchiol (o) - 细支气管

bronch (o) -, bronchi (o) - 支气管

diaphragmat (o) -, phren (o) - 膈

mediastin (o) - 纵膈

pharyng (o) - 咽

pleur (o) - 胸膜

pneum (o) -, pneumon (o) - 肺, 气

pulmon (o) -, pulm (o) - 肺

spir (o) - 呼吸

steth (o) -, thorac (o) - 胸

trache (o) - 气管

7. 消化系统 (digestive system)

例7

abdomin (o) -, celi (o) -, lapar (o) - 腹

appendic (o) - 阑尾

cec (o) - 盲肠

cholangi (o) - 胆管炎

chol (o) -, chol (e) -, bil (i) - 胆汁

col (o) -, colon (o) - 结肠

dent (i) -, dent (o) -, odont (o) - 牙

duoden (o) - 十二指肠

enter (o) - 肠

esophag (o) - 食管

gastr (o) - 胃

gluc (o) -, glyc (o) -, sacchar (o) - 糖

hepat (o) - 肝

ile (o) - 回肠

jejun (o) - 空肠

labi (o) -, cheil (o) - 唇

lingu (o) -, gloss (o) - 舌头

lip (o) -, steat (o) - 脂肪

or (o) -, stomat (o) - 口

pancreat (o) - 胰腺

pept (i) -, peps (i) - 消化

rect (o) - 直肠

saliv (a) -, sial (o) - 唾液

sigmoid (o) - 乙状结肠

8. 泌尿系统 (urinary system)

例8

cyst (o) - 膀胱

glomerul (o) - 肾小球

pyel (o) - 肾盂

ren (o) -, nephr (o) - 肾

ureter (o) - 输尿管

urethr (o) - 尿道

ur (o) -, uri (o) - 尿

vesic (o) - 囊泡

9. 生殖系统 (reproductive system)

例9

andr (o) - 雄性, 男性

embry (o) - 胚胎

genit (o) - 生殖器

gravid (o) - 妊娠

gyn (o) -, gynec (o) - 女性

mamm (o) -, mast (o) - 乳房

men (o) - 月经

obstetr (o) - 生产, 助产

ovari (o) -, oophor (o) - 卵巢

ov (o) -, ov (i) -, o (o) - 卵子

pen (o) -, phall (o) - 阴茎

placent (o) - 胎盘

prostat (o) - 前列腺

sperm (o) -, spermat (o) - 精子

test(o)-, orchid(o)- 睾丸　　　　umbilic(o)-, omphal(o)- 脐

uter(o)-, hyster(o)-, metr(o)- 子宫　　vagin(o)-, colp(o)- 阴道

10. 内分泌系统(endocrine system)

例10

adren(o)- 肾上腺　　　　　　cortic(o)- 皮质

gluc(o)- 葡萄糖　　　　　　　hormon(o)- 激素

pituitar(i)- 脑垂体　　　　　　secret(o)- 分泌

thym(o)- 胸腺　　　　　　　　thyr(o)-, thyroid(o)- 甲状腺

11. 其他

例11

bacteri(o)- 细菌　　　　　　　carcin(o)- 癌

cyt(o)-, cellul(o)- 细胞　　　　chrom(o)- 颜色

hered(o)- 遗传　　　　　　　　hist(o)-, histi(o)- 组织

hydr(o)- 水　　　　　　　　　hypn(o)-, somn(i)- 睡觉

immun(o)- 免疫　　　　　　　luc(o)-, phot(o)- 光

nucle(o)- 细胞核　　　　　　　onc(o)- 肿瘤

ox(o)-, oxy- 氧　　　　　　　　path(o)- 病理

pharmac(o)- 药　　　　　　　psych(o)-, ment(o)- 心理

radi(o)- 放射　　　　　　　　surgic(o)- 外科

tox(o)-, toxic(o)- 毒　　　　　vir(o)- 病毒

1.1.1.2　医学词缀

医学词缀是与词根结合构成新的语词的词素,按其在单词中的位置,可分为前缀和后缀。

1. 医学前缀

在普通英语中,前缀是指位于单词前部的一个单一字母或字母组合,其作用在于改变或修饰词义,但不能独立成词。在医学英语中,医学前缀具有同样的功能,改变或调整医学单词的意义,但其位置更灵活,既可置于词首,也可位于词的中段。如"肌萎缩"对应的英语单词有两个,即amyotrophy 和 my(o)atrophy,表达否定概念的前缀 a-位置就比较灵活。

前缀按照表述的意义主要分为以下几类:

(1) 表示空间方位的前缀

例12

ante-, antero-, pre- 前　　　　　sinistro- 左

retro-, postero- 后　　　　　　dextro- 右

e-, ec-, exo-, extra- 外　　　　　hyper-, hypso-, super- 上,高

intra-, endo-, eso- 内　　　　　sub-, hypo-, infra- 下

centr-, inter-, meso- 中间　　　　circum-, peri- 周围

in-, en- 里, 内　　　　　　　　　contra- 相反

epi- 上, 外　　　　　　　　　　　dia-, trans-, per- 通过, 穿过

re- 再, 又　　　　　　　　　　　sub- 下

co-, syn-, sym- 合, 共　　　　　anti- 相反

tele- 远　　　　　　　　　　　　para- 近, 旁

（2）表示否定的前缀

例13

a-, an-; anti-; de-; ab-; dis-; il-, im-, in-, ir-; non-; un--

（3）表示数量的前缀

例14

mono-, uni-, haplo- 单一　　　　bi-, di-, diplo-, twi-, du- 双, 二

tri-, triplo- 三　　　　　　　　　tetra-, quadri-, quart- 四

pent-, penta-, quinque- 五, 戊　　hex-, hexa- 六, 己

hepta-, sept- 七, 庚　　　　　　oct- 八, 辛

nona-, noni- 九　　　　　　　　deca-, deka- 十

hecto- 百　　　　　　　　　　　kilo- 千

deci- 十分之一　　　　　　　　　centi- 百分之一

milli- 千分之一, 毫　　　　　　　micro- 百万分之一, 微量

hemi-, semi- 半　　　　　　　　mega- 百万, 兆

macro- 多, 巨大　　　　　　　　poly- 多, 复合

mero- 部分　　　　　　　　　　nulli- 零, 无

hyper-, over-, super-, supra-, ultra- 过多, 超过

hypo-, oligo-, sub- 少, 小, 不足

（4）表示颜色的前缀

例15

leuko-, leuco-, albo-, albumo- 白色

melano-, nigro- 黑色　　　　　　glauco-, polio- 灰色

erythro-, rubo- 红色　　　　　　chloro- 绿色

cyano- 蓝色　　　　　　　　　　xantho- 黄色

（5）其他

例16

homo-, iso- 同　　　　　　　　　hetero-, allo-, para- 异

neo- 新　　　　　　　　　　　　dys-, mal- 不良, 障碍

auto- 自动　　　　　　　　　　　brachy- 短

brady- 慢　　　　　　　　　　　tachy- 快

pseudo- 假, 伪

2. 医学后缀

医学后缀是指位于医学词根之后,用以改变词义或改变词性的一类词素。对于一个医学单词而言,通常后缀是不可或缺的。后缀一般位于词尾,且后面不能再接其他词素。按照后缀的构成形式,医学后缀可分为简单后缀和复合后缀两大类。简单后缀是指由不可再分的单一词缀构成的后缀。如后缀-er(指人或物)和-itis(炎症)。复合后缀是指由词根与简单后缀复合而成的后缀。如后缀-pathy(疾病),是由词根 patho-(疾病、病痛)与后缀-y(表状态、过程、行为等)复合而成的。有些复合后缀还可能是由前缀、词根与简单后缀共同复合而成。如后缀-ectomy(外科上的切除),是由前缀 ec-(去除)、词根 tom-(切)与后缀-y(表状态、过程、行为等)共同复合而成的。

按照语法功能(词性),后缀主要分为以下几类:

(1)名词性后缀

例17

-er,-or,-ist,-ant,-ee,-ent,-an 人,者

-action,-tion,-sion,-ion 表状态

-let 片剂　　　　　　　　　　　　-ity,-ness 表状态,属性

-ary 人或地点　　　　　　　　　　-escence 表状态

-ics 研究,学科　　　　　　　　　-ism 机制,行为,结果

-itis 炎症　　　　　　　　　　　　-oma 肿瘤,病态生长

-osis 异常的或病理的状态

(2)动词性后缀

例18

-ate,-en,-(i)fy,-ize(ise)

(3)形容词性后缀

例19

-ed,-ful,-ish,-less,-like,-ly,-y,-able,-ible,-ive,-ative,-sive,-al,-ic,-ac,-ar,

-eal,-ary,-ous,-oid

(4)副词性后缀

例20

-ly,-ward(s),-wise

按照意义所属类别,后缀主要分为以下几类:

(5)表生理的后缀

例21

后缀	意义	例词
-cele	腔,空洞	blastocele 囊胚腔,分裂腔
-cyte	细胞	monocyte 单核细胞
-esthesia	感觉,感情,意识	anesthesia 感觉缺失

续表

后缀	意义	例词
-genesis	形成,生成	angiogenesis 血管生成
-blast	成……细胞	osteoblast 成骨细胞
-clast	破……细胞	osteoclast 破骨细胞
-stasis	抑制,保持常态	bacteriostasis 抑菌作用

（6）表病理的后缀

例22

后缀	意义	例词
-algia	疼,痛	gastralgia 胃痛
-cele	疝	cystocele 膀胱膨出
-ectasia -ectasis	扩张,膨胀	arteriectasia 动脉扩张
-emia	血症	leukemia 白血病
-iasis	形成,存在	nephrolithiasis 肾结石形成
-lysis	溶解,水解	myolysis 肌溶解
-malacia	软化	osteomalacia 骨软化
-megaly	肿大	hepatomegaly 肝肿大
-dynia	疼,痛	cardiodynia 心痛
-oma	瘤	sarcoma 肉瘤
-pathy	疾病	adenopathy 腺病
-penia	缺乏,不足	leukocytopenia 白血球减少
-philia	异常的瘾,嗜,亲	hydrophilia 亲水性
-phobia	畏惧,恐怖症	hydrophobia 恐水症(狂犬病)
-plegia	中风,麻痹,瘫痪	thermoplegia 热射病,中暑
-ptosis	下垂	blepharoptosis 眼睑
-rrhea	分泌,排出	diarrhea 腹泻
-rrhagia	大量流出	gastrorrhagia 胃出血
-rrhexis	破裂	hepatorrhexis 肝破裂
-schisis	畸形,裂	cheiloschisis 唇裂
-sclerosis	硬化	arteriosclerosis 动脉硬化
-spasm	痉挛	enterospasm 肠痉挛
-stenosis	狭窄	laryngostenosis 喉狭窄

（7）描述治疗的后缀

例23

后缀	意义	例词
-centesis	外科穿刺	thoracentesis 胸腔穿刺术
-clysis	冲洗	bronchoclysis 支气管灌洗
-desis	外科包扎	arthrodesis 关节固定术
-ectomy	切除（术）	appendectomy 阑尾切除术
-gram	记录的结果	electrocardiogram 心电图
-graph	记录的仪器	thermograph 温度记录器
-meter	测量仪器	thermometer 温度计
-metry	测量	pelvimetry 骨盆测量术
-iatry, -iatrics	治疗，医学学科	podiatry 足医术，pediatrics 儿科
-pexy	固定	hepatopexy 肝固定术
-plasty	修复，成形	osteoplasty 骨成形术
-rrhaphy	缝合，修复	nephrorrhaphy 肾缝合术
-scopy	镜检查	cystoscopy 膀胱镜检查
-stomy	造口术、吻合术	gastrostomy 胃造口术
-tomy	切开术	craniotomy 颅骨切开术
-tripsy	研磨	lithotripsy 碎石术
-logy	研究过程，学科	pharmacology 药理学

1.1.1.3 连接元音

在医学术语的构成中，还有另一类重要的词素，即连接元音（combining vowel）。顾名思义，连接元音即在构词中起到连接作用的元音。当两个词根连接时，需保留连接元音。当词根与后缀连接时，如果后缀的首字母是元音，则词根的连接元音应省略。如单词 aden / o / carcinoma（腺瘤）中，o 即是连接元音。又如 gastr / o / duoden / o / stomy（胃十二指肠吻合术）中，词根 gastr- 和 duoden- 之间的 o 即是连接元音，词根 duoden- 和后缀 -stomy 之间的 o 也是连接元音。在医学单词的连接元音中，o 是使用频率最高的，其次还有元音 i，e 和 a。词根和连接元音结合后形成的词素被称为连接形式（combining form）。如前例中的 adeno-（aden + o）。对于各前缀和连接元音的搭配，更多的例子可参见前文 1.1.1.1 中的词根列表。

1.1.2　医学术语的构成形式

1.1.2.1　医学术语的构成类型

　　医学术语的构成成分包括词根、前缀、后缀和连接元音,其中前面三类词素为基本成分。医学术语根据一般遵循的规律可分为特定的类型。了解这些类型有助于分析理解术语的形成及意义的产生。以词根、前缀和后缀为基准,医学术语的构成类型主要可分为以下五种类型。

　　类型一　词根

　　gene → 基因

　　类型二　词根+后缀

　　hepat + itis → hepatitis

　　（肝）（炎症）（肝炎）

　　词根+连接元音+后缀

　　therm + o + meter → thermometer

　　（热）　　（测量仪器）　　（温度计）

　　词根+连接元音+词根+连接元音+后缀

　　gastr + o + enter + o + logy → gastroenterology

　　（胃）　　　（肠）　（研究）　　（胃肠病学）

　　词根+连接元音+词根+后缀

　　labi + o + dent + al → labiodental

　　（唇）　　（牙）　　　（唇齿的）

　　类型三　词根+词根

　　sial + aden → sialaden

　　（唾液）（腺）（唾液腺）

　　词根+连接元音+词根

　　troph + o + blast → trophoblast

　　（营养）　　（胚芽）　　（滋养层）

　　类型四　前缀+词根+后缀

　　epi + gastr + ic → epigastric

　　（上）（胃）　　　（上腹部的）

前缀+连接元音+词根+后缀

hom + o + gen + ous → homogenous

（同）　　（产生）　　　　（同种／质的）

前缀+前缀+词根+后缀

sub +　　　 peri + oste + al → subperiosteal

（下，亚）（周围）（骨）　　　　（骨膜下的）

前缀+词根+连接元音+后缀

dys +　　　 men + o + rrhea → dysmenorrhea

（坏，不良）（月）　　　（流）　　　（痛经）

类型五　前缀+后缀

para +　　centesis →　　paracentesis

（旁）　　（穿刺）　　　（穿刺术）

1.1.2.2　医学术语构成成分的顺序

根据派生法，医学术语的构成是相当灵活的。常见的构成类型就多达十多种，生成的单词数量巨大。在此情况下，医学术语构成成分的排列顺序就显得重要起来。因为同样的词素以不同的顺序排列，可能产生完全不同的意义。如 blastocyte 和 cytoblast。两词都是由 blast 和 cyt(o)-合成，前者意指"胚细胞"，后者则为"细胞核"，且后者已经被另外的新词取代，不再使用。又如 phagocyte 和 cytophagy，前词为"吞噬细胞"，后词指"吞噬作用"。更有甚者，不同的排列顺序生成一个毫无意义且根本就不存在的单词，如 podagra 指"（足）痛风"，agropod 则是个错误的单词。又如 lithotripsy 为"碎石术"，然而 tripsolith 这个词则根本不存在。因而，掌握医学术语的构成成分及类型，有助于分析和理解医学单词，但切不可使用这些知识来生造或臆造术语。在不确定时，仍需要查阅专业字典或其他工具书。对于追求严谨的医学，这一点是尤其重要的。

1.1.2.3　医学术语的对抗形式

医学术语大量使用希腊语和拉丁语，并且构词灵活，这就使得单词中大量存在拼写或意义类似的词素。这些词素被称作医学术语的对抗形式（competing form）。医学术语的对抗形式主要有以下三类：

1. 含有共同词根但使用不同连接元音的词素

例24

| pneum / a / type | 呼气像 | pneum / o / cele | 肺膨出 |
| sperm / i / cide | 杀精子剂 | sperm / o / lyt / ic | 溶解精子的 |

2. 同一词根的不同拼写形式

例25

| hem / o / rrhage | 出血 | hemat / o / logy | 血液学 |

gangli / ec / tomy　　神经节切除术　　　ganglion / ec / tomy　神经节切除术

mega / cocc / us　　　巨型球菌　　　　　megal / o / cephaly　巨头畸形

3. 表达相同意义的希腊语和拉丁语词素

例26

意义	拉丁语	希腊语
身体	corpus	soma
肠	intestine	enter(o)-
呼吸	spir(o)-	pneum(o)-
牙	dent(i)-	odont(o)-
脂肪	adip(o)-	lip(o)-
心	cor-	cardi(o)-
手	manu-	cheir(o)-，chir(o)-
关节,连接	articul(o)-	arthr(o)-
肾	ren(o)-	nephr(o)-
泪	lacrim(o)-	dacry(o)-
口	or(o)-	stomat(o)-
红色	rub(o)-	erythr(o)-
皮肤	cutis	derm(o)-
舌头	lingu(o)-	gloss(o)-
血管	vas(o)-	angi(o)-
女性	fem-	gyn(o)-
阴道	vagin(o)-	colp(o)-

1.1.3　医学术语的拼读和复数规则

1.1.3.1　医学术语的拼读规则

1. 医学术语的拼写

医学术语的正确拼写是正确使用医学术语的重要基础。对拼写的掌握不仅能反映使用者对术语的理解,也能反映其对知识的严谨态度。同时最重要的是,错误的拼写也许会造成重大的理解错误,带来不可挽回的损失。医学术语使用了大量的外来语语素,但长期以来的英语化趋势使其与普通英语在拼写上越来越趋同。因而,在此仅强调以下几点。

（1）名词概念与其对应的连接形式

对名词概念和其对应的连接形式而言，表述基本词意部分的拼写有时会出现不同。

例27

名词概念	连接形式	例词
pharynx	pharyng(o)-	pharyngeal
thorax	thorac(o)-	thoracopathy
pancreas	pancreat(o)-	pancreatitis

（2）同化现象

语言学中，语流中两个邻近的不同的音，其中一个受到另一个的影响而变得与之相同或相近的现象称为同化。医学术语的各构成成分在组合时，拼写和发音也会出现同化现象。如：appendectomy 由 ad-、pend-和-ectomy 组合而成，当词素 ad 与 pend 相连时，字母 d 与 p 发生同化，拼写变为 append-。类似的词汇还有：

例28

affusion ← ad + fus + ion

collapse ← con + lapse

compress ← con + press

（3）音、形不一致

记忆英语单词时，人们普遍认为按音记词是一种有效的方法。在此情况下，对于某些音形不一致的词，应特别注意。

① 某些双辅音和辅音组合中的个别字母不发音，在拼写时易漏掉。

例29

rheumatosis [ˌruːməˈtəusis]中的 h

cnemitis [niːˈmaitis]中的 c

pneumonia [njuːˈməuniə]中的 p

② 某些单词具有相同的读音，但却有不同的拼写形式和意义，即所谓的同音词。

例30

[saiˈtɔlədʒi]对应 cytology(细胞学) 和 sitology(饮食学、营养学)

[ˈiliæk]对应 ileac(回肠的、肠梗阻的) 和 iliac(髂骨的)

（4）简化趋势

随着语言的演变发展，医学术语的拼写出现了简化趋势，具体体现为某些元音字母、辅音字母或它们相互间的组合，由于发音简便和拼写的需要而被省略掉。

例31

aetiology → etiology(病因学)

oulorrhagia → ulorrhagia(龈出血)

adrenalopathy → adrenopathy(肾上腺病)

megagastria → megastria（巨胃）

appendicectomy → appendectomy（阑尾切除术）

（5）连字符构词

当前缀或词根与另一词根相连时，如果前缀或词根以元音结尾，则有时会使用连字符连接这些构词成分。如 multi-infection（多重感染），ultra-acoustics（超声学），mega-esophagus（巨食管）。目前，连字符具有被省略掉的趋势，如 microorganism（微生物）。

（6）同义演变

医学术语中存在着一些同义词，是由部分词素拼写变化形成的。

例32

c →k　　　leucocyte → leukocyte（白细胞）

ph →f　　　sulphonamide → sulfonamide（磺胺）

y →i　　　bacilysin → bacillisin（杆菌溶素）

2. 医学术语的读音

医学术语中存在大量的外来语素，一般遵从源语的发音规则，会很特别。实际上随着语言的发展演变，读音已经逐步适应了现代英语的规则，与普通英语无异，只是在某些辅音的发音和重读音节的选择上，还应该遵循一些特定的规则。

（1）特定辅音

① 单辅音

c 在字母 a、o、u 前发 [k]，如 cardiac、coagulation 和 culture；在 e、i、y 前发 [s]，如 placenta、cilium 和 emergency。

g 在字母 a、o、u 前发 [g]，如 gastrocele、gonad 和 anticoagulant；在 e、i、y 前发 [dʒ]，如 analgesia、gingivitis 和 gynopathy。

x 在词首发 [z]，如 xerosis 和 xerodermia，在词的其他位置则发 [ks]，如 anthrax 和 staxis。

② 双辅音

ch、ph 和 rh 是双辅音，在单词中它们被视为一个整体，在发音时不受组合辅音的影响，作为一个整体发音。

ch 常发作 [k]，如 cholesterol 和 chromosome，也可发作 [tʃ]，如 chest 和 chin。

ph 组合发音为 [f]，如 phlebitis 和 phagocyte。

rh，rrh 发 [r]，如 rheumatism 和 hemorrhage。

③ 辅音组合

辅音组合如 cn、gn、mn、pn、ps 和 pt，置于词首时，第一个辅音不发音；位于词中时，两个辅音均独立发音。

例33

cnidoblast [ˈnaidəblæst] 和 gastrocnemius [ˌgæstrɔkˈniːmiəs]

gnathostatics [næθəuˈstætiks] 和 prognosis [prɔgˈnəusis]

mnemonics [niːˈmɔniks] 和 amnesia [æmˈniːziə]

pneumonia [nju:ˈməuniə] 和 apnea [æpˈni:ə]

pseudopodia [sju:dəuˈpəudiə] 和 apselaphesia [ˌæpseləˈfi:ziə]

pteridine [ˈterəˌdi:n] 和 hemoptysis [hiˈmɔptisis]

（2）重音

由派生法形成的医学术语包含大量的外来语素，尤其是希腊语和拉丁语素，且构成复杂，通常形成的单词偏长。因而要读准医学术语，正确找出其重读音节和次重读音节是非常重要的。

总体来说，医学术语遵从拉丁语的重读规则，一般规则如下：

① 单音节词无重读音节，如 cell [sel] 和 heart [hɑ:t]。双音节词的第二个音节一般不能是重读音节，故重音一般在词首，如 system [ˈsistəm] 和 hippo [ˈhipəu]；

② 对于多音节词，如果倒数第二个音节包含一个长元音或双元音，则重音在倒数第二个音节上。如 epidermis [ˌepiˈdə:mis] 和 appendicitis [əˌpendiˈsaitis]；

③ 对于大多数的多音节词，如果倒数第二个音节包含一个短元音，则重音在倒数第三个音节上，这是医学术语读音中最常见的。如 biology [baiˈɔlədʒi] 和 pharmacotherapy [ˌfɑ:məkəuˈθerəpi]。

医学术语主要借助大量的后缀派生构成单词，后缀的大量使用使得医学术语的重读情况复杂多样，但仍有规律可循。现总结如下：

① 重音在倒数第二个音节

例34

类别	后缀	例词	音标	意义
疾病后缀	-itis	gastritis	[gæˈstraitis]	胃炎
	-ia	anemia	[əˈni:miə]	贫血
	-osis	sclerosis	[skliəˈrəusis]	硬化
	-oma	adenoma	[ˌædiˈnəumə]	腺瘤
	-iasis	elephantiasis	[ˌelifənˈtaiəsis]	象皮肿
物质	-ic	antibiotic	[ˌæntibaiˈɔtik]	抗生素
	-in	gentamycin	[ˌdʒentəˈmaisin]	庆大霉素
	-ion	solution	[səˈlu:ʃn]	溶液
	-ium	bacterium	[bækˈtiəriəm]	细菌
其他	-ian	pediatrician	[ˌpi:diəˈtriʃn]	儿科医生
	-ious	infectious	[inˈfekʃəs]	感染的
	-escent	alkalescent	[ˌælkəˈlesənt]	弱碱性的

② 重音在倒数第三个音节

例35

类别	后缀	例词	音标	意义
学科	-logy	cardiology	[ˌkɑːdiˈɔlədʒi]	心脏病学
诊断	-graphy	angiography	[ˌændʒiˈɔgrəfi]	血管造影术
	-meter	thermometer	[θəˈmɔmitə]	温度计
	-metry	psychometry	[saiˈkɔmitri]	精神测定法
	-scopy	endoscopy	[enˈdɔskəpi]	内窥镜检查
手术	-tomy	laparotomy	[ˌlæpəˈrɔtəmi]	剖腹术
	-stomy	colostomy	[kəˈlɔstəmi]	结肠造口术
	-ectomy	appendectomy	[ˌæpenˈdektəmi]	阑尾切除术
有机化合物	-ate	carbonate	[ˈkɑːbəneit]	碳酸盐
	-ide	monosaccharide	[ˌmɔnəuˈsækəraid]	单糖
	-oid	carotenoid	[kəˈrɔtənoid]	类胡萝卜素
	-ose	amylose	[ˈæmləus]	直链淀粉
	-ase	transaminase	[trænˈsæmineis]	转氨酶

③ 重音在倒数第一个音节

例36

后缀	例词	音标	意义
-rrhea	diarrhea	[ˌdaiəˈriə]	腹泻
-ine	vaccine	[vækˈsiːn]	疫苗
-ee	trainee	[treiˈniː]	受训者

④ 重音从原

单音节的自由词素位于词尾时，重音应从原词尾前的那个词素。

例37

后缀	例词	音标	意义
-cele	enterocele	[ˈentərəsiːl]	肠疝
-cyte	spermatocyte	[ˈspəmətəˌsait]	精母细胞
-blast	spermatoblast	[ˈspɜːmətoublɑːst]	精子细胞
-gram	electrocardiogram	[ɪˌlektrouˈkɑːrdiougræm]	心电图
-graph	encephalograph	[enˈsefələgrɑːf]	脑 X 线照像仪

续表

后缀	例词	音标	意义
-phage	bacteriophage	[bæk'tɪərɪəfeidʒ]	噬菌体
-scope	esophagoscope	[iː'sɔfəgəskəup]	食道镜
-therm	poikilotherm	[pɔɪ'kɪləuθɜːm]	变温动物
-tome	osteotome	['ɒstɪətəum]	骨凿刀

医学术语是由医学词根、前缀、后缀和连接元音组成,这有助于分析和理解词的构成和意义,但医学术语读音中音节的划分以及重读音节的确立,遵循的却是另外一套完全不同的规则。因此,在分析医学术语的读音时,切不可按照构成成分来发音,因为这极有可能造成误读,如 bronch / o / pathy 正确读音为 [brɒŋ'kɒpəθi],hemat / o / ly / sis 正确读音为 [ˌhiːmə'tɔlisis]。

医学术语的发音固然不简单,但也是有规律可循的,特别是对于重读音节的确立,大多数情况下重音都置于倒数第三个音节上。对于一个新单词,如若实在无把握其正确读音,则需借助于查阅词典。

1.1.3.2　医学术语的复数规则

医学术语大多数都是名词,其复数形式一般取决于词源。由于医学术语的外来词源多是希腊语和拉丁语,尽管英语化的趋势使某些词以在词尾加上 -(e)s 作为复数形式,仍有大部分词使用它们对应的希腊语或拉丁语复数形式。具体如以下两表:

例38

希腊词源的复数

单词词尾		例词		
单数	复数	单数		复数
-ma	-mata / -mas	sarcoma derma lymphoma	肉瘤 皮肤 淋巴瘤	sarcomata / sarcomas dermata / dermas lymphomata / lymphomas
-on	-a	phenomenon protozoon ganglion	现象 原生动物 神经节	phenomena protozoa ganglia
-is	-es	analysis arthrosis psychosis	分析 关节病 精神病	analyses arthroses psychoses

续表

单词词尾		例词		
单数	复数	单数		复数
-is	-ides	epididymis	附睾	epididymides
		glottis	声门	glottides
-ax	-aces	thorax	胸腔	thoraces
-inx	-inges	meninx	脑膜	meninges

例39

拉丁词源的复数

单词词尾		例词		
单数	复数	单数		复数
-a	-ae	maxilla	上颌骨	maxillae
		corona	冠	coronae
		vertebra	椎骨	vertebrae
-um	-a	medium	媒介	media
		flagellum	鞭毛	flagella
		labium	唇	labia
-us	-i	bronchus	支气管	bronchi
		fungus	真菌	fungi
		thrombus	血栓	thrombi
-us	-era	genus	种类,属	genera
-us	-ora	stercus	粪便	stercora
		corpus	体	corpora
-ex	-ices / -exes	apex	顶点	apices / apexes
		pollex	拇指	pollices / pollexes
-ix	ices / -ixes	appendix	阑尾	appendices / appendixes
		cervix	颈部	cervices / cervixes
		varix	静脉曲张	varices
-s	-sa	vas	管	vasa

需要指出的是,有些医学术语的复数只有英语规则的变化形式,比如:virus 的复数形式只有 viruses,electron 的复数形式只有 electrons。有些医学术语的复数则两者兼有,即:既可以采用它们对应的希腊语或拉丁语复数形式,也可以采用英语规则的复数形式,比如:fungus 的复数形式有 fungi 和 funguses 两种,vertebra 的复数形式有 vertebrae 和 vertebras 两种,appendix 的复数形式有 appendices 和 appendixes 两种。

1.2 医学专业特异性词汇

医学专业词汇的一个主要分支是第一节中讲述的医学术语。除此之外,还有四种常见的医学专业特异性词汇,即:英语词汇、医学冠名术语、缩略语和形象性描述语。

1.2.1 英语词汇

医学专业特异性词汇并非全部都是源于希腊语和拉丁语的医学术语,还有一类大量存在的词汇,即能够表达医学相关内容的英语词汇。随着英语成为世界性语言,大量的英语词汇开始描述医学现象。

比如用来描述人体器官的一些英语单词 heart(心脏)、brain(大脑)、lung(肺)、liver(肝脏)、kidney(肾脏)、bladder(膀胱) 源自中古英语或古英语。用来描述人体症状或疾病的一些英语单词 fever(发烧,发热)、cough(咳嗽)、disease(疾病)、cancer(癌症)、tumor(肿瘤)、fracture(骨折) 源自中古英语。其他的单词或单词组合,比如描述血细胞三大组成成分的 red blood cell(红细胞)、white blood cell(白细胞) 和 platelet(血小板) 均源自中古英语。

1.2.2 冠名术语

医学英语中,表述解剖结构、疾病、手术、临床检验、病毒、细菌、新原理等的术语常被冠以人名、地名或事件名。这类术语被称作医学冠名术语。尽管这种命名方法并不能准确形象地描述和说明对象,但也能直观、简明地陈述由于科学、物质水平所限不能探明和确定的对象,有些甚至能传达某种历史文化深义。

1.2.2.1 以医生或患者姓名冠名的医学术语

有些医学术语以医生的姓名冠名,目的在于纪念这些医学从业人员对某一医学研究领域或医学事业的整体发展所作出的贡献。如 Parkinson's disease(帕金森病) 以英国内科医生詹姆斯·帕金森(1755—1824) 冠名,以纪念他于 1817 年首次发文描述此病,此病亦称震颤麻痹。如 Alzheimer's disease (阿尔茨海默病) 以德国神经病学家 Alois Alzheimer (1864—1915) 冠名,以纪念他首先发表了"老年痴呆症"的病例以及在神经病学领域所做的贡献。又如 hippocratic face(死相,预后不良) 以被西方尊为"医学之父"的希腊医生希波克拉底(Hippocrates) 冠名,只因这种提示预后不良的面部表情(瘦削的,痛苦而苍白的面容) 是由他最初描述的。此外,还有一些医学术语是以患者姓名冠名的,如 Hela cells(海拉细胞) 得名于美国患者 Henrietta Lacks,又名"人宫颈癌传代细胞",只因该细胞最初是从她的子宫颈癌中分离的癌细胞株培养所得,故以病人姓名组合命名。

这类医学术语一般由两部分构成,前一部分是医生或患者的姓名,后一部分由普通的或专业的医学术语构成,如 syndrome(综合征)、disease(病)、operation (术)、therapy(疗法)、test(试验)、method(法)、reagent(剂)、reaction (反应)、point(点)、duct(导管)、fascia(筋

膜)、ganglion(神经节)、anemia(贫血)等。其中,syndrome 构成的术语最多。

1.2.2.2　以神话或文学中的人物或事件冠名的医学术语

神话在人类认识世界的意识形成中扮演了重要角色,由于医学词素大量吸收希腊语、拉丁语成分,希腊罗马神话也成为了医学冠名术语的重要来源。这种冠名方式同时也赋予了术语强烈的文化色彩。

Achilles 是希腊神话中骁勇善战的英雄。出生时,母亲海洋女神 Thetis 握着他的脚踝将他浸泡在冥河水中,使他全身刀枪不入,唯有脚踝例外,成为致命的部位。一系列术语以此命名,如 Achilles tendon(跟腱)、Achilles jerk(跟腱反射)。又如 Proteus 是希腊神话中的水神,可随意改变形状。Proteus syndrome(普鲁透斯综合征)就借用此意来指一种具有多种表征的罕见的先天性疾患。

医学术语还有一种冠名方式,即以文学作品或其塑造的人物形象冠名。Pickwickian syndrome(匹克威克综合征)得名于英国小说家狄更斯作品《匹克威克外传》中主人公胖小孩的形象,即形貌矮小、肥胖、嗜睡等;Lear complex(李尔王恋女情结)得名于莎士比亚的悲剧《李尔王》。

1.2.2.3　以地名冠名的医学术语

医学术语中还有一类是以地名冠名,通常是以某一疾病或病毒等的首发报道地或某一项技术的研发地而冠名。

例40

Borna disease(博纳病),以德国萨克森州 Borna 地区命名,实指该地区流行的一种病毒所致的马、牛、羊的致命性地方性脑炎。

Chagres fever(恰格尔斯热),因首发于巴拿马恰格尔斯流域而得名,实为一种恶性疟疾。

Chiba needle(千叶针),是由日本千叶大学研发的抽吸细针,用于经皮肝胆管造影。

Keshan disease(克山病),因首发于中国克山地区的儿童而得名,实为一种微量元素缺乏引起的致命性充血性心肌病。

类似的例子还有 Mediterranean anemia(地中海贫血),schistosoma Mekongi(湄公河血吸虫)和 West Nile virus(西尼罗河脑炎病毒)。

随着医学事业不断发展进步,人们对疾病等的认识不断加深,医学冠名术语也呈现出了一些新的发展趋势。如 disease 取代 syndrome,某些病症在尚未探明或确定时,通常冠以 syndrome,一旦确定,则以 disease 代之。

例41

Addisonian syndrome(艾迪生综合征)→ Addisonian disease(艾迪生病)肾上腺皮质功能减退;

Meniere's syndrome(梅尼埃综合征)→ Meniere's disease(梅尼埃病)耳性眩晕病;

当病症被完全探明,相应的专业描述术语产生,或取代前者,或二者共存意指同一对象。

如 Martin Bell syndrome = fragile X syndrome（马-贝综合征，脆性 X 染色体综合征），Degos' disease = malignant atrophic papulosis（德格斯病，恶性萎缩性丘疹病）。

1.2.3　缩略语

在英语词汇中，缩略语是指由单词进行部分简化或省略构成的新词。医学是使用缩略语最活跃的领域之一，无论是在诊疗室、病房、化验室或是各种研究机构，缩略语都很常用。缩略语可极大地提高工作效率、降低材料消耗。医学领域中使用的缩略语按照构成类型，主要包括拼缀词、截短词和首字母缩略词。

1.2.3.1　拼缀词

拼缀词是指由两个词的某些部分结合在一起，或其中一词与另一词的某些部分结合起来构成的新词，常见的有以下两种：

1. 词首+词尾

例42

metabolism + genomics → metanomics（代谢组学）

nutrition + pharmaceutical → nutraceutical（营养药物）

2. 词首+单词

例43

medical + care → medicare（医疗保险）

cesarean + section → C-section（剖宫产术）

1.2.3.2　截短词

截短词是指把原来较长的单词截掉部分后形成的新词，截掉的部分可以是词首或词尾，也可以是二者都去掉，还可以是词中的部分。

例44

influenza → flu（流感）

poliomyelitis → polio（小儿麻痹症）

laboratory → lab（实验室）

weight → wt（重量）

1.2.3.3　首字母缩略词

首字母缩略词在此被视作一个广义的概念，泛指将单词的第一个字母结合起来，或由第一个字母或字母组合与词的其他部分结合构成的新词。常见的有以下几种构词形式：

1. 所有单词（通常指实词）的首字母结合构成的新词

这种类型又包括两种亚型：

① 合成新词按字母逐个拼读

例45

blood pressure → BP(血压)

growth hormone → GH(生长激素)

magnetic resonance imaging → MRI(磁共振成像)

chief complaint → CC(主诉)

② 合成新词作为一个单词拼读

例46

acquired immune deficiency syndrome → AIDS(获得性免疫缺陷综合征)

Journal of American Medical Association → JAMA(美国医学会杂志)

severe acute respiratory syndrome → SARS(严重急性呼吸综合征)

2. 由复合词或单词的一部分的字母构成的新词

例47

deoxyribonucleic acid → DNA(脱氧核糖核酸)

Medical Clinics of North America → Med Clin NA(北美内科学)

Medical Subject Headings → MeSH(医学主题词)

tuberculosis → TB(肺结核)

3. 由构词成分的首字母结合构成的新词

例48

ultraviolet → UV(紫外线的)

intravenous → i.v.(静脉内的)

out-patient → OP(门诊病人)

electrocardiogram → ECG(心电图)

4. 由单词的首字母倒置结合构成的新词

例49

Doctor of Medicine → MD(医学博士)

diabetic index → ID(糖尿病指数)

doctor of optometry → OD(验光医师)

manifest hypermetropia → HM(显性远视)

5. 由首字母缩略词与其他单词连用构成的新词

例50

sinoatrial node → SA node(窦房结)

Eastern Equine Encephalomyelitis virus → EEE virus(东方马脑脊髓炎病毒)

left long leg brace → LLL brace(左长腿支具)

oral-facial-digital syndrome → OFD syndrome(口-面-指/趾综合征)

需要指出的是,有些医学术语的命名可能综合采用了上述两种或多种构词类型,比如,2019 年发现的新型冠状病毒,于 2020 年 1 月 12 日被世界卫生组织命名为 2019-nCoV,这个医学英语新名词的全称是 2019 novel coronavirus,综合采用了拼缀法和首字母缩略法。同年 2 月 11 日,世界卫生组织将新型冠状病毒感染的肺炎命名为 COVID-19,这个医学英语新名词来源于 corona(冠状)、virus(病毒)以及 disease(疾病)三个词,而 19 则代表这个疾病出现的年份为 2019 年。

1.2.4　形象性描述语

形象性描述语因表意生动鲜明,在文学语言及日常用语中广泛使用。在追求表意严谨准确的医学用语领域,有时医务工作者为追求表述的有效性,也会借助日常事物来表达医学信息。在意义转换过程中,各种修辞手法,如借喻、借代、类比等起到了重要的作用,从而形成了医学术语中特殊的形象性描述语。

医学术语中的形象性描述语多用来表述一些形状相似的概念。表示人体结构各部分的名称多数都借用了形状相似的概念,如 bridge of nose(鼻梁),drumstick finger(杵状指),wallet stomach(袋状胃),leopard heart(豹斑心)。有时,由于文化上的差异,英汉两种语言在表述同一对象时,使用的概念也会有所差异,如 pigeon chest(鸡胸),goose flesh(鸡皮疙瘩)。在表述某些疾病概念时,由于形似,形象性描述语也被广泛使用,用意在于直观地描述体征,如 rose spot(玫瑰疹),dumb-bell tumor(哑铃状瘤)。

在医学术语中,形象性描述语也被用于指称一些在功能、性状等方面相似的概念。如 target cell(靶细胞),envelope antigen(包膜抗原,包被抗原),bottle-feeding(人工喂养),cocktail therapy(鸡尾酒疗法)。对于某些特定疾病,人们对它们的认识已经足够清晰,并赋予了准确的科学命名,但为使表意形象,也使用形象性描述语,从而使得同一疾病的两种命名同时存在,如 bovine spongiform encephalopathy(BSE,牛海绵状脑病),又俗称 mad cow disease(疯牛病)。对于人类历史上曾大规模流行的瘟疫和病毒,人们也常借用修饰语概念来描述其巨大的危害及带来的严重损伤,如 black death(黑死病)。

1.3　生物医学英文文献的文体特点

生物医学英文文献在语言特点方面与文学等其他文献有很大的差别。在生物医学英文文献的写作过程中,必须充分了解并实现其语篇特点,具体包括语气正式、陈述客观、语言规范、文体质朴、术语丰富。

1.3.1　语气正式

生物医学英文文献语气正式的一个表现是很多英语句子缺少人称主语。人具有主观性,所以无人称便是语气正式的一个特点。生物医学英文文献,特别是教科书、专著等包含的都是无人称主语的句子,这主要是由于其所描述和讨论的是医学原理和医学现象。下例选自英文教科书,从中可以看出生物医学英文文献语气正式的特点。

例51

The circulatory system is a network of blood vessels that bring nutrients and other essential elements to the cells throughout the body and carry away wastes. The heart is the pump that circulates the blood throughout this network of blood vessels. Blood enters the two upper chambers of the heart, the atria and leaves through the two lower chambers, the ventricles. Blood leaving the left ventricle of the heart travels to all parts of the body (called systemic circulation) whereas blood leaving the right ventricle travels to the air sacs of the lungs to be oxygenated (called pulmonary circulation). As the blood leaves the left ventricle, it passes through the aorta, the largest artery in the body. At the aorta the process of branching off into smaller arteries begins almost immediately and continues until every area of the body is reached.

译文：循环系统是一个血管网络，输送营养物质和其他重要成分至全身细胞，并排出废物。心脏是血管网络中的泵，推动血流运行。血液从心房（心脏上方两腔室）流入心室（心脏下方两腔室），从下部两心室流出。血液离开左心室流向全身各个部位（称为体循环），而离开右心室到肺泡中氧合（称为肺循环）。血液从左心室流出到达主动脉——全身最大的动脉。然后从此处，血管开始进行连续不断地分枝，成为大大小小的血管，直达全身各处。

值得一提的是，无人称这种情况不是绝对的。有时由于行文等需要，如研究论文中，涉及研究者和研究对象的描述，往往也使用含人称主语的句子，如下例。

例52

The RECORD study has been described in detail previously. We recruited patients for the study from April 2001 through April 2003. Eligible patients had type 2 diabetes, as defined by criteria of the World Health Organization; were between the ages of 40 and 75 years; had a body mass index (the weight in kilograms divided by the square of the height in meters) of more than 25.0; and had a glycated hemoglobin level of more than 7.0% and less than or equal to 9.0% while receiving maximum doses of metformin or a sulfonylurea.

译文：我们以前曾对 RECORD（评估罗格列酮对心血管转归和血糖调节的影响）研究做过详细描述。我们从 2001 年 4 月至 2003 年 4 月为该研究招募患者。合格的病人患有世界卫生组织定义的 2 型糖尿病，年龄在 40~75 岁，体重指数（体重的公斤数除以身高米数的平方）>25.0，接受最大剂量二甲双胍或磺脲类药物治疗时的糖化血红蛋白水平>7.0%，但≤9.0%。

1.3.2　陈述客观

生物医学英文文献反映客观医学事物，其陈述必须客观、准确。生物医学英文文献中被动语态使用广泛，是其客观性的体现，因为被动语态不强调动作的主体。

例53

Bronchiectasis is defined by the presence of permanent and abnormal dilation of the bronchi. This usually occurs in the context of chronic airway infection causing inflammation. The main clinical manifestation is a productive cough. Bronchiectasis is currently nearly always diagnosed using high-resolution computed tomography（HRCT）scanning. The main diagnostic features are：1）internal diameter of a bronchus is wider than its adjacent pulmonary artery；2）failure of the bronchi to taper；and 3）visualization of bronchi in the outer 1-2 cm of the lung fields. This review will describe the pathophysiology of noncystic fibrosis bronchiectasis. With the widespread availability of HRCT it has been realized that bronchiectasis remains a common and important cause of respiratory disease. It has been estimated that there are at least 110,000 adults in the United States with this condition. In addition, there is overlap with chronic obstructive pulmonary disease（COPD）with two studies reporting an incidence of bronchiectasis in COPD as being 29% and 50%, respectively. Bronchiectasis is characterized by mild to moderate airflow obstruction that tends to worsen over time.[①]

说明：此例选自一篇关于支气管扩张病理生理学的综述文章，共有 10 句话，其中有 5 句话使用了被动语态。文章的主题是支气管扩张（bronchiectasis），故文章中有 3 句话以 bronchiectasis 为主语使用了被动语态，以突出生物医学英文文献陈述客观的语言特征。另外，医学英语文献中，常使用 it has been realized/estimated that 的句式，其中作为 be 动词现在完成时的表述 has been 会有时态上的变化。

译文：支气管扩张是指支气管永久性异常扩张，常见于可引起炎症的慢性气道感染。其主要临床表现是排痰性咳嗽。目前支气管扩张几乎总是借助于高分辨计算机断层扫描来诊断。其主要的诊断特征是：（1）支气管内管径比其毗连的肺动脉宽；（2）支气管未能逐渐变细；（3）肺野外带 1~2 厘米处支气管可见。本综述将对非囊性纤维化支气管扩张的病理生理学进行描述。随着高分辨计算机断层扫描的广泛使用，学界已认识到支气管扩张依然是呼吸道疾病的一种常见且重要的病因。据估计，美国至少有 11 万成年人患有支气管扩张。另外，此病与慢性阻塞性肺病常共病，因为两项研究发现，慢性阻塞性肺病患者支气管扩张的发病率分别为 29% 和 50%。支气管扩张表现为有轻度到中度的气流阻塞，并日益加重。

1.3.3 语言规范

规范的医学语言，能准确表达医学信息，利于医学资料的编纂、收录、检索和利用，促进国际间的学术交流等。规范的医学语言，主要体现为使用正式规范的医学术语和行业表达。

例54

A 22-year-old man who was a known heroin abuser was admitted to an emergency department comatose, with shallow respirations. Routine laboratory studies and chest X-ray

---

① 例子源自王兰其、王玉安，《医学英语新教程》（上册），上海：复旦大学出版社，2012 年，第 168-169 页。

studies were done after the patient was aroused. He was then transferred to the ICU. He complained of left-sided chest pain. Examination of the chest film showed three fractured ribs on the right and a large right pleural effusion. Further questioning of a friend revealed that he had fallen and struck the corner of a table after injecting heroin.

The diagnosis was traumatic hemothorax secondary to rib fractures, and a chest tube was inserted into the right pleural space. No blood could be obtained despite maneuvering of the tube. Another chest X-ray showed that the tube was correctly placed in the right pleural space, but the fractured ribs and pleural effusion were on the left. The radiologist then realized that he had reversed the first film. A second tube was inserted into the left pleural space, and 1500 ml [6 to 7 cups] of blood was evacuated.[①]

说明：此例选自一篇病例报告，其中使用了 chest X-ray（胸部 X 线检查）、ICU（重症监护病房）、hemothorax（血胸）、pleural effusion（胸腔积液）等专业的医学术语，以及 admitted to（收治）、transferred to（转诊至）、complain of（主诉）、secondary to（继发）等医学行业的规范表达。

译文：患者，男，22 岁，海洛因滥用者，因昏迷、呼吸浅，收治入急诊室。患者苏醒后进行实验室常规检查和胸部 X 线检查。然后，被转诊至重症监护病房。主诉左侧胸痛。胸片检查显示右侧有三处肋骨骨折，右侧胸腔积液较多。进一步询问朋友后得知，注射海洛因后摔倒并撞到桌角。

诊断为由肋骨骨折继发的创伤性血胸。将胸管插入其右侧胸膜腔，尽管插管完成，但未抽到胸腔中的积血。胸部 X 线检查显示，插管正确置于右侧胸膜腔内，但肋骨骨折和胸腔积液位于左侧。放射科医生随即意识到自己之前将胸片放颠倒了。将第二个插管置入左侧胸膜腔，并抽出 1500 ml[6 至 7 杯]血液。

1.3.4　文体质朴

生物医学英文文献的主要目的是传达信息，因此在文体方面，呈现出文风质朴、句子结构直截了当的特点。这种质朴的文体主要表现为语言简洁、语句平衡、不累赘拖沓。

生物医学英文文献文体质朴的特点从前面所有的例子中都有所体现，又如下面一篇医学综述文献的摘要部分。

例55

Most cancers arise in individuals over the age of 60. As the world population is living longer and reaching older ages, cancer is becoming a substantial public health problem. It is estimated that, by 2050, more than 20% of the world's population will be over the age of 60—the economic, healthcare and financial burdens this may place on society are far from trivial. In this Review, we address the role of the ageing microenvironment in the promotion of tumour progression. Specifically, we discuss the cellular and molecular changes in non-

---

① 例子源自 Davi-Ellen Chabner, The language of Medicine (11th Edition), St. Louis, Missouri：Elsevier，2017 年，第 485 页。

cancerous cells during ageing, and how these may contribute towards a tumour permissive microenvironment; these changes encompass biophysical alterations in the extracellular matrix, changes in secreted factors and changes in the immune system. We also discuss the contribution of these changes to responses to cancer therapy as ageing predicts outcomes of therapy, including survival. Yet, in preclinical studies, the contribution of the aged microenvironment to therapy response is largely ignored, with most studies designed in 8-week-old mice rather than older mice that reflect an age appropriate to the disease being modelled. This may explain, in part, the failure of many successful preclinical therapies upon their translation to the clinic. Overall, the intention of this review is to provide an overview of the interplay that occurs between ageing cell types in the microenvironment and cancer cells and how this is likely to impact tumour metastasis and therapy response.

说明:此例选自 2019 年发表在 Nat. Rev. Cancer 上的一篇名为 *How the ageing microenvironment influences tumour progression* 的综述文章,是其摘要部分。写作特点表现为语言简洁、语句平衡、不累赘拖沓。

译文:大多数癌症发生在 60 岁以上的人群中。随着世界人口寿命的延长和老龄化,癌症正成为一个重大的公共卫生问题。据估计,到 2050 年,超过 20% 的世界人口将超过 60 岁,这可能给社会带来严重的经济、医疗和财政负担。本综述讨论了衰老微环境对肿瘤进展的促进作用。我们具体讨论了非肿瘤细胞在衰老过程中的细胞和分子变化,以及这些变化如何促成有利于肿瘤生长的微环境。这些变化包括细胞外基质的生理改变,分泌因子和免疫系统的变化。因为衰老可预测治疗结局(包括存活),我们还讨论了这些变化对癌症治疗效果的影响。然而,临床前研究大多选择 8 周大的小鼠建模,而不是与疾病年龄匹配的老年小鼠,因此衰老微环境对疗效的影响在很大程度上被忽略了。这在一定程度上就可以解释为什么许多成功的临床前治疗方案在应用到临床后会失败。总之,本综述旨在概述微环境中衰老细胞类型和癌细胞之间的相互作用,以及这种作用对肿瘤转移和疗效的影响机制。

1.3.5 术语丰富

医学术语是构成医学信息的语言基础,其语义具有严谨性和单一性。生物医学英文文献中术语丰富,表意严谨,也因此表现出严格的专业性。

例56

Diagnosis, the determination of the nature of a disease, is based on many factors, including the signs, symptoms, and, often, laboratory results. Laboratory tests include such familiar procedures as urinalysis, blood chemistry, electrocardiography, and radiography. New diagnostic-imaging techniques such as computerized tomography (CT scan), radiology, ultrasound, and nuclear medicine provide a visualization never before possible. Diagnostic procedures used in determining various diseases are discussed for each system. A physician also derives information for making a diagnosis from a physical examination, from interviewing the patient or a family member, and from a medical history of the patient and family. The physician, having made a diagnosis, may state the possible prognosis of the disease, or the predicted course, and outcome of the disease.[1]

说明：此例选自一篇关于疾病介绍的文献，其中出现了大量的医学相关术语，比如：sign（体征）、symptom（症状）、urinalysis（尿液分析，尿常规检查）、blood chemistry（血液化学）、electrocardiography（心电描记术）、radiography（射线照相术）、computerized tomography（计算机体层摄影）、radiology（放射学）、ultrasound（超声）、nuclear medicine（核医学）、physical examination（体格检查）、medical history（病史）、prognosis（预后）等。

译文：诊断，即确定疾病性质，需要基于多种因素，如体征、症状及实验室检查结果等。实验室检查包括我们熟悉的检查项目，比如：尿液分析（尿常规检查）、血液化学、心电描记术和射线照相术。新的诊断成像技术如计算机体层摄影（CT 扫描）、放射学检查、超声和核医学则提供了前所未有的可视化信息。每个系统相关疾病的诊断过程也有分别论述。医生还可借助体格检查、与病人及其家属的交谈、病人及其家族的病史获得信息、作出诊断。医生在作出诊断后可说明疾病可能的预后（即预期的病程）和疾病的结局。

总体来说，生物医学英文文献的语言特征可主要归纳如下：

第一，生物医学英文文献使用的词汇来源多样，包括大量源于希腊语和拉丁语的医学术语、英语词汇、冠名术语、缩略语和形象性描述语。

第二，生物医学英文文献在文体方面语气正式，注重客观陈述、语言规范、文体质朴、且含有丰富的术语。

第三，生物医学英文文献在表达方面力求准确无误，清楚易懂；在篇章结构方面，层次清楚、组织严谨、逻辑性强。

总之，生物医学英文文献是一种语体正式，但又文风质朴的体裁。掌握生物医学英文文献的语言特征，对于写作者而言，有助于克服生物医学英文文献写作过程中的语言障碍；对于医学学科和专业而言，则有利于医学信息的传播与交流。

---

[1] 例子源自王兰其、王玉安，《医学英语新教程》（下册），上海：复旦大学出版社，2013 年，第 7 页。

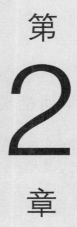

第

2

章

生物医学期刊
英文论文写作
的选词原则：
忠实医学内容，
符合约定表达

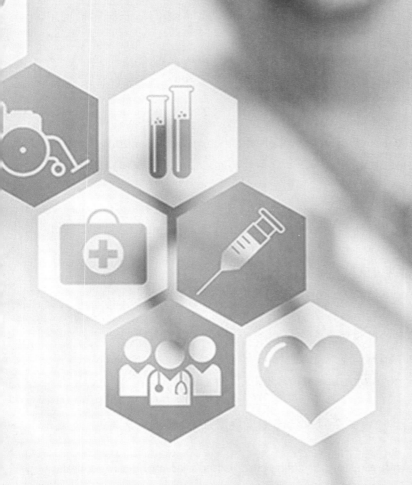

2.1　医学两栖英语词汇

　　医学两栖词汇并不是一类新词,而是某些普通词汇用于医学语境时具有特定的涵义。对于普通词汇的医学意义,即使借助字典,有时也较难正确把握。这就要求论文作者具备一定的医学常识和借助上下文进行理解的能力。

　　医学两栖词汇中存在一些约定俗成的概念,它们由普通词构成,但表达的却是确定的医学意义。如词组 culture medium,对于单个单词,culture 一般理解为"文化",medium 则是"媒介"。构成词组后,词组的意义与这二者出入很大,意为"培养基"。同样,词组 trace elements 中,trace 常指"足迹、踪迹",element 则为"元素、因素"。当二者结合在一起,则是特指"微量元素"。单个单词的使用也类似。形容词 fast 本义为"快速的",在医学语境中,特指"抗……的",如 acid-fast(抗酸的)。

例1

　　心脏杂音一般对身体没有影响,也可能不会引起症状;当血液在心脏流动的速度比正常情况更快时(如运动,怀孕或儿童生长期),就会发生杂音。

　　译文:<u>Heart murmur</u> can be harmless, which may not cause symptoms and can happen when blood flows more rapidly than normal through the heart such as during exercise, pregnancy, or rapid growth in children.

例2

　　老年肝炎患者往往**并发**急性与亚急性肝坏死。

　　译文:Acute and sub-acute hepatic necrosis more often <u>complicates</u> hepatitis in the elderly.

　　儿童和老年人中,流感常常**并发**细菌性肺炎。

　　译文:The bacterial pneumonia may <u>complicate</u> flu at both extremes of age.

例3

　　麦氏点**压痛**和肠鸣音减弱是诊断急性阑尾炎的重要依据。

　　译文:<u>Tenderness</u> in the McBurney's point and decreased bowel sound are given considerable weight in the diagnosis of acute appendicitis.

例4

　　56 岁男性患者,曾患结肠炎,**主诉** 3 个月来背部僵直逐渐加重,最近两天发热、无痛性血便。

　　译文:A 56-year-old male with a history of colitis <u>complained</u> of 3 months of worsening back stiffness and 2 days of fever and painless bloody stool.

例5

　　交感神经属于自主神经系统,可在**应激状态**下通过减慢消化速度、增加心率、呼吸和血压来调节身体。

译文：The <u>sympathetic</u> nerve，belongs to autonomic nervous system，could regulate the body for <u>stress</u> by slowing digestion and increasing the heart rate，respiration，and blood pressure.

更多两栖词汇见下表：

单词	常用公共英语释义	常用医学英语释义	单词	常用公共英语释义	常用医学英语释义
abortion	夭折、失败	流产、堕胎	administration	管理、行政	用药、给药
angry	生气	发炎肿痛的	attack	攻击	（疼痛）发作、（疾病）侵袭
bypass	旁路、小道	搭桥术	calf	小牛	小腿、腓肠区
cataract	大瀑布、暴雨	白内障	colon	冒号	结肠
complication	复杂、混乱	并发症	consumption	消耗、消费	结核病
convulsion	震动、灾变	惊厥、抽搐	cramp	夹、钳	绞痛、痛性痉挛
delivery	发送、交付	分娩、生产	depression	沮丧、压抑	抑郁症
disorder	混乱、无序	病症、功能紊乱、失调	dressing	穿衣、梳妆	敷料
eminence	卓越、显赫	隆起、凸出	fit	合适的	（病痛的）阵发、痉挛
foreign	外国的、陌生的	异物的、外来的	gum	口香糖	牙龈
history	历史	病史	host	主人、主持人	宿主
indication	指示	指征	insufficiency	不足	功能不全
intervention	干涉、干预	介入疗法	knit	编织、联合	接合骨折
labor	体力劳动	分娩、生产	mass	质量、群众	肿块
murmur	嘀咕	（心脏）杂音	portal	入口	门静脉的
pulp	果肉、纸浆	牙髓	rash	急躁的	皮疹
reduction	减少	（骨骼）复位	resident	居民	住院医师、住院患者
secondary	次要的	继发性的	sign	标记	体征

续表

单词	常用公共英语释义	常用医学英语释义	单词	常用公共英语释义	常用医学英语释义
stroke	敲打	中风	sympathetic	同情的	交感神经的
tenderness	柔软	压痛	topical	热门话题的	局部的
trunk	树干	躯干、大血管、神经主干	ward	保卫	病房

2.2 医学特异性固定表达

语言规范是生物医学期刊英文论文的重要文体特点之一。在写作时,作者要注意词汇、短语、句子表达是否符合医学习惯。比如,"假实验组"并非 false group 而应该是 sham group;"无创和微创手术"在医学领域用 minimally invasive and non-invasive surgery 表达;"天然血凝素"中的"天然"用 native 描述。因此,这类表达不能仅停留在字面上的语言转化,要确保符合规范、正式和专业的医学表达要求。更多例子如下:

例6

本研究的病例为 102 例有**早产**史和 107 例有**足月分娩**史的女性。

说明:在妇产学科中分娩一词"delivery"有很多固定搭配 preterm delivery(早产), term delivery(足月分娩), post-term delivery(过期产), difficult delivery(难产), normal delivery(平产)等。

译文:Cases in this study were 102 women who had a history of **preterm delivery** and 107 women who had a history of **term delivery**.

例7

有效的护理不仅可以及时发现不良反应、避免严重后果,而且可以提高患者的**从医性**,达到更好的治疗效果。

说明:"从医性"一般不用 follow the doctor's advice 表达。

译文:Efficient nursing can not only detect adverse reactions in time and avoid serious consequences, but also promote patients' **compliance with doctor's advice** and achieve better therapeutic effect.

例8

总之,这本书为**健康促进**计划的制定者提供了有用的详细指南。

说明:"健康促进"是预防医学中的专业术语,有固定表达,即 health promotion。

译文:In summary, this book provides a useful detailed guide to planners of **health promotion** programs.

例9

取 10 只雄性 SD 大鼠随机分配到**溶媒对照组**和药物（脱氢表雄酮）组。

说明：基础实验中所涉及的"溶媒"一般多用 vehicle 而不是 medium or solvent。

译文：Ten Sprague-Dawley（SD）male rats were randomly divided into **vehicle control group** and DHEA-treated group.

例10

研究表明，阿托珠单抗和化疗相结合的**联合疗法**能够将滤泡淋巴瘤患者死亡风险有效降低 34%。

说明：医学领域中，联合疗法多用 combined therapy 而不是 joined therapy。

译文：Studies show that **combined therapy** with atozumab and chemotherapy can effectively reduce the risk of death by 34% in patients with follicular lymphoma

例11

在此，我们讨论了心血管（CV）结局试验中**联合终点**的必要性，阐明了它们的演变过程，描述了两种最常用的评估动脉粥样硬化心血管（CV）疾病结局的联合终点，并强调了其优缺点。

说明：联合终点多用 composite end points 而不是 combined end points 来表示。

译文：Herein, we discuss the necessity of **composite end points** in CV outcome trials, illustrate their historical evolution, describe the two most commonly used composite end points for assessment of atherosclerotic CV disease outcomes, and highlight their key strengths and weaknesses.

例12

对于重症监护室的腹内脓毒症患者，采用开腹手术治疗并根据血液培养和敏感性测试结果给予抗生素治疗后可有效控制其**急腹症状**。

说明：急腹症是临床专业术语，可统称为 acute abdomen，需手术治疗的急腹症称为 surgical abdomen。

译文：Intra-abdominal sepsis management of patient in an intensive care unit with open abdomen treatment and antibiotics given based on blood culture and sensitivity results enables successful management of difficult **surgical abdomen.**

例13

本文探讨了对尊重患者**知情同意**权的必要性和内容以及具体的实施细节。

说明：临床试验描述中获得受试者的"知情同意"用固定表达 informed consent 而不是 known agreement。

译文：This paper discussed the necessity and contents of respecting patient's right of **informed consent** and how to specifically implement it.

例14

由于临床研究受多种因素干扰，深入研究**心脏骤停**和心肺复苏的病理生理机制存在一定难度。

说明："心脏骤停"的专业表达为 cardiac arrest 而不是字面上理解的 cardiac stop。

译文：Due to influence of many factors in the clinical investigation, it is difficult to conduct a profound pathophysiologic study regarding **cardiac arrest** (CA) and cardiopulmonary resuscitation (CPR).

例15

临终关怀并非是一种治愈疗法，而是一种专注于在患者将要逝世前的几个星期甚至几个月的时间内，减轻其疾病的症状、延缓疾病发展的医疗护理。

说明：护理学中专业术语"临终关怀"一般不用 ending care 而是 terminal care 或 hospice care。

译文：**Hospice care** is not a treatment, but a medical care focused on reducing the symptoms and delaying the disease progression during the weeks and even months before patient's death.

2.3 非医学特异性表达

生物医学期刊英文论文除使用大量高度科学化、专业化和专一化的纯医学术语外，对非医学词汇的选择也有较高要求。因为若选择不够准确、或不符合医学领域写作规范和表达习惯，信息传递的清晰性、准确性和可读性就会受影响。例如，total, overall, whole, general, collective 从词义来看都含有"总"的意思，但在不同的语境中英文表达固定且含义灵活多变：total RNA 是"总 RNA"；overall survival 表示"总生存率"；general peritonitis 表示"弥漫性腹膜炎"；whole blood 表示"全血"。更多例子见下表：

例16

人工	人工喂养（bottle-feeding）、人工呼吸（artificial respiration）、人工引产（induced labor）
易感	易感人群（susceptible population）、易感基因（predisposing gene）、易感因素（predisposing factor）
全	全食，即普通饮食（full diet）、全血（whole blood）、全适供血者（universal donor）、全子宫切除术（complete/total hysterectomy）
治疗	个体化治疗（individualized treatment）、康复治疗（rehabilitation management）、家庭保健治疗（home health care）
general	general anesthesia（全麻）、general check-up（身体全面检查）、general hospital（综合性医院）、general practitioner（全科医生）、general peritonitis（弥漫性腹膜炎）、general health condition（整体健康情况）、general surgery（普外）

续表

heavy	heavy smoker / drinker（嗜烟或酗酒的人）、heavy eater（食量大的人）、heavy food（难消化的食物）、heavy hurt（重创）
primary	primary prevention（初级预防）、primary infection（原发性感染）
discharge	nasal discharge（鼻涕）、discharge from hospital（出院）、partial discharge（局部放电）

　　这类词汇种类繁多，需要长期积累并灵活掌握。为此，医学论文作者除了提高自身业务素质和英文水平外，还应广泛涉猎国际权威医学刊物，熟知最新国际医学写作和用词规范；多积累、多总结、多对比才能更好地进行信息传递和国际间交流。

2.4　复合形容词

　　英语中，两个或两个以上的单词组成的复合形容词常用来修饰名词。组成复合形容词的每个单词之间要用连字符连接以避免混淆和词不达意。由复合形容词构成的词可以扼要地表达繁复的概念，言简意赅。一些论文作者为了让读者对论文印象深刻，使用多余从句、后置定语等冗词赘语，使得行文晦涩难懂。这种情况可以尝试使用复合形容词，比如… the group which was treated by propofol 可以用 the propofol-treated group 简化，更多分类及例子如下：

例17

类型	中文	英文
numeral + noun 数词+名词	两个小时的实验	2-hour experiment
	三个月的治疗 / 持续三个月之久的症状	3-month treatment / symptoms
	四室结构	4-room structure
	双向通道	two-way direction pathway
numeral + noun + *adj.* 数词+名词+形容词	4 岁大的	4-year-old
	6 英寸高的	6-inch-tall
	350 克重的	350-gram-weight
	800 米长的	800-meter-long

续表

类型	中文	英文
adj. + n. // *n. + adj.* 形容词+名词 // 名词 +形容词	中期分析 / 期末分析	mid / final-term analysis
	一流的 / 高规格的	first-rate / high-class
	大规模调查	large-scale investigation
	终身的	life-long
	全国范围内的	nation-wide
	无蛋白质的 / 脱脂的 / 无糖的	protein / fat / sugar-free
	色盲儿童	color-blind kid
	剂量限制性（毒性）	dose-limiting（toxicity）
	化疗难治性（癌症）	chemotherapy-refractory（cancer）
*adj. + n.*ed 形容词+名词 ed 形式	睡眼惺忪的	sleepy-eyed
	有远见的	long-sighted
	目光短浅的	short-sighted
	远视的 / 近视的	far-sighted / near-sighted
	肤色深的,皮肤黝黑的	dark-skinned
*adj. + v.*ing 形容词+动词 ing 形式	影响深远的	far-reaching
	长期忍受的	long-suffering
*n. / adj. + v.*ed 名词 / 形容词 +动词 ed 形式	现成的	ready-made
	新生的	new-born
	以病人为本	patient-oriented
	标记物标记的	tracer-marked
	用乙醚麻醉的	ether-anesthetized
	实验室培养的	lab-grown
	妊娠性的	pregnancy-induced

续表

类型	中文	英文
n. + *v.*ing 名词 + 动词 ing 形式	颌动瞬目（综合征）	jaw-winking（syndrome）
	引人注目的，显著的	eye-catching
	排除故障的	trouble-shooting
	战胜疾病的	disease-fighting
	致病的	disease-causing
	威胁生命的	life-threatening
	长时间持续的	long-running
	救命的	life-saving
others 其他	标准的	up-to-standard
	高于或低于平均水平	higher / lower-than-average
	首次用于人类的	first-in-human
	难以治疗的	hard-to-treat

Exercise

Translate the following sentences with underlined words into English.

1. SARS 的 CT 基本影像表现为磨玻璃样密度（ground-glass opacities）影像和肺实变影像。

2. 我们将 54 只首次用于实验的大鼠随机分成 3 组，每组 18 只。

3. 研究初步证实，使用不卫生的奶瓶是婴幼儿腹泻的一个主要危险因素，如果父母停止使用奶瓶喂养可将腹泻发病率降低 73.7%。

4. 这些因素对妊娠性高血压病的发生、进展、严重程度及脐动脉血流阻力指数（umbilical artery resistance index）可能有重要影响。

5. 酸中毒是缺血的一个常见特征，常常导致脑损伤，但其机制尚不明确。

6. 手术后 4 周、8 周、12 周分批处死家兔，并行气管 CT、内镜、组织病理及扫描电镜检查。

7. 本研究进行耐药监测共 3761 例，原发性耐药率为 27.7%（958 / 3459），继发性耐药率为 41.1%（124 / 302）。

8. 接受孕激素以预防和治疗先兆流产有益于有复发性流产史的孕妇。

9. 酒依赖者的特点包括精神依赖性、身体依赖性、戒断综合征及耐受性。

10. 除了肾功能受损外，我们不能确定其他乳酸酸中毒（lactic acidosis）的诱发因素。

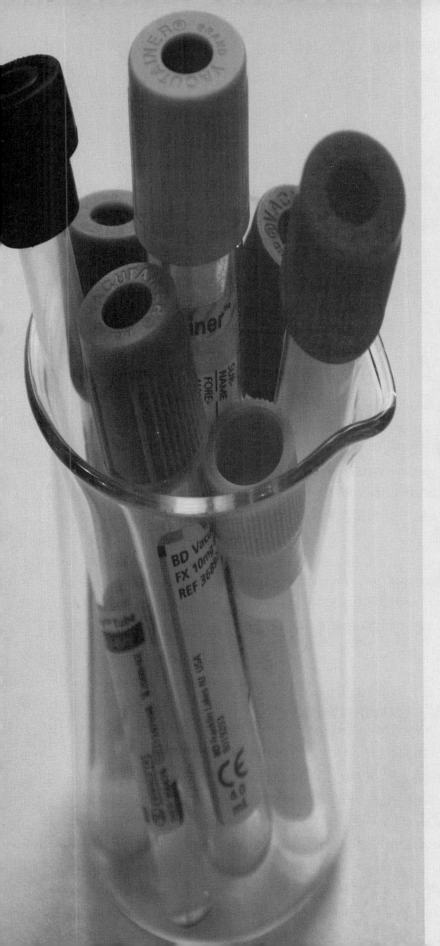

第
3
章

生物医学期刊
英文论文写作
的造句原则：
比照汉语，贴
近英语

3.1 准确表达主谓信息

句子的各成分中,主语和谓语通常是表意的核心部分,准确表达句子的主谓信息不仅是句子写作的基本要求,对于医学论文的写作而言,它的重要性还体现在表意的直截了当和重点突出。

3.1.1 突出句子的重心

医学论文写作应注意句子表达的重心。句子的重心常在主语,写作应选择重点强调的内容作为句子的主语,反映句子的主题。

例1

原句:If pulmonary vascular resistance does not decrease, the newborn will have syndrome of persistent pulmonary hypertension, often leading to death.

说明:原句没有语法错误,但句中主语的选择不恰当。应强调发生的疾病,而非患者。

修改句:If pulmonary vascular resistance does not decrease, the syndrome of persistent pulmonary hypertension, often leading to death, occurs in the newborn.

译文:如果肺血管阻力未降低,新生儿将发生通常可导致死亡的持续性肺动脉高压综合征。

例2

原句:Literature search was performed with PubMed, using the term as "acute necrotizing encephalopathy" with the filter of adult 19+ years.

说明:原句选择 literature search 作为主语不仅使动作的表达弱化,还未能突出表达的重点,即数据库 PubMed。

修改句:PubMed was searched for literature, using the term as "acute necrotizing encephalopathy" with the filter of adult 19+ years.

译文:采用 PubMed 进行文献检索,使用检索词"急性坏死性脑病"并筛选 19 岁以上成人。

例3

原句:Significant improvements in PaO_2 : FiO_2 were observed in the methylprednisolone group on days 3 and 14 after enrollment. Plateau pressure was significantly lower in the methylprednisolone group on days 4, 5, and 7 after enrollment, as compared with the placebo group, whereas respiratory-system compliance was significantly improved on days 7 and 14.

说明:原表述中的两句在陈述对比结果时分别使用了观察结果(significant improvements）和观察指标（plateau pressure 与 respiratory-system compliance）作为主语。通常指标应作为重点内容加以强调，因而对第一句进行修改。此外，在此类句子的表达中，还应注意主语部分在观察指标和观察对象之间做取舍时，也应选择观察指标，参见例 4。

修改句：The ratio of PaO$_2$ to FiO$_2$ was significantly improved in the methylprednisolone group on days 3 and 14 after enrollment. Plateau pressure was significantly lower in the methylprednisolone group on days 4，5，and 7 after enrollment，as compared with the placebo group，whereas respiratory-system compliance was significantly improved on days 7 and 14.

译文：纳入研究后 3 天和 14 天，甲泼尼龙组病人的 PaO2／FiO2 比显著改善。纳入研究后 4 天、5 天和 7 天，甲泼尼龙组病人的平台压显著低于安慰剂组，而 7 天和 14 天的呼吸系统顺应性显著改善。

例4

原句：Patients receiving monotherapy had a lower all-cause mortality than those receiving combination therapy.

说明：原句的主语不是最佳选择，因为句子陈述的是对照研究的结果。一般情况下强调的内容应是观察指标，而不是观察对象。

修改句：All-cause mortality was lower among patients receiving monotherapy than among those receiving combination therapy.

译文：单药治疗组的全因死亡率低于联合治疗组。

3.1.2　实义动词代替抽象名词

在传统论文写作中，用动词的分词形式或动词演变的名词构成句子成分，另以动词搭配组成句子的情况并不少见，这种写作的弊端是句子表达晦涩呆板。相反，如果使用实义动词代替抽象名词，句子则会充满活力，变得自然、简洁、明了。

例5

原句：A significant decrease in the blood pressure occurred during the surgery.

说明：原句中动词 occurred 不能真正表达该句的行为。而真正的行为却被不恰当地表达为主语。另外，如前所述，本句的重心，即主题应为 blood pressure，应调整为句子的主语。

修改句：The blood pressure decreased significantly during the surgery.

译文：术中血压明显下降。

例6

原句：Resection of the aneurysm was accomplished.

说明：本句的重心应该是 aneurysms，即描述的对象，应作主语。原主语 resection 是发生的事件，应作谓语。

修改句：The aneurysm was resected.

或：We resected the aneurysm.

译文：动脉瘤被切除。

例7

原句：The results indicate that immunization and irradiation both cause stimulation of lysosomal enzyme activity in macrophages.

说明：在原句中，宾语从句中的宾语 stimulation 含动词意义，cause stimulation 这样的表述繁琐，且表意效果弱化，因而应该直接使用实义动词 stimulate。

修改句：The results indicate that immunization and irradiation both stimulate lysosomal enzyme activity in macrophages.

译文：结果表明免疫和辐射均能激发巨噬细胞的溶酶体酶活性。

例8

原句：Injection of the protein was more difficult of achievement in older animals due to frequency of occurrence of thrombosis.

说明：这句话使用了 3 个含动作意义的名词，即 injection，achievement 和 occurrence。在语法意义上，表意毫无问题，但原句中 injection 和 occurrence 所在的介词短语表意效果明显不如实义动词，achievement 所在的结构则过于书面化，属于无意义的重复。此外，本句表意调整为形式主语句更符合英语的表达习惯，且简洁易懂。

修改句：It was more difficult to inject the protein into older animals because thrombi often occurred.

译文：在老年动物体内注射蛋白更难，原因在于经常发生血栓。

例9

原句：There was a prompt reversion of the serum creatinine-level.

说明：原句使用了 reversion 与 there be 句型搭配，语法上正确。但 there be 句型表意较弱，与抽象名词搭配就进一步弱化了语意的表达效果。

修改句：The serum creatinine-level promptly reverted to normal.

译文：血清肌酐迅速恢复正常。

3.1.3 强调动词表意的准确

在写作句子时，除强调实义动词代替抽象名词外，还应仔细思考其中表达的行为，对动词的选择力求准确、具体，以更好地实现表意的目的。

例10

原句：The cardiac fibroblasts were exposed to a hypoxia chamber.

说明：本句突出了主谓信息，但谓语动词的选择不够准确。暴露一词的表意不符合实验的具体操作方式，即在特定环境中孵化，故而将动词 exposed 更换为 incubated。

修改句：The cardiac fibroblasts were incubated in a hypoxia chamber.

译文：心脏成纤维细胞在低氧舱中孵化培养。

例11

原句：Consuming 4 cups / d of caffeinated coffee for 24 wk was associated with a modest reduction in urinary creatinine concentrations.

说明：如前所述，句子的最佳谓语应为实义动词，表达直接了当，信息明了突出。因此，将本句中隐于介词结构中的 reduction 一词确定为谓语。

修改句：Consuming 4 cups / d of caffeinated coffee for 24 wk modestly reduced urinary creatinine concentrations.

译文：每日饮用含咖啡因咖啡 4 杯、持续 24 周可轻微降低尿肌酐浓度。

3.2　合理使用前置修饰语

前置修饰语是实现表意准确的重要方法，常见的前置修饰语包括形容词、副词和名词。在论文写作中，前置修饰语的使用要注意简洁，避免类似修饰语的重复出现。同时，在使用多个前置修饰语，特别是名词作为修饰语时，还应注意清晰表达修饰关系，避免出现修饰对象不明。

3.2.1　前置修饰语的简洁性

例12

原句：The present research cannot fully and unambiguously explain the potentially underlying mechanism of this disease.

说明：mechanism 前的修饰语 potentially underlying 存在表意重复，可将修饰作用较弱的 potentially 去掉。同时，谓语动词 explain 前的 fully 和 unambiguously 也有类似的问题，可去其一。

修改句：The present research cannot fully explain the underlying mechanism of this disease.

译文：目前研究不能充分解释这种疾病的潜在机制。

例13

原句：The impressive and clinically and statistically significant data are of great and unique importance to this rather poorly researched field of Alzheimer's disease and will substantially improve the understanding of it.

说明：原句 data 的前置修饰语较长，既包括直接修饰词 impressive 和 significant，还包括修饰 significant 的 clinically 和 statistically，不仅没能加强表意效果，反而使表达啰嗦、意义重复。并且，在此句中，对 data 的描述既包括前置修饰语又包括主系表句子结构中的表语，故而可做取舍，考虑删减表意重复部分以体现语言的简洁性。

修改句：The statistically significant data in clinic substantially improve the current understanding of Alzheimer's disease.

译文：这些临床上具有统计学意义的数据极大地提升了目前对阿尔兹海默症的认识。

3.2.2　名词性修饰语的合理性

许多医学术语是由一个或多个名词组成的复合词语。这些复合词语为医学界公认，可以广泛使用而不引起混淆，例如：blood flow（血流），protein metabolism（蛋白质代谢），liver function（肝功能），ion concentration（离子浓度），glucose tolerance test（葡萄糖耐量测试），和 growth hormone deficiency syndrome（生长激素缺乏综合症）等。但对于非公认的名词性复合词语，使用时须谨慎。使用两个以上的名词修饰语，或名词词组前加形容词修饰语时，应该避免因修辞语堆砌或误置造成理解困难甚至歧义，需用恰当的介词结构加以调整以达到准确表达。

例14

原句：Our study was to discuss the protective effects of Fuyuan capsule on the pig serum induced liver fibrosis rat.

说明：原句中 pig serum induced liver fibrosis rat 受中文表达影响，由多个名词堆砌而成，中间还穿插一个过去分词修饰语。应该重新安排，使各成分关系表达清楚，更加符合英语的表达规范。

修改句：Our study was to discuss the protective effects of Fuyuan capsule on the rat with liver fibrosis induced by pig serum.

译文：我们的研究旨在检测复元胶囊对猪血清所致肝纤维化大鼠的保护作用。

例15

原句：Normal and traumatic brain injury microglial activation were assessed.

说明：原句中主语因修饰语，特别是名词修饰语的堆叠使"normal"的修饰对象表达不清，应按照表意目的进行调整，并添加信息。

修改句：The microglial activation in normal subjects and patients with traumatic brain injury were assessed.

译文：评估正常人和外伤性脑损伤患者小胶质细胞的激活情况。

例16

原句：T4 stimulated choline incorporation into primary fetal lung cell cultures.

说明：此句中 primary 既可以理解为 fetal lung cells 的修饰语，也可理解为 cultures 的修饰语，造成理解上的混淆。应该用恰当的介词结构 fetal lung cells in primary cultures 表达修饰关系。

修改句：T4 stimulated incorporation of choline into fetal lung cells in primary cultures.

译文：T4 刺激胆碱合成原代培养物中的胎儿肺细胞。

3.3　恰当使用代词

代词能代替名词、名词短语和句子，使语句表达简练，并具有较强的表意功能。这就使得在论文写作中代词的使用必须正确,否则就易出现表意不清。在使用代词时,应重点注意以下两方面。

3.3.1　避免代词指代不明

例17

原句：Namely, hepatic cell carcinoma is related to genetic changes in injured hepatocytes. They result from the effect of HBV and chemical carcinogen, but the exact mechanism is unknown.

说明：原句中 they 指代不明,既可指紧邻的 injured hepatocytes,又可指 genetic changes。要使意思明确,需要重复所指代的内容。

修改句：Namely, hepatic cell carcinoma is related to genetic changes in injured hepatocytes. The genetic changes were caused by HBV and exposure to chemical carcinogen, but the exact mechanism is unknown.

译文：也就是说,肝细胞癌与受损肝细胞的基因改变有关。基因改变由乙肝病毒和接触化学致癌物所致,但具体机制尚不清楚。

例18

原句：Stroke represents a syndrome rather than a single disease, and is caused by a number of distinct pathologies. The majority of those are caused by cerebral ischemia resulting in infarction.

说明：原句中 those 一词指代不明,从其复数形式及相邻位置可能是 pathologies,然而根据上下文,它实际所指的应该是 stroke。故而此处代词使用不当,应重复所指代的名词。

修改句：Stroke represents a syndrome rather than a single disease, and is caused by a number of distinct pathologies. The majority of strokes are caused by cerebral ischemia resulting in infarction.

译文：卒中是综合征而不是单一的疾病,由多种不同的病理机制所致。多数卒中是由引起梗塞的脑缺血所致。

3.3.2　避免先行词缺失

代词使用中另一种常见的错误是用代词指代前句中的某些概念,而不是前句中的具体名词。这就会导致句子意义含糊不清,通常的解决方法是在代词后重复前句中的一个概念词或是根据前句增加一个类别词。

例19

原句：

The relationship between these factors and AKI could not be established in our study. We speculate that this might be due to some pathophysiological differences between western and eastern populations.

说明：原句中的 this 指代不明，在前文未出现先行词。需要根据前文表达或隐含的概念，总结提炼出一个概念词。根据句意，this 表达的是隐含在前句里的一个概念："本研究与先前研究的不一致性"，应该用"this inconsistency"予以明确。

修改句：The relationship between these factors and AKI could not be established in our study. We speculate that this inconsistency（between our study and previous studies）might be due to some pathophysiological differences between western and eastern populations.

例20

原句：The study combined radiation therapy and androgen-deprivation therapy. As a result of this, the survival among some men with an intact prostate was prolonged.

说明：虽然代词 this 暗指 combination 这一疗法，但语法上原文没有对应的所指名词，因此需要基于上文明确这一概念词。

修改句：The study combined radiation therapy and androgen-deprivation therapy. As a result of this combination（therapy）, the survival among some men with an intact prostate was prolonged.

译文：本研究将放射疗法与雄激素阻断疗法相结合。结果表明这种联合疗法延长了一些前列腺完整的男性患者的生存期。

3.4　正确使用平行结构

平行结构是指由连词连接的两个或两个以上重要性和逻辑性相当的词、词组、短语或句子，在结构上必须完全对等、相互平行，同时要求它们的数、格、时态也都必须一致。常用的连接词有：and, but, or, both... and, either... or, neither... or, not only...but also, than, as well as 等。使用平行结构的目的是使读者关注句子表达的内容而非形式，从而使阅读更快捷有效。在论文写作中应重点关注以下两方面。

3.4.1　平行结构表达形式的一致性

例21

原句：To help prevent the spread of respiratory viruses, the public were instructed to avoid close contact with people who are sick, and they should wash hands often with soap and to water for at least 20 seconds.

说明：原句中 instructed 的宾语有不定式和从句形式，不平行。

修改句：To help prevent the spread of respiratory viruses, the public were instructed to avoid close contact with people who are sick, and to wash hands often with soap and water for at least 20 seconds.

译文：为了防止呼吸道病毒的传播，要求大众避免与病人密切接触，并经常用肥皂和水洗手至少 20 秒。

例22

　　原句：The systolic pressure decreased by 10%, but 5% increase was found for the diastolic pressure.

　　说明：but 连接的两个句子表对比，语意平行，形式上也应保持一致。

　　修改句：The systolic pressure decreased by 10%, but the diastolic pressure increased by 5%.

　　译文：收缩压下降了 10%，而舒张压上升了 5%。

例23

　　原句：The neutralizing antibody level in children of 6–12 months was found to be the lowest, the group of 13–14 years old showed a higher level while the level in the group of 8–9 years old was the highest.

　　说明：本句中有三个并列分句介绍三个年龄组的中和抗体含量，重要性和逻辑性相当。然而用三种不同的句式来表达影响读者快捷有效地获取信息。

　　修改句：The neutralizing antibody level was found to be the lowest in children of 6-12 months, higher in those of 13-14 years, and the highest in those of 8-9 years.

　　译文：中和抗体的含量在 6~12 个月的婴儿组最低，13~14 岁的年龄组较高，而 8~9 岁年龄组最高。

3.4.2　避免平行结构的错误表达

例24

　　原句：For prevention of death caused by hemorrhage, tranexamic acid was as efficacious but cheaper than antibiotics.

　　说明：原句中描述 tranexamic acid 属性的两个修辞语 efficacious 和 cheaper 并不是平行的结构，所以不能简单地罗列在一起。

　　修改句：For prevention of death caused by hemorrhage, tranexamic acid was as efficacious as antibiotics, but was cheaper.

　　译文：对于预防出血导致的死亡，氨甲环酸和抗生素一样有效，但成本较低。

例25

　　原句：The department was responsible for recruiting, monitoring and analyzing the data.

　　说明：介词 for 后的三个动名词搭配的宾语并不都是 data，表达平行结构时应明确不同的宾语。

　　修改句：The department was responsible for recruiting the patients, monitoring the trial, and analyzing the data.

　　译文：该部门负责招募患者、监控试验以及分析数据。

3.5 注意句子的可读性

生物医学期刊英文论文写作的准确性特点决定了行文中表意的复杂性和多层次性，这就使得论文中句子的表达相对较长。然而，长句并不符合人们的阅读习惯。因而，在写作中，作者应注意句子长度的可读性。请对照阅读下面三个小段①。

例26-1

Two canine（犬的）cadavers（尸体）with orthopedic（矫形的）abnormalities were identified which included a first dog that had an unusual deformity secondary to premature closure of the distal ulnar physis（尺骨骨骺）and a second dog that had a hypertrophic nonunion of the femur（股骨），and the radius（桡骨）and femur of both dogs were harvested and cleaned of soft tissues.

说明：此例共 1 句，有 54 个词，表达了大量的信息。句子过长，不利于读者阅读和获取信息。

例26-2

Two canine cadavers with orthopedic abnormalities were identified. The first dog had an unusual deformity. It was secondary to premature closure of the distal ulnar physis. The second dog had a hypertrophic nonunion of the femur. The radius and femur of both dogs were harvested. They were cleaned of soft tissues.

说明：此例将上一句的信息拆分到了 6 个句子，共用词 51 个。每个句子平均包含 8.5 个词。这种短句表达过于碎片化，造成句间信息不连贯，也不利于阅读。

例26-3

Two canine cadavers with orthopedic abnormalities were identified. The first dog had an unusual deformity secondary to premature closure of the distal ulnar physis; the second, a hypertrophic nonunion of the femur. The radius and femur of both dogs were harvested and cleaned of soft tissues.

说明：此例用了 3 个句子，共 46 个词表达以上语意。每个句子平均包含 15.3 个词，是较理想的句子长度，且各句信息表达完整。

增加句子的可读性，应注意以下两个方面。

3.5.1 合理省略句子成分

表现为平行结构的并列句，在写作时可以省略部分相同句子成分，使表达简洁。省略常见三种形式，以下例句中省略部分用括号标出。

第一种形式是相同主谓语，重复出现的主谓语应省略。

---

① 例文摘引自 Matthews, Janice R and Matthews, Robert W. *Successful Scientific Writing：a step-by-step guide for the biological and medical sciences*. New York：Cambridge University Press，third edition，2008，pp.110-111.

例27

原句：The overall survival rate at 12 years was 76.3% in the bicalutamide group, and the overall survival rate at 12 years was 71.3% in the placebo group.

说明：and 连接的两个句子是在陈述两组人群的同一指标，重复的主谓语应省略。但在省略后为使表意更准确，可加上副词"respectively"。如存在比较的意味，也可进一步修改为比较句。

修改句：The overall survival rates at 12 years were 76.3% and 71.3% in the bicalutamide group and the placebo group, respectively.

或：The overall survival rate at 12 years was 76.3% in the bicalutamide group, as compared with 71.3% in the placebo group.

译文：比卡鲁胺组 12 年总生存率为 76.3%，而安慰剂组为 71.3%。

第二种形式是相同主语不同谓语，重复出现的主语应省略。

例28

原句：The rats were injected with 100 μl of normal saline in the tail vein once every day for four consecutive days, and then the rats were treated with allantoin (200 mg/kg, po) for 8 weeks.

说明：原句是对实验大鼠操作步骤的描述，主语均为大鼠，所以无需重复陈述。同时，由于两个谓语都是被动语态，重复的系动词也应一并省掉。

修改句：The rats were injected with 100 μl of normal saline in the tail vein once every day for four consecutive days, and then treated with allantoin (200mg/kg, po) for 8 weeks.

译文：对大鼠每天尾静脉注射 100 μl 生理盐水 1 次，连续 4 天；随后再用尿囊素（按体重每公斤用量 200 毫克，口服）处理 8 周。

第三种形式是不同主语相同谓语，重复的谓语应被省略。

例29

原句：Adverse events with a maximum grade of 1 were reported in 93 patients (33%) in the osimertinib group and in 15 (11%) in the platinum-pemetrexed group, and adverse events with a maximum grade of 2 were reported in 117 (42%) and in 56 (41%), respectively.

说明：原句 and 连接的两个句子主语不同，但谓语都为 were reported。为使表达简洁，可省掉后一句的谓语。

修改句：Adverse events with a maximum grade of 1 were reported in 93 patients (33%) in the osimertinib group and in 15 (11%) in the platinum-pemetrexed group, and adverse events with a maximum grade of 2 in 117 (42%) and in 56 (41%), respectively.

译文：奥西米替尼组 93 名患者（33%）和铂培美曲塞组 15 名患者（11%）报告了最高分级为 1 的不良事件，两组中分别有 117 名（42%）和 56 名（41%）报告了最高分级为 2 的不良事件。

写作中还切忌出现另一个极端，即表达过于简单化，受中文影响却不考虑英语句子表达的语法需要。

例30

原句：Injection of ethanol（17 cases）：recurrence 2 cases（11%）．Open surgery（48 cases）：recurrence 4 cases（8.3%）．Laparoscopic surgery（21 cases）：recurrence 1 case（4.8%）．

修改句：Of 17 cases of ethanol injection，2 cases of complication occurred．Of 48 cases of open surgery，4 cases of recurrence occurred．Of 21 cases of laparoscopic surgery，1 case of recurrence occurred．

译文：无水乙醇注射治疗 17 例，出现并发症 2 例；开腹手术 48 例，复发 4 例；腹腔镜手术 21 例，复发 1 例。

3.5.2　避免写作长难句

生物医学论文写作强调语言表达的简洁性和可读性，论文写作者应纠正句子信息越丰富、越能体现其价值的错误观念。非必需的堆叠修饰语以及表达多层语意所构建的长难句不仅会增加阅读难度，严重时还会导致语意表达不清。因而，在表达复杂意义时，写作者应学会拆分，避免长难句。

例31

原句：To examine the effect of gut microbiota in a mouse model of rheumatoid arthritis that develops atherosclerosis，we created three groups of K／BxN female mice that were positive for the anti-glucose-6-phosphate isomerase antibody to carry out the serological tests and histological analysis．

说明：原句中包含了三层信息，即实验目的、实验对象和实验方法。虽然没有语法错误，但众多重要信息在一个句子中呈现不仅会造成读者阅读困难，也易造成重要信息被忽略。应将句子按信息层进行拆分。

修改句：The purpose of the study was to examine the effect of gut microbiota in a mouse model of rheumatoid arthritis that develops atherosclerosis．For this purpose，we created three groups of K／BxN female mice that were positive for the anti-glucose-6-phosphate isomerase antibody．The serological tests and histological analysis were used to determine the effects．

译文：本研究旨在检测肠道微生物群在类风湿关节炎形成动脉粥样硬化小鼠模型中的作用。为此，我们建立了三组抗葡萄糖-6-磷酸异构酶抗体阳性的 K／BxN 雌性小鼠。本研究使用血清学检验和组织学分析方法。

值得注意的是，生物医学期刊英文论文中长句是屡见不鲜的，长句存在的必要性是因为在这些句子中有主要信息和支撑信息构成一个逻辑严密、形式严谨的信息整体，而这时如果使用松散零碎的短句也会使表达显得中文化，不符合英文写作的要求。

例32

原句：Five cases of chyluria were treated by retroperitoneoscopic renal pedicle lymphatic disconnection from 2005 to 2007. Three are males and 2 females. Their age was from 38 to 68 years. The average age was 48 years.

修改句：Five patients with chyluria were treated by retroperitoneoscopic renal pedicle lymhatic disconnection from 2005 to 2007，among whom 3 were males and 2 females，ranging in age from 38 to 68 years，with the average of 48 years.

译文：2005 年至 2007 年我院经后腹腔镜肾蒂淋巴管结扎术治疗乳糜尿患者共 5 例，其中男性 3 例，女性 2 例，年龄 38~68 岁，平均 48 岁。

3.6　避免常见语法错误

在进入论文写作阶段，写作者一般具有一定的英语写作能力，对语法掌握较好。然而，在写作时也会因为不仔细或受中式思维的影响犯一些语法错误。最常见的是以下两种，应尽量避免。

3.6.1　主谓不一致

例33

原句：The past medial history, family history and social history of patient was checked.

说明：主语和谓语的单复数形式不一致。

修改句：The past medial history, family history and social history of patient were checked.

译文：检查了病人的既往病史、家族病史和社会史。

例34

原句：Neither the experiment group nor the control group were informed of the test results.

说明：neither… nor 表达了对两项内容的否定，按照语法规则，谓语的单复数形式由 nor 的宾语决定，所以原句谓语应修改为单数。

修改句：Neither the experiment group nor the control group was informed of the test results.

译文：实验组和对照组都没有被告知测试结果。

例35

原句：Few data has showed an inverse association between serum lipid levels and EOC severity.

说明："数据"这一概念在使用时通常指称复数，对应 data。这就使得写作者常忽略其还有单数形式 datum，类似的还有 criteria（criterium），media（medium）等。

修改句：Few data have showed an inverse association between serum lipid levels and EOC severity.

译文：很少有数据显示血脂水平与 EOC 严重程度呈负相关。

例36

原句：Comorbidities such as depression was likely to contribute to the development of CI.

说明：尽管离系动词最近的概念是单数的 depression，但句子的真正主语是复数的comorbidities。

修改句：Comorbidities such as depression were likely to contribute to the development of CI.

译文：抑郁症等共病可能导致 CI 的发展。

句子主谓不一致的问题除体现在单复数上，受汉语被动句无主语表达的影响，英文被动句的写作也常出现主语（动作实施对象）选择不当的情况，表现为主谓表达意义不一致。

例37

原句：The Sprague-Dawley rats were peritoneally injected endotoxin（3mg／kg），recorded the time and amount of coma rats within 12h later, determined the blood plasma ammonia concentration, counted the apoptosis cells and GFAP positive cells, and western blots of GS.

说明：此句受汉语被动句无主语表达的影响，与其他句子并列使用时在语法上就表现为主谓不一致的错误。鉴于本句包含信息多，且为互不关联的独立信息，修改时应该在每表达一个新主题和信息时重启一个句子，使信息重点突出，层次分明。

修改句：The Sprague-Dawley rats were peritoneally injected with endotoxin（3mg／kg）. The duration of coma and the number of coma rats were recorded within 12h. The ammonia concentration in blood plasma was determined. The apoptosis cells and GFAP positive cells were counted. GS were analyzed by western blotting.

译文：腹腔注射内毒素（3mg／kg），记录 12h 内 Sprague-Dawley 大鼠昏迷间期和发生昏迷大鼠的只数，测定血氨浓度，对凋亡细胞和 GFAP 阳性细胞计数，用免疫印迹法分析 GS。

3.6.2 游离短语

游离短语是指句中的某些表述与结构和句子的其他内容在语法上不构成关联，从而处于游离的状态。故而，游离短语的出现应被视为语法错误。常见的有以下两种形式。

第一种形式是悬垂分词，即逻辑主语与所处句子的主语不一致的动词现在分词或过去分词。

例38

原句：Modifying the operation rules, the research results were satisfied.

说明：原句中现在分词短语 modifying the operation rules 的主语应理解为 researchers，与句子主语不一致，变成了游离短语。修改时可明确分词短语的主语，或运用抽象名词弱化施动者。

修改句：The research results were satisfied after researchers modified the operation rules 或：The research results were satisfied after modification of the operation rules.

译文：研究者调整操作规范后，研究结果令人满意。

例39

原句：Based on previous study, the majority of patients in need of a hematopoietic-cell transplant do not have a matched related donor.

说明：原句中过去分词短语的主语应是抽象的 knowledge 或 information，与句子的主语不一致。

修改句：On the basis of the previous study, the majority of patients in need of a hematopoietic-cell transplant do not have matched related donors.

译文：根据之前的研究，大多数需要造血细胞移植的患者没有匹配的相关供体。

值得注意的是，在不产生歧义的情况下，生物医学期刊英文论文中也开始出现以悬垂分词充当状语的句子，如 Sth. was done by doing sth.，以及 Sth. was done using…。详见以下摘选自期刊 *Cell* 的例子。

例40

Approximately 20% stretch was achieved by first removing the mesentery and pinning the gut taught (but unstretched) to the agarose bed, measuring the length of the midgut segment between the pins, and then removing one of the pins and placing it at an increased distance to change the length and thus stretch the midgut by about 20% of its original length.

译文：大约 20% 的拉伸是通过以下方法实现的。首先切除肠系膜、将调校好的（但未拉伸的）肠管钉在琼脂糖床上，测量两针之间中肠段的长度，然后取出其中一个针，将其放置在更远的点以改变长度，从而将中肠拉伸约 20% 的原始长度。

第二种形式是短语结构，常见形容词构成的短语结构。

例41

原句：Although not typical in symptoms, CT scanning confirmed the infection.

说明：形容词短语 not typical in symptoms 的主语应理解为 patients，与主句主语 CT scanning 不一致，成为游离短语。

修改句：Although not typical in symptoms, the patient was confirmed with infection by CT scanning.

译文：尽管症状不明显，CT 扫描确诊患者感染。

Exercise

Find out the faulty sentence structures in the following sentences and correct them.

1. After treatment, the patient was found an increase in the blood oxygen saturation.

2. Evaporation of ethanol from the mixture takes place rapidly.

3. Measurements of blood pH were made with a radiometer capillary electrode.

4. There are still three main shortcomings: 50% acute closure, 35% late restenosis, and another 50% of cases unsuitable to be treated with PTCA.

5. We performed a seventh intercostal space anterior lateral thoracotomy on the patient.

6. The course of the patient's illness was followed after leaving the hospital.

7. Each of the 41 fecal specimens were treated as described in the text.

8. Ataxia telangiectasia may be associated with DNA repair deficiency of the damage caused by ionizing radiation.

9. We should like to point out, however, that lipid peroxidation may still be involved somehow in the inception of atherosclerosis or in forwarding its progress.

10. Pulse rate decreased by 40 beats/min, systolic blood pressure decreased by 50 mmHg, and cardiac output decreased by 18%.

11. The preparation of the cardioplegic solution should meet the following requirements: (1) maintain a proper concentration of potassium ion, (2) contain all principal electrolytes existing in the normal myocardium, (3) keep an appropriate osmolarity, and (4) the solution must be easy to prepare and stable.

12. Our approach aimed to pave the way toward a systematic unveiling of the human microbiome chemical repertoire.

13. We recently observed bronchospastic reactions in an asthmatic patient after ingesting this drug.

14. None of the groups were found side effects.

15. Deaths occurring within 30 days of operation were considered early mortalities, and deaths occurring after 30 days of operation were considered late mortalities.

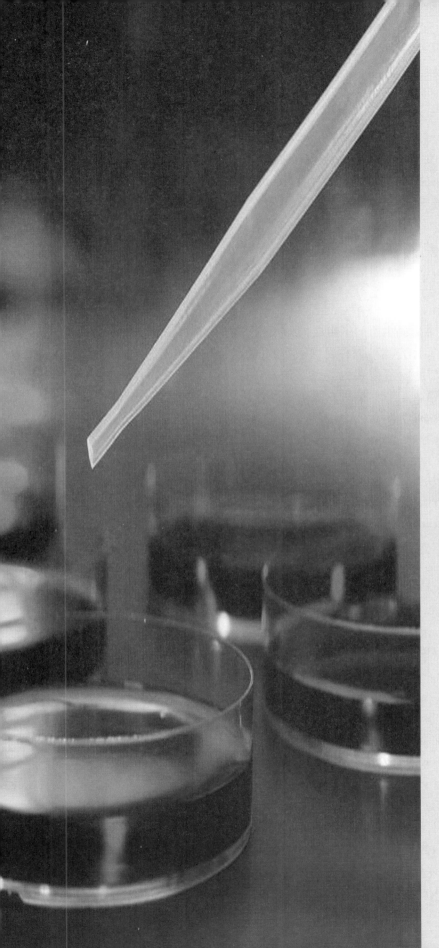

第
4
章

生物医学期刊
英文论文写作
的成段原则：
逻辑连贯有序，
语言简洁易懂

生物医学期刊英文论文每一个段落都应有良好的组织结构和连贯性,突出重点内容,清楚阐明信息。每一个段落必须要有明确的主题,以及合乎逻辑的连贯叙述来阐述这一主题。这样,不管读者是否具备论文相关领域的专业知识,都能借助清晰的写作思路理解文章大意。写好一个清楚的段落,必须掌握以下基本原则:段落结构有序、句子连贯清晰、重点内容突出。下面分别加以叙述。

4.1 段落结构有序

一个段落由围绕一个主题的多个句子组成,目的是汇集与主题相关的信息,从而传递一个明确的中心思想。多种写作方式可以实现这一目的,最常用和最清晰的方式是首先阐述段落的概要,然后提供细节。段落概要的典型写法是在段落开始部分写作主题句(topic sentence),提示段落的主题或信息。然后在段落中写作用以支持主题句、进行细节描述的其他句子,即支持句(supporting sentence)。

例1

(S1) Throughout the years, mice have proven to be invaluable model organisms for biomedical research, allowing researchers to investigate disorders by manipulating the environment or the genome. (S2) Unlike their human counterparts, mice can be studied in a carefully controlled environment. (S3) It is also relatively easy for researchers to manipulate diet composition, food availability, exercise, and other environmental factors that can contribute to differences in physiological outcomes in mice. (S4) In addition to being relatively inexpensive, fast to reproduce, and easy to maintain compared to other mammalian models, mice are also remarkably similar to humans in terms of their physiology and genetics. (S5) Mice and humans share approximately the same number of genes and exhibit extensive synteny. (S6) Because of their genetic similarity to humans, mice have been used to pioneer genetic manipulation technologies, such as gene overexpression and gene knockout and knockdown models at the whole-organism level or in specific tissues. (S7) These technological breakthroughs in genetics research have fueled several decades of rapid discovery and knowledge expansion in many biomedical fields. (S8) The ability to manipulate both genetic and environmental variables with relative ease has made mice one of the most widely used in vivo models in biomedical research today.

说明:第1句为主题句;第2~7句为支持性句子。最后一句呼应主题句,重述该段落的要点。

译文:(S1)多年来,小鼠已被证明是进行生物医学研究的宝贵模型生物,使研究人员可以通过操纵环境或基因组来研究疾病。(S2)与人类不同的是,小鼠研究可以在精心控制的环境中展开。(S3)研究人员相对容易控制饮食构成、食物供应、运动和其他可能导致小鼠生理结局差异的环境因素。（S4）与其他哺乳动物模型相比，小鼠不仅成本相对低廉、繁殖速度快、易于喂养，而且其在生理和遗传方面与人类也非常相似。（S5）小鼠和人类的基因数量大致相同，并表现出广泛的共线性。（S6）由于小鼠与人类的遗传相似性，它们已被用于开发基因操作技术，如在整个生物体水平或特定组织中的基因过表达、基因敲除和敲除模型。（S7）遗传学研究中的这些技术突破推动了许多生物医学领域几十年的快速发现和知识扩展。（S8）遗传和环境变量相对易控的特性已使小鼠成为当今生物医学研究中使用最广泛的体内模型之一。

在生物医学期刊英文论文写作中，段落中的支持句按照一定的逻辑关系展开。常见的展开方式有以下几种：一是按重要性大小的顺序，先主后次或先次后主；二是按主题句交代的顺序；三是正反论证；四是按时间顺序；五是问题-解答或解答-问题模式；六是漏斗模式。①

4.1.1　按重要性大小的顺序

按重要性大小的顺序（importance order），也就是从最重要到不重要或不重要到最重要的顺序来组织段落。支持句可以通过例证、比较和对比、因果关系等方式展开。写作时将表达段落主旨信息的主题句置于段首，然后按重要性顺序添加支持性的细节。

例2

（S1）There was no association of PiB SUVR or change in PiB SUVR with changes in MMSE score, UPDRS-III score, or RCF-measured visual-perceptual performance.（S2）A potential explanation is lower statistical power or relatively narrow range of values in DLB group.（S3）Additionally, cognitive fluctuations may contribute to both short-term and long-term variability in clinical and cognitive evaluations.（S4）Moreover, the MMSE might not be an optimal measure of global cognitive decline in DLB, although some studies have suggested otherwise.（S5）Most importantly, these clinical and cognitive measures may be influenced by other pathologies, such as NFT-tau or α-synuclein, or by other neurologic and functional factors, such as mood or daytime sleepiness.

说明：第1句是主题句；第2~5句为支持句，支持句按照重要性大小排列，从次重要到最重要；标记语 Most importantly…出现在段落的最后一句。

译文：（S1）PiB SUVR 或 PiB SUVR 变化与 MMSE 评分、UPDRS-III 评分或 RCF 测量的视觉-感知能力的变化之间无相关性。（S2）一种可能的解释是 DLB 组的统计功效较低或值范围相对较窄。（S3）此外，认知波动可能会导致临床和认知评估的短期和长期差异。（S4）再者，MMSE 可能不是衡量 DLB 整体认知能力下降的最佳指标，尽管一些研究表明并非如此。（S5）最重要的是，这些临床和认知指标可能受其他病理因素（例如 NFT-tau 或 α-突触核蛋白）和神经性和功能性因素（例如情绪或白天嗜睡）的影响。

---

① Mimi Zeiger, *Essentials of Writing Biomedical Research Papers*. U.S.A.：The McGraw-Hill companies, Inc., second edition, 2000, p. 55.

例3

（S1）Many factors contributing to the impairment of renal function in patients with HF have been proposed, including reduced cardiac output, intra-abdominal pressure and CVP, sympathetic overactivity, a maladaptive RAA system, oxidative injury, endothelial dysfunction, and anemia. （S2）Reduced cardiac output in HF is considered to be the main factor leading to a decrease in renal function. （S3）However, data analysis from the Evaluation Study of Congestive heart failure And Pulmonary artery catheterization Effectiveness trial（ESCAPE）showed that cardiac output was not the only risk factor causing impaired renal function, and a weak correlation between the cardiac index and eGFR was shown. （S4）Nonetheless, CVP level can affect eGFR and mortality. （S5）Damman et al. reported that increased CVP was associated with impairment of renal function and independently associated with all-cause mortality during a 10-year follow-up period in patients with CVD. （S6）In addition, a high CVP level has been reported to be the most important hemodynamic factor leading to renal dysfunction in decompensated patients with advanced HF. （S7）A previous clinical study reported that, when the intra-abdominal venous pressure increased up to approximately 20 mmHg, the GFR decreased by 28%. （S8）Therefore, the appropriate use of diuretics may reduce renal venous pressure and thus improve GFR. （S9）RV dysfunction may also contribute to central venous congestion and impairment of renal function, and thus improving RV function may decrease the extent of renal dysfunction. （S10）Along with the hemodynamic factors, HF can activate the RAA system that would subsequently increase sodium reabsorption, water retention, sympathetic overactivity, peripheral vascular contraction, and LV remodeling. （S11）Renal function may decline after RAA system activation. （S12）Previous studies have shown that ACEIs and ARBs can protect against the deterioration of renal function in diabetic nephropathy.

说明：第 1 句是主题句；第 2～12 句为支持句，支持句按照重要性大小排列，从最重要到次重要。

译文：（S1）已有研究提出导致心衰患者肾功能受损的诸多因素，包括心输出量减少、腹腔内压力和 CVP、交感神经过度活跃、RAA 系统适应不良、氧化性损伤、内皮功能障碍和贫血。（S2）心衰患者心输出量减少被认为是导致肾功能下降的主要因素。（S3）然而，充血性心力衰竭和肺动脉插管有效性试验评估研究的数据分析表明，心输出量并不是导致肾功能受损的唯一风险因素，并且心脏指数与 eGFR 之间呈弱相关（如图所示）。（S4）尽管如此，CVP 水平会影响 eGFR 和死亡率。（S5）Damman 等人报道，在对 CVD 患者的 10 年随访期内，CVP 升高与肾功能受损有关，并且与全因死亡率独立相关。（S6）此外，据报道，高 CVP 水平是导致晚期失代偿性心衰患者肾功能异常的最重要的血液动力学因素。（S7）以往的一项临床研究表明当腹腔内静脉压力增加至约 20 mmHg 时，GFR 降低了 28%。（S8）因此，合理使用利尿剂可以降低肾静脉压力，进而改善 GFR。（S9）RV 功能障碍也可能导致中央静脉充血和肾功能损害，因此，改善 RV 功能可降低肾功能损害的程度。**(S10)** 除了血液动力学因素外，心衰还可以激活 RAA 系统，从而增加钠的重吸收、液体潴留、交感神经过度活跃、外周血管收缩和左室重构。**(S11)** RAA 系统激活可能导致肾功能下降。**(S12)** 既往研究表明 ACEIs 和 ARBs 可以预防糖尿病肾病患者肾功能的恶化。

4.1.2　按主题句交代的顺序

段落也可以按照主题句中对多个小主题陈述的先后顺序组织（announced order）。也就是支持句按照主题句中陈述的多个小主题展开，展开的顺序与主题句中交代的几个小主题的排列顺序相同。

例4

(S1) Human MSCs and HUVECs were used in this study. **(S2)** Human MSCs were isolated from commercially-acquired bone marrow mononuclear cells（MNC）（Lonza, Belgium）using a conventional attachment isolation protocol（adapted from D'Ippolito et al. [40]）. **(S3)** The MSCs were cultured using proliferative / basal medium consisting of low glucose（1 g / l）Dulbecco's Modified Eagle Medium（DMEM）（Lonza, Belgium）, 10% foetal bovine serum（FBS）（Lonza, Belgium）, 1% antibiotic-antimycotic solution（A+A）（SigmaeAldrich, UK）, 1% non-essential amino acids（NEAA）（SigmaeAldrich, UK）and 2 mM l-glutamine（Lonza, Belgium）. **(S4)** The cells were maintained at 37 ℃ and 5% CO_2, and were used for experiments at passage 4. **(S5)** The HUVECs（Life Technologies, UK）were cultured using Medium 200（Life Technologies, UK）supplemented with 2% low serum growth supplement（LSGS）（Life Technologies, UK）at 37 ℃ and 5% CO_2[41]. **(S6)** The cells were used at passage 4.

说明：本段落选自论文的方法部分。第 1 句是主题句，介绍了本研究中使用的两种材料：Human MSCs 和 HUVECs。第 2～5 句是支持句，展开的顺序与主题句中两种材料的排列顺序相同。

译文：(S1) 本研究选用人骨髓间充质干细胞（MSCs）和人脐静脉内皮细胞（HUVECs）。**(S2)** 采用常规附着分离技术（由 D'Ippolito 等人分离技术改进）从市售骨髓单核细胞 MNC（Lonza，比利时）中分离出人 MSCs。**(S3)** 用含低葡萄糖（1g / l）Dulbecco 改良 Eagle 培养基（DMEM）（Lonza,比利时）、10%胎牛血清（FBS）（Lonza, 比利时）、1%抗生素-抗真菌溶液（A+A）（SigmaeAldrich,英国）、1%非必需氨基酸（NEAA）（SigmaeAldrich，英国）和 2mM l-谷氨酰胺（Lonza，比利时）组成的增殖／基础培养基培养 MSCs。**(S4)** 细胞培养维持 37 ℃和 5% 浓度 CO_2 环境，第 4 代细胞用于实验。**(S5)** HUVECs（Life Technologies, 英国）用添加 2%低血清生长添加剂（LSGS）（Life Technologies，英国）的培养基 200（Life Technologies, 英国）在 37 ℃和 5% CO_2 条件下培养。**(S6)** 使用第 4 代细胞。

4.1.3 正反论证

正反论证（pro-con）是结合正面支持论据与反面反驳论据的论证方法，其结论的成立（至少在论证者看来）源于正面论据的逻辑力量经过权衡战胜反面论据。在正反论证的段落中，支持性证据的位置灵活，可在开篇，也可在结尾；其组织由论点和论据质量决定。对主要信息的正反两方面进行论证，目的在于突出正面论证。

例5

（S1）Intranasal administration of naloxone confers several advantages over intramuscular administration. （S2）Intranasal administration removes the possibility of needlestick injury, and intramuscular administration typically requires higher levels of training than intranasal drug delivery, particularly for people unfamiliar with injection（such as noninjecting family members of people who inject drugs）. （S3）One exception here is a naloxone autoinjector, which is easy to use but is dramatically more expensive than other preparations.

说明：本段落选自论文的讨论部分。第1句是主题句；第2句为支持论据；第3句是反面论据，语言标记是 exception，但从句中标记语 but 的出现构成对反面论据的反驳，实为支持论据。

译文：（S1）纳洛酮鼻内给药与肌肉给药相比，具有多个优点。（S2）鼻内给药避免了针刺损伤；与鼻内给药相比，肌内给药要求施药人员接受更高水平的训练，特别是不熟悉注射的人员（如不熟悉注射操作的患者家属）。（S3）纳洛酮自动注射器是一个例外，其使用虽然方便，但比其他制剂昂贵得多。

在论证相关主题时，除联合使用正反论证外，单独使用正方论证或反方论证也是有效的论证方法。

1. 正方论证

正方论证（pros），是指先陈述本研究的结果，然后用数据或先前的研究结果等来支持本研究发现。

例6

（S1）Our results showed that both the complex（SM extract）and its main active constituent（SB）, cotreated with MMS, exerted protective effects by reducing the amount of DNA in the comet tail by 42.49% and 34.20% respectively, when compared to positive control（MMS）. （S2）Previous studies also demonstrated the protective effects of SM and SB. （S3）In particular, SM and SB significantly decreased point mutations based on the Ames test and reduced the proportion of micronucleated polychromatic erythrocytes based on the mice bone marrow assay [29]. （S4）Furthermore, SB was demonstrated to exert protective effects against γ-radiation-induced strand breaks in plasmid DNA, reduce DNA damage and micronuclei formation in human lymphocytes and rat leukocytes, and reduce mouse mortality and DNA damage in blood leukocytes following whole-body γ-exposure in mice [16, 30].

　　说明：第 1 句是主题句,陈述主题;第 2~4 句是支持证据,引用文献对主题句论断给予有力支持。

　　译文：**(S1)** 我们的结果表明,经 MMS 共处理后的复合物（SM 提取物）及其主要活性成分（SB）通过降低彗星尾部的 DNA 含量发挥保护作用（与阳性对照 MMS 相比,分别降低了 42.49% 和 34.20%）。**(S2)** 先前的研究也证明了 SM 和 SB 的保护作用。**(S3)** 尤其是埃姆斯测验表明 SM 和 SB 使点突变显著减少,小鼠骨髓检测显示 SM 和 SB 可使微核多色红细胞的比例降低。**(S4)** 此外,SB 可保护质粒 DNA 免于 γ-辐射诱导的链断裂,减少人淋巴细胞和大鼠白细胞的 DNA 损伤和微核形成,降低小鼠死亡率和减少小鼠全身 γ-辐射后血白细胞的 DNA 损伤。

　　2. 反方论证

　　反方论证（cons）,是指通过报道文献中相反的研究结果来反对或不支持本研究结果。

例7

　　(S1) Unexpectedly, we found an inverse association between red meat intake and endometrial cancer; this association was not attenuated by adjustment for known risk factors, such as body mass index or menopausal hormone therapy, or by fine control for smoking, which has been inversely associated with this malignancy [28]. **(S2)** Previous studies have reported null [29, 30] or positive relations [31] between red meat and endometrial cancer. **(S3)** We also observed inverse associations between processed meat intake and leukemia and melanoma. **(S4)** In contrast to our findings, childhood leukemia has been positively associated with intake of processed meats in a case-control study [32].

　　说明：第 1,3 句是主题句,unexpectedly 为信息标记语;第 2,4 句是支持句,提供不支持主题句的证据。

　　译文：**(S1)** 出乎意料的是,我们发现红肉摄入量与子宫内膜癌发生之间呈负相关。调整已知危险因素（体重指数或绝经期激素治疗）或严格控烟后这一关联性并未减弱,事实上,严格控烟已被发现与子宫内膜癌呈负相关。**(S2)** 以往研究报告红肉摄入与子宫内膜癌发生之间无相关或正相关。**(S3)** 我们还观察到加工肉类摄入与白血病和黑色素瘤发生呈负相关。**(S4)** 与我们的结果相反,一项病例对照研究发现儿童白血病发生与加工肉类摄入呈正相关。

4.1.4　按时间顺序

　　段落也可以按时间先后顺序（chronological order）进行组织。时间顺序被认为是最直接的段落组织方式,常含有表示时间的副词如 after,before, then,as soon as 等。按发生时间先后顺序组织的段落主要出现在方法和结果部分,不过也同样适用于示例、描述或任何其他段落。

例8

（S1）For lung distension, we ventilated the fetus's lungs with a gas mixture that preserved normal fetal blood gas content. （S2）First, we opened the two polyvinyl tubes connected to the tracheal tube and allowed the tracheal fluid to drain by gravity. （S3）Then we balanced a mixture of nitrogen, oxygen, and carbon dioxide to match the fetal blood gases obtained during the baseline experiment. （S4）The gas mixture was about 92% nitrogen, 3% oxygen, and 5% carbon dioxide. （S5）Then we connected the tubing to a specially designed respirator and adjusted ventilation as described previously（12）. （S6）Ventilatory settings are presented in Table 1.

说明：第 1 句是主题句；第 2~5 句是支持句，使用了 first，then，then 等时间副词。

译文：（S1）为了实现肺膨胀，用气体混合物对胎羊进行肺通气，以保持正常的胎羊血气含量。（S2）首先，打开连接气管的 2 根聚乙烯软管，重力引流出气管内液体。（S3）随后，平衡调制含氮、氧、二氧化碳的混合气体，以匹配基线实验中所获胎羊血气。（S4）此混合气体成分为 92% 的氮气，3% 的氧气和 5% 的二氧化碳。（S5）然后，将软管连至一特殊设计的呼吸机，并且按之前文献所述方法调节通气。（S6）通气装置见表 1。

4.1.5　问题-解答或解答-问题模式

问题-解答（problem-solution）或者解答-问题（solution-problem）模式，即：先陈述问题，然后给出答案；或者先给出答案，然后再陈述问题。这种段落的展开方式多见于方法学论文、序贯设计研究论文的结果部分。

例9

（S1）To determine whether human HSCs require MLLT3, two validated *MLLT3* short hairpin RNAs were tested in an HSPC expansion culture system using the OP9M2 stromal stem-cell line 4. （S2）Both of the shRNAs resulted in premature depletion of fetal liver HSPCs（FL-HSPCs）in vitro（Fig. 1b, c, Extended Data Fig. 1g-j）. （S3）When FL-HSPCs transduced with MLLT3-knockdown（KD）or control vector were transplanted into immunodeficient NSG（NOD-SCID *Il2rg*-null）mice, only the control cells showed multilineage（myelo/lymphoid）human haematopoietic reconstitution（Fig. 1d, e, Extended Data Fig. 1k, Supplementary Table 1）, which indicates an important regulatory function for MLLT3.

说明：本例是问题-解答模式。第 1 句陈述问题，提出研究目的和检测方法，使用了标记语 To determine whether…；第 2~3 句是研究发现，即结果，第 3 句中包含标记语 indicate 的 which 从句则表明研究答案。

译文：（S1）为了确定人 HSC 是否需要 MLLT3，使用 OP9M2 基质干细胞系在 HSPC 扩展培养系统中对两个经过验证的 *MLLT3* 短发夹 RNA（shRNA）进行了测试。（S2）两种 shRNA 均导致胎肝 HSPC（FL-HSPC）在体外提前耗竭（图 1b,c,扩展数据图 1g-j）。（S3）当用 MLLT3-敲除（KD）或对照载体转导的 FL-HSPC 被移植到免疫缺陷的 NSG（NOD-SCID *Il2rg*-null）小鼠中时，只有对照细胞显示出多谱系（骨髓/淋巴）人类造血重建（图 1d, e, 扩展数据图 1k,补充表 1），这表明 MLLT3 具有重要的调节功能。

4.1.6　漏斗模式

漏斗模式（funnel model）由三部分构成：宏观命题和具体命题的已知信息、具体命题的未知信息、以及由已知和未知信息之间的差异产生的问题和/或研究方案。漏斗模式主要用于引言部分。

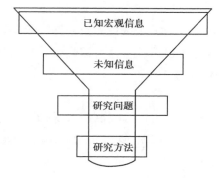

例10

（S1）The occurrence of a thermal transition in human serum lipoprotein depends on the triglyceride-cholesteryl ester ratio and the size of the lipoprotein particle. （S2）The triglyceride-cholesteryl ester ratio is known to correlate negatively with the peak temperature of the thermal transition of intact low density lipoprotein. （S3）However, it is not yet known how low a triglyceride-cholesteryl ester ratio and how small a particle size are necessary for the occurrence of the thermal transition in triglyceride-rich lipoproteins from human serum. （S4）To answer these questions, we assessed the triglyceride-cholesteryl ester ratio and the particle size in two classes of triglyceride-rich lipoproteins whose ratios of triglyceride to cholesteryl ester and whose particle size are between those of low density lipoproteins and very low density lipoproteins.

说明：第 1~2 句表述已知信息，使用了标记语… is known；第 3 句表述未知信息，使用了标记语 However, it is not yet known…；第 4 句表述研究问题和研究方法，使用了标记语 To answer these questions,we assessed…。

译文：(S1)人血清脂蛋白热转换的发生取决于甘油三酯-胆固醇酯的比率和脂蛋白颗粒的大小。(S2)已知甘油三酯-胆固醇酯的比率与完整的低密度脂蛋白热转换的最高温度呈负相关关系。(S3)然而,对于人血清中富含甘油三酯的脂蛋白颗粒在热转换时所需甘油三酯-胆固醇酯的最低比率和颗粒的最小程度却尚未清楚。(S4)为了回答这些问题,我们评估了在两类富含甘油三酯的脂蛋白中甘油三酯-胆固醇酯的比率和蛋白颗粒的大小。这两类脂蛋白甘油三酯-胆固醇酯的比率和蛋白颗粒的大小介于低密度和极低密度脂蛋白之间。

4.2　句子连贯清晰

　　段落结构有序是生物医学期刊英文论文写作的基本要求,而句子的连贯性,即句子间的清晰关系,是阐明科学信息的更高要求。句子的连贯性主要通过以下六种技巧实现:重复关键词、使用连接语表明信息间的关系、保持一致的叙述顺序、保持一致的视角、并列结构表达并列内容、标记段落内的小主题。下面分别举例说明。①

4.2.1　重复关键词

　　重复关键词(repeating key terms)是保持句子连贯性最重要的方法。关键词既可以是论文中反映主题的专业词汇,如:凋亡、灭活;也可以是表达信息的非专业词汇,如:上调、增加等,以实现清晰、准确、专一的内容表达。

例11

　　(S1) The use of dual antiplatelet therapy (a P2Y12 inhibitor plus aspirin) after percutaneous coronary intervention (PCI) reduces the risk of ischemic or atherothrombotic events, including stent thrombosis, recurrent myocardial infarction, and cardiovascular death.[1] (S2) Approximately 5% to 7% of patients with coronary artery disease who are undergoing PCI have an indication for long-term oral anticoagulant therapy.[2] (S3) The use of antiplatelet agents in combination with anticoagulation results in an increased risk of bleeding events, as shown recently in a nationwide Danish cohort study.[3] (S4) As a consequence, the selection of the most effective antithrombotic treatment for patients with atrial fibrillation and stable coronary artery disease is a clinical challenge requiring careful assessment of the risks of ischemia and bleeding in each patient.

　　说明:第1句为主题句,第2~3句为支持句,第4句为结论句。段落中多个关键词的重复,如:antiplatelet therapy 与 antiplatelet agents, ischemic 与 ischemia, PCI, anticoagulant therapy 与 anticoagulation,使段落写作流畅,信息连贯。

　　译文:(S1)经皮冠状动脉介入治疗(PCI)后使用双重抗血小板治疗(P2Y12 抑制剂加阿司匹林)可降低缺血或动脉粥样硬化血栓事件的风险,包括支架血栓形成、复发性心肌梗死和心血管死亡。(S2)在接受 PCI 治疗的冠心病患者中,5%~7%的患者有长期口服抗凝药物的指征。(S3)抗血小板药物联合抗凝血治疗增加出血事件的风险,这一发现在最近一项丹麦国家队列研究中得以证实。(S4)因此,为房颤和稳定型冠心病患者选择最有效的抗血栓治疗是临床面临的一大挑战,需要对每位患者的缺血和出血风险进行仔细评估。

---

① Mimi Zeiger, *Essentials of Writing Biomedical Research Papers*. U.S.A.: The McGraw-Hill companies, Inc., 2000, second edition, p. 58.

4.2.2　使用连接语表明信息间的关系

连贯性除了句子间自然的逻辑顺序外，还需要借助连接语来实现（using transitions to indicate relationship between ideas）。连接语包括连接词、连接短语、连接从句，其中除下面列举的常用连接词外，for wide spectrum screening，for macrophage staining，in our trial，to explain these findings 等介词结构性的连接短语是生物医学期刊英文论文中表达句子间逻辑关系的重要手段。

常用的连接词有：

递进关系：again，and，also，besides，equally important，first（second，etc.），further，furthermore，in addition，moreover，next，too

举例：for example，for instance，in fact，specifically，that is，to illustrate

比较：although，and yet，at the same time，but，despite，even though，however，in contrast，in spite of，nevertheless，on the contrary，on the other hand，still，though，yet

总结：all in all，in conclusion，in other words，in short，in summary，on the whole，that is，therefore，to sum up

时间：after，afterward，as long as，as soon as，at last，before，during，earlier，finally，formerly，immediately，later，meanwhile，next，since，shortly，subsequently，then，thereafter，until，when，while

地点方位：above，below，beyond，close，elsewhere，farther on，here，nearby，opposite，to the left（north，etc.）

因果关系：accordingly，as a result，because，consequently，for this reason，hence，if，otherwise，since，so，then，therefore，thus

例12

In accordance to the current study, Bassyouni et al. [42] have demonstrated that all of the Lactobacillus isolates obtained from Egyptian dairy product had a strong antibacterial effect against E. coli and Salmonella typhimurium. **However**, among the results that were revealed by the same author, 3 isolates had the most potent antimicrobial activity against the tested pathogenic microorganisms with the inhibition zone ranged from 17 to 21 mm in diameters. **In agreement to** this study, Tadesse et al. [5] have verified that all the LAB isolates（n = 118）originated from Borde and Shamita belonging to the genera Lactobacillus, Lactococcus, Leuconostoc, and Streptococcus were found to inhibit the growth of the test strains such as S. aureus, Salmonella spp., and E. coli O157：H7 with inhibition zones that ranged from 15 to 17 mm in diameters. **In line with** this, Choi et al. [43] have reported that out of the 4 strains of LAB, the Lactobacillus strain has completely inhibited the growth of food-borne pathogens, E. coli O157：H7 ATCC 35150, Salmonella enteritidis KCCM 12021, Salmonella typhimurium KCTC 1925, and S. aureus. [16] Tigu et al. have also revealed that out of the 11 probiotic LAB isolated from traditional Ethiopian fermented condiments, namely, Datta and Awaze, 2 Lactobacillus isolates inhibited the growth of Salmonella typimurium and Escherichia coli with inhibition zones ranging from 10. 3 to 14.3 mm in diameters. **In line with** this, Haghshenas et al. [37] have reported that among the selected 8 LAB isolated from Iranian fermented dairy products, Lactobacillus species, particularly Lb. plantarum 15HN, showed the most efficient antagonistic activity against Staphylococcus aureus, Listeria monocytogenes, Salmonella typimurium, and Escherichia coli with inhibition zones of 11. 7, 13. 7, 12. 3, and 12. 3 mm diameters, respectively. **Likewise**, Rajoka et al. [34] have verified that all the Lactobacillus rhamnosus isolated from human milk inhibited the growth of Staphylococcus aureus, Salmonella typimurium, and Escherichia coli using the agar-well diffusion method with variable diameters (6 mm to 14 mm).

说明：本段使用多个连接词,如 In accordance to, In agreement to, In line with, Likewise,使得句子之间的逻辑关系清楚明白。

译文：根据目前的研究,Bassyouni 等人已证明从埃及乳制品分离出的所有乳酸杆菌对大肠杆菌和鼠伤寒沙门氏菌具有很强的抗菌作用。然而,同一作者的研究结果表明,有 3 种分离物对被检测病原微生物具有最强的抗菌活性,其抑菌圈的直径范围为 17 至 21 mm。与这项研究一致,Tadesse 等人也已证实所有来自 Borde 和 Shamita 的实验室乳杆菌属、乳球菌属、白串珠菌属及链球菌属分离菌株 (n = 118) 均对试验菌株(例如金黄色葡萄球菌、沙门氏菌属和大肠杆菌 O157：H7)的生长有抑制作用,其抑制区的直径范围为 15~17 mm。与此相符,Choi 等人发现在 4 种实验室菌株中, 乳酸杆菌菌株完全抑制了大肠埃希菌 O157：H7 ATCC 35150、肠炎沙门氏菌 KCCM 12021、伤寒沙门氏菌 KCTC 1925、金黄色葡萄球菌等食源性致病菌的生长。Tigu 等研究者还发现,从传统埃塞俄比亚发酵调味品 (名称为 Datta 和 Awaze) 中分离出的 11 种益生菌中,有 2 种乳酸杆菌分离菌株对伤寒沙门氏菌和大肠杆菌的生长有抑制作用,抑菌圈范围直径为 10.3~14.3 mm。与此相符,据 Haghshenas 等人报道,在从伊朗发酵乳制品中分离出的 8 种实验室分离菌中,乳酸菌属,尤其是 Lb. 植物乳酸菌 15HN,对金黄色葡萄球菌、单核细胞增生性李斯特菌、鼠伤寒沙门氏菌和大肠埃希氏菌具有最有效的拮抗作用,其抑菌圈直径分别为 11.7、13.7、12.3 和 12.3 mm。同样,Rajoka 等人已证实采用不同直径 (6 毫米至 14 毫米) 的琼脂井扩散法从人乳中分离出的所有鼠李糖乳杆菌均能抑制葡萄球菌、金黄色葡萄球菌、沙门氏菌和大肠杆菌的生长。

4.2.3 保持一致的叙述顺序

保持一致的叙述顺序 (keeping consistent order),是指如果主题句列举了几个有待说明的事项,支持句的顺序就应当按照列举事项的先后顺序安排。此外,支持句展开的细节只限于主题句提及的事项,不能随意增加另外的内容。同时,为确保支持句中交代的信息与主题句中一致,需遵循准确重复关键词的原则。

例13

（S1）The aggregates used here consisted of MSC／HUVEC co-cultures that were formed using two different methods：suspension culture aggregation and pellet culture aggregation.（S2）The suspension culture method comprised a simple F127-coated hydrophilic environment that encouraged the cells to remain in suspension［42］.（S3）Once suspended, the cells were free to aggregate and self-assemble into spheroidal structures.（S4）The pellet culture method, on the other hand, forced the cells into a cell pellet that subsequently aggregated and became spheroidal.（S5）The suspension culture method is considered to be a less severe method of aggregation with the cells self-aggregating and self-assembling.

说明：第 1 句为主题句，提到两种不同的方法；第 2～4 句为支持句，说明的顺序与主题中列举的顺序一致；第 5 句为总结句。

译文：（S1）所使用的聚集体由 MSC／HUVEC 共培养组成，共培养采用两种不同的方法：悬浮培养聚合法和颗粒培养聚合法。（S2）悬浮培养法包括一个简单的 F127 包被的亲水环境，该环境促使细胞保持在悬浮状态。（S3）一旦悬浮，细胞就可以自由聚集并自我聚合成球状结构。（S4）另一方面，颗粒培养法是通过迫使细胞进入细胞颗粒，随后聚集并变成球形。（S5）悬浮培养法被认为是一种较不严格的聚合法，这种方法中，细胞进行自我聚合和自我组装。

4.2.4　保持一致的视角

如前所述，句子的主语应该表达句子的主题，同样，如两个或多个句子的主题一致，则应使用相同的主语。保持一致的视角（keeping a consistent point of view）即是两个或多个句子阐述同一主题时，各句的主语应该使用同一或相同类型的关键词。在生物医学论文中，处理因素（自变量）和观察因素（因变量）是最常见的两种视角。

例14

（S1）Figure 1A shows that intraperitoneal injection of 100 or 1, 000 mg／kg potassium oxonate could significantly increased the serum uric acid levels in tree shrews, within 2 h.（S2）In the group treated with 1, 000 mg／kg potassium oxonate, the serum uric acid level increased from 133.54 ± 26.39 μmol／l at 0 h to 453.01 ± 96.94 μmol／l in 2 h and reached 480.57 ± 60.76 μmol／l by 4 h.（S3）The serum uric acid levels of the tree shrews treated with 100 mg／kg potassium oxonate dose increased from 141.89 ± 39 μmol／l to 431.24 ± 18.36 μmol／l at 2 h after injection.（S4）The serum uric acid levels in both the groups were higher than the uric acid crystallization point（417 μmol／l）.（S5）There were significant differences in serum uric acid levels between the potassium oxonate-treated groups and the control group（[**] $P<0.01$）.（S6）There were no changes in the levels of serum urea nitrogen or serum Cr（Figs.1B and 1C）.

说明：第 1 句是主题句，引出因变量 the serum uric acid level；第 2～4 是支持句，都采用了相同的主语 the serum uric acid level 以保持一致的视角。第 5～6 句描述补充信息。

译文：(S1) 图 1A 显示腹腔内注射 100 mg 或 1000 mg／kg 的草酸钾可在 2 小时内显著增加树鼠血清尿酸水平。(S2) 草酸钾治疗组 (1000 mg／kg) 注射后 2 小时血清尿酸水平从 133.54 ± 26.39 μmol／l 升高到 $453.01 \sim 96.94$ μmol／l，4 小时内达到 480.57 ± 60.76 μmol／l。(S3) 草酸钾治疗组 (100 mg／kg) 注射后 2 小时，血清尿酸水平从 141.89 ± 39 μmol／l 升高到 431.24 ± 18.36 μmol／l。(S4) 两组血清尿酸水平均高于尿酸结晶点 (417 μmol／l)。(S5) 草酸钾治疗组与对照组血清尿酸水平有显著性差异 ($^{**}P < 0.01$)。(S6) 血清尿素氮或血清 Cr 水平没有变化 (如图 1B 和 1C 所示)

4.2.5　并列结构表达并列内容

并列内容 (parallel ideas) 是指相同类型的信息；并列结构 (parallel form) 则是指一致的结构形式，是利用语法形式的重复来表达一系列等价的概念。应用并列结构表达并列的内容时，需要保持一致的视角，并使用完全相同的句子结构，其目的是有效地展示同一主题不同信息之间的异同之处。

例15

(S1) Eligible patients in the two trials were randomly assigned to receive either a prophylactic dose of low-molecular-weight heparin (treatment group) or no anticoagulant therapy (control group). (S2) In the POT-KAST trial, low-molecular-weight heparin was administered once daily for the 8 days after arthroscopy; the first dose was administered postoperatively but before discharge on the day of surgery. (S3) In the POT-CAST trial, low-molecular weight heparin was administered for the full period of immobilization; the first dose was administered in the emergency department. (S4) In both trials, patients in the treatment group received nadroparin or dalteparin (according to the preference at the hospital), administered subcutaneously; a dose of 2850 IU of nadroparin or 2500 IU of dalteparin was used for patients who weighed 100 kg or less, and a double dose (in one daily injection) was used for patients who weighed more than 100 kg.

说明：第 1 句是主题句，第 2～4 句为支持句；第 2 和第 3 句为并列的内容用并列结构表述，第 4 句中分号之后的后半句也是两个并列结构的句子。

译文：(S1) 两项试验中符合标准的患者被随机分配至接受预防剂量的低分子肝素治疗 (治疗组) 或不接受抗凝剂治疗 (对照组)。(S2) 在 POT-KAST 试验中，患者在关节镜术后 8 日内每日 1 次低分子肝素注射；首剂注射在术后当天出院前完成。(S3) 在 POT-CAST 试验中，患者在制动的全程阶段均接受低分子肝素注射；首剂在急诊科注射。(S4) 在两项试验中，治疗组中的患者皮下注射那曲肝素或达肝素 (依从医院的选择)。患者体重若 ≤ 100 kg，则使用 2850 IU 那曲肝素或 2500 IU 达肝素；患者体重若 > 100 kg，则注射剂量翻倍 (每日 1 次)。

4.2.6　标记段落内的小主题

段落主题最好在段首的主题句中写作；同样，段落中的小主题也应在句子开始以关键词的方式加以标记（signaling the subtopics for a paragraph）。小主题主要体现为句子的主语，也可以是连接短语的宾语，如上例中：In the POT-KAST trial，In the POT-CAST trial，In both trials。

例16

（S1）In this study of trends in the use of cardiovascular diagnostic testing among fee-for-service Medicare beneficiaries from 1999 to 2016，we found that the overall rate of testing increased from 1999 to 2008 and then steadily declined through 2016. （S2）High-value testing among eligible patients hospitalized for AMI and HF steadily increased for both cohorts throughout the study period，approaching 90% for the AMI cohort and 80% for the HF cohort. （S3）Low-value testing before low-risk surgery was performed infrequently but increased from 2000 to 2008 and declined thereafter，returning by 2015 to the 2000 level. （S4）Low-value testing after PCI or CABG slightly increased from 2000 to nearly 50% in 2003，but then steadily declined to approximately 30%.

说明：第 1 句是主题句，主题信息是 cardiovascular diagnostic testing；第 2～4 句分别阐述三个小主题，用主题词 High-value testing，Low-value testing 和 Low-value testing 作为语言标记开启一个新句子；每个主题词都包含 testing 这一关键词。

译文：（S1）一项针对按需付费医疗保险受益人在 1999 年至 2016 年期间使用心血管诊断检测的趋势研究发现，总体测试率在 1999 年至 2008 年期间呈上升趋势，继而稳步下降直至 2016 年。（S2）在整个研究期间，两个队列中符合纳入条件的 AMI 和 HF 住院患者高价项目检测率稳步上升，AMI 队列接近 90%，HF 队列接近 80%。（S3）低风险手术前的低价项目检测很少进行，但从 2000 年到 2008 年呈上升趋势，此后有所下降，到 2015 年恢复到 2000 年的水平。（S4）PCI 或 CABG 后的低价项目检测从 2000 年开始略有增加，到 2003 年增加了近 50%，但随后稳步回落到 30% 左右。

4.3　重点内容突出

除结构有序、信息连贯之外，生物医学论文的段落写作还应分清主要信息和次要信息。可以通过以下六种技巧突出重要信息：浓缩或省略次要的信息；将重要信息置于段落的突出位置；将次要的信息置于段落的次要位置；标记重要信息；重复重要信息；直接阐明而非隐含重要信息[①]。下面就其中四种予以叙述。

---

① Mimi Zeiger, *Essentials of Writing Biomedical Research Papers*. U.S.A.：The McGraw-Hill companies, Inc., 2000, second edition, p. 98.

4.3.1　浓缩或省略次要的信息

突出重点内容最重要的技巧之一是浓缩或省略次要信息（condensing or omitting less important information），其目的是避免繁杂且不重要的多余信息掩盖与主题密切相关的重要信息。

例17

（S1）Stock-out events and vaccine manufacturing capacity have been problematic for particular vaccines, even in high-income countries. （S2）Manufacturers emphasize the time needed to build and commission a factory[71]. （S3）Although manufacturers in middle-income country are now supplying most low-cost vaccines globally, they face low profit margins, ferocious tenders, and often unpredictable procurement schemes. （S4）More efficient and modular production technologies may enable decentralized production with lower capital costs.

说明：第 1 句是主题句，主题信息是 problematic，因此放在最醒目的位置。第 2~4 句是支持句，其中信息表达精炼，逻辑清楚。

译文：（S1）即使在高收入国家，某些疫苗存在缺货情况和生产能力不足的问题。（S2）制造商强调建造和启用工厂所需要的时间。（S3）尽管中等收入国家的疫苗厂商供应着全球范围内大多数低成本疫苗，但他们面临利润率低、招标激烈、以及采购计划通常无法预知的问题。（S4）更高效率和模块化的生产技术可以实现分散生产，降低资本成本。

4.3.2　将重要的信息置于段落的突出位置

突出重点内容还需将重要的信息置于段落的突出位置（placing important information in a power position）。突出的位置在句子的开始和结尾部分，开始部分最为突出。主题句表达段落最重要的信息，因此通常被置于段落的开始位置；同样，如果主题句中的主语能表达整个段落的主题，主题句的信息就变得尤为突出。

例18

（S1）The duration of ARDS before study entry and procollagen peptide type III levels at baseline were found to interact with treatment and mortality. （S2）Treatment with methylprednisolone was associated with a significantly increased mortality rate among patients who had had ARDS for more than 13 days before enrollment and a significantly decreased mortality rate among those with higher-than-median levels of procollagen peptide type III in bronchoalveolar-lavage fluid at baseline （Table 2 and Table 3）. （S3）None of the other interactions, including tidal volume （$P = 0.63$）and date of enrollment （$P = 0.34$）, were significant. （S4）There were no significant differences between the group enrolled 7 to 13 days after the onset of ARDS and the group enrolled at least 14 days after the onset of ARDS, other than in the percentage of men and the positive end-expiratory pressure at baseline（13.3+5.0 and 10.8+5.1 cm of water，respectively；P = 0.004）（Table 4 of the Supplementary Appendix）．

说明：第 1 句和第 2 句是段落最醒目的位置，报道最重要的结果；而第 3 句和第 4 句是段落的次要位置，报道次重要的结果。

译文：（S1）入选前 ARDS 病程及基线 Ⅲ 型前胶原肽水平，与甲泼尼龙治疗及病死率存在相互作用。（S2）甲泼尼龙治疗使入选前 ARDS 超过 13 天的患者死亡率显著升高，但使支气管肺泡灌洗液中 Ⅲ 型胶原蛋白基线水平高于中值的患者死亡率显著降低（表 2 和表 3）。（S3）其他相互作用，如潮气量（P = 0.63）和纳入研究日期（P = 0.34），均不显著。（S4）ARDS 发病后 7~13 天纳入研究组与 ARDS 发病后 ≥14 天纳入研究组比较，除男性患者比例和基线呼气末正压有明显差异外 [（13.3±5.0）厘米水柱和（10.8±5.1）厘米水柱，P = 0.004]，其余方面无显著差异（见补充附录表 4）。

4.3.3 标记重要信息

标记重要信息（labeling important information）也是突出重点内容的一种技巧。在生物医学期刊英文论文写作中，标记语通常被用来标记引言和讨论部分的重要内容，例如，One of the major insights to emerge from the study is…；This is the first study to our knowledge…；… remains an important unsolved problem；Surprisingly，there is little evidence that…等。

例19

（S1）One of the most striking findings in our small and large pre-clinical animal studies is that CBSCs（cortical bone derived stem cells）treated animals showed a significant smaller infarct sizes after cardiac injury. （S2）Cardiac fibroblast plays a vital role in wound healing after myocardial injury and affects multiple aspects of wound healing response including deposition of extracellular matrix proteins to wound angiogenesis and scar maturation. （S3）Following acute MI，cardiac fibroblasts in the heart become activated and rapidly proliferate. （S4）In rodent hearts，peak cardiac fibroblast numbers are achieved within 7-14 days after permanent ligation of the LAD53 and within 3 days of IRI54 . （S5）Many laboratories using multiple stem cell types have reported the persistence or presence of stem cells during the same time window after transplantation. （S6）Consequently，it is extremely important to study the role and interaction of transplanted cells with the fibroblast to uncover how scar formation and maturation occur after cell therapy. （S7）As mentioned above CBSCs treated animals showed a significant smaller infarct sizes，there is a need to better understand their relationship with the cell type（fibroblast）that is a key player in scar formation and maturation as an important arm in wound healing.

说明：第 1 句以这样的标记语开始：One of the most striking findings in… is that…，第 6 句中也使用了 it is extremely important to…对段落内的重要信息进行标记。

译文：（S1）我们进行的小样本和大样本临床前动物研究中最引人注目的发现之一是：在心脏损伤后，皮质骨源性干细胞（CBSCs）处理后的动物梗塞面积明显较小。（S2）心肌成纤维细胞在心肌损伤后伤口愈合中起着重要作用，并影响伤口愈合反应的多个方面，包括细胞外基质蛋白的沉积、伤口血管生成与瘢痕成熟。（S3）急性心肌梗死后，心脏成纤维细胞被激活并迅速增殖。（S4）在啮齿动物心脏中，心脏成纤维细胞的数量在 LAD 永久结扎后 7~14 天内以及 IRI 后 3 天内达到峰值。（S5）许多使用多种干细胞类型的实验室报告了干细胞在移植后同一时间窗内的持续存在或出现。（S6）因此，研究移植细胞作用及与成纤维细胞的相互作用对了解 CBSCs 处理后瘢痕的形成和成熟的过程具有重要意义。（S7）如上所述，CBSCs 处理后动物的心肌梗死面积明显较小，因此有必要进一步了解其与细胞类型（成纤维细胞）的关系，因为成纤维细胞在伤口愈合过程中对疤痕形成和成熟至关重要。

4.3.4　重复重要信息

生物医学期刊英文论文中有关研究命题的信息是最重要的信息，重要信息需要重复强调（repeating important information）。重复的信息可以贯穿整个论文，如引言中关于研究问题、研究背景的信息可以在讨论部分加以强调；结果部分的主要发现、主要结局也可以在讨论部分加以重复。同样，段落中的重要信息首先在段首的主题句中陈述，还可以在段尾的主题句中重复。

例20

Although mortality inequalities are largely associated with socioeconomic factors, we found that NCD mortality in the South showed similar trends across counties of different income levels, suggesting that the influence of high-income status on reducing the NCD burden had not reached the disadvantaged geographic pattern. For example, people living in high-income counties tend to have higher Medicare reimbursements but less access to NCD treatment and prevention programs if they reside in the South, which leads to higher risk of NCD death. Moreover, among 19 states that did not join Medicaid expansion, 10 of them were in the South.[37] Lack of Medicaid expansion may obstruct access to health care, especially for people with low socioeconomic status in the South. A prior study showed that income difference may be associated with delayed and forgone health care.[38] In addition, southern counties have higher proportions of black people, which may relate to other county-level factors（eg, health behaviors, health care access, and physical environment）.[39] Thus, it appears that improving income status would not be enough to reduce the NCD burden in a racially disadvantaged population.

说明：段落的重要信息在段首的主题句中陈述，该重要信息同时在段落结束时的第二个主题句中重复。

译文：尽管死亡率不均衡在很大程度上与社会经济因素有关，但我们发现南方的 NCD 死亡率在不同收入水平的区县之间出现相似的趋势，这提示高收入状况对减轻 NCD 负担的影响尚未惠及偏远的地区。例如，生活在高收入县的人往往有较高的医疗保险报销，但是南部地区的居民获得 NCD 治疗和预防计划的机会较少，这会导致 NCD 死亡的风险较高。此外，在没有加入医疗补助扩大计划的 19 个州中，有 10 个位于南部。缺少医疗补助扩大计划可能会减少人们获得医疗保健服务的机会，尤其是南方社会经济地位较低的人口。一项既往研究表明，收入差异可能与延误和放弃医疗服务有关。此外，南部县的黑人比例较高，这可能与其他县级因素有关（例如，健康习惯、医疗服务机会和自然环境）。因此，改善收入状况似乎不足以减轻弱势民族群体的 NCD 负担。

Exercise

Analyze the writing techniques in the following passages.

1. Temperate countries and Asia have different patterns of virus circulation. In temperate countries, the pattern of virus circulation is well established, with the main activity during the winter. In contrast, in Asia, two different patterns occur: year-round circulation with no clear peak of activity or peaks that coincide with cool or rainy seasons.

2. We tested whether pretreatment with American ginseng and one of its active antioxidant constituents, ginsenoside Re, could counter cisplatin-induced emesis using a rat pica model (reflecting nausea and vomiting in the rat). A significant dose-response relationship was observed between increasing doses of pretreatment with ginseng and reduction in cisplatin-induced pica. Pretreatment with ginsenoside Re also significantly decreased pica. *In vitro* studies demonstrated a concentration-response relationship between ginseng and its antioxidant ability. Thus, ginseng has a potential value for the treatment of chemotherapy-induced nausea and vomiting.

3. Purified T cells from DO11.10 and DO11.10p27 mice (10 106 cells/ml) were labeled for 30 min at 37 ℃ with the intracellular fluorescent dye CFSE. Then, cells were washed twice with cold RPMI 1640 medium containing 10% FCS, resuspended in PBS and transferred intravenously into BALB/c mice (5 106 cells per mouse). Syngeneic hosts were left untreated (naive) or treated with PBS followed by immunization with OVA (323-339) as described above. Then, 3 days later, lymphocytes were isolated from the draining lymph nodes of the BALB/c hosts.

4. Limitations to this study include sporadic stooling patterns associated with prematurity, which did not permit standardized collection times. Furthermore, not all NEC samples were obtained, as there is often decreased stooling with acute illness. However, given the noninvasive nature of stool collection, this process offers clear clinical advantages over serological testing that can lead to iatrogenic blood loss in infants.

5. CD31 staining was used to identify the presence and spatial distribution of HUVECs

located in and / or around the aggregates. The sample sections were incubated for 30 minutes in 10% FBS (diluted in phosphate buffered saline (PBS)) to prevent non-specific background staining (blocking). The samples were then incubated for 1 hour in the primary antibody, mouse anti-human CD31 (Dako, UK), at a dilution of 1 : 20 in PBS. The samples were then incubated for 1 hour in the secondary antibody, alexa-fluor 594- conjugated goat anti-mouse IgG1 (Life Technologies, UK), diluted 1 : 200 in PBS. DAPI staining was carried out using a DAPI-conjugated mounting medium without further adjustment. The samples were then ready for imaging.

6. The Maf transcription factor family is a homolog of the v-Maf oncogene, which was identified from the AS42 virus and causes musculoaponeurotic fibrosarcoma in chicks. The Maf transcription factor is separated into two subfamilies. Large Maf family proteins have a basic domain and a leucine zipper domain (b-Zip) that mediate dimerization and DNA binding and an acidic domain to regulate target gene transcription. In contrast, the small Maf family only contains a b-Zip domain and lacks an acidic domain. Homodimers of small Mafs inhibit target gene transcription, whereas heterodimers regulate target gene transcription depending on the partner protein (Fig. 1). In mammals, four large Maf proteins (MafA, MafB, c-Maf, and NRL) and three small Maf proteins (MafK, MafG, and MafF) have been identified. All Maf proteins bind to the Maf recognition element (MARE), which is a palindromic sequence, or a MARE half-site in the promoter region of their target gene (Fig.1b).

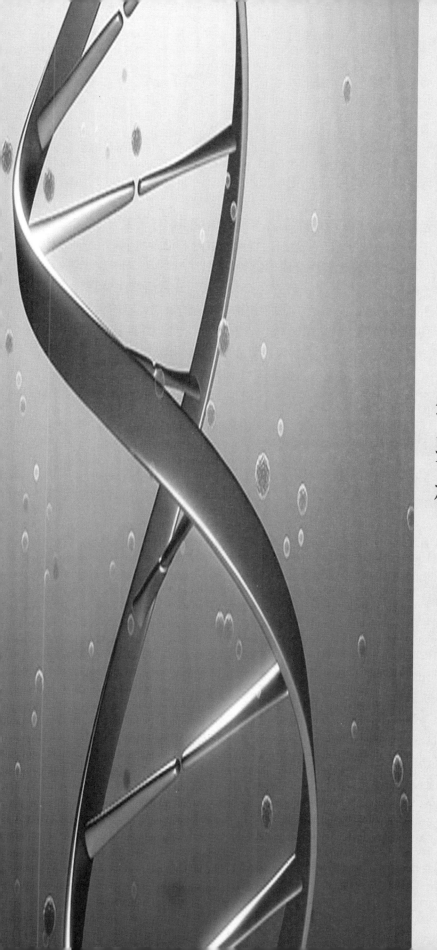

第

5

章

生物医学期刊
英文论文写作
概述

5.1 何谓生物医学期刊英文论文

生物医学是一门前沿交叉学科,综合了医学、生命科学等学科知识与研究方法,旨在解决生命科学命题,特别是与医学相关的问题。作为一门快速发展的前沿学科,学界人员之间的交流是必要和必须的。生物医学期刊是实现交流的重要平台,生物医学期刊英文论文便是交流内容的重要载体。一般来讲,生物医学期刊英文论文是指讨论或研究生物医学学术问题并议论说理的文章。凡是直接阐述生物医学研究中客观事物的道理、反映医学事物的本质与规律,以表明作者见解和学术观点的文章,都称为生物医学论文。为实现学术交流的广泛化,全球重要的生物医学期刊大都使用英文发表论文。故而,生物医学期刊英文论文是生物医学科研工作者用英语撰写,在英、美生物医学期刊或非英语国家英文版生物医学期刊上发表的学术论文。

5.2 生物医学期刊英文论文的分类

生物医学期刊英文论文按不同的标准有如下分类:

按医学学科及课题性质分为四类:基础医学论文、临床医学论文、预防医学论文和康复医学论文。

按论文的研究内容分为五类:实验研究论文、调查研究论文、实验观察论文、资料分析论文和经验体会论文。

按论文的论述体裁分为:论著、文献综述、述评、临床分析、疗效观察、病例报告和医学科普论文等。

以下就上述提及的一些概念进行说明。

实验研究 一般为病因、病理、生理、生化、药理、生物、寄生虫和流行病学等实验研究。主要包括:对各种动物进行的药理、毒理实验,外科手术实验;对某种疾病的病原或病因的体外实验;某些药物的抗癌、抗菌、抗寄生虫实验;消毒、杀虫和灭菌的实验。

临床分析 对临床上某种疾病病例(百例以上为佳)的病因、临床表现、分型、治疗方法和疗效观察等进行分析讨论,总结经验教训,并提出新建议新见解,以提高临床疗效。

疗效观察 使用某种新药、新疗法治疗某种疾病,对治疗的方法、效果、剂量、疗程及不良反应等进行观察研究,或设立对照组对新旧药物或疗法的疗效进行比较,对比疗效的高低、疗法的优劣、不良反应的种类及程度,并对是否适于应用提出评价意见。

病例报告 主要报告罕见病及疑难重症。适用于虽然曾有少数类似报道但尚有重复验证或加深认识的必要情况。

病例(理)讨论 临床病例讨论主要是对某些疑难、复杂、易于误诊的病例,在诊断和治疗方面进行集体讨论,以求得正确的诊断和有效的治疗。临床病例讨论对少见或疑难疾病的病理检查、诊断及相关内容以讨论为主。

调查报告　在一定范围的人群里,不施加人工处理因素,对某一疾病(传染病、流行病、职业病、地方病等)的发病情况、发病因素、病理、防治方案等提出建议。

文献综述　作者从一个学术侧面,围绕某个问题收集一定历史时期内有关文献资料,以自己的实践经验为基础,进行消化整理、综合归纳、分析提炼而成的概述性、评述性专题学术论文。

5.3　生物医学期刊英文论文的特点

生物医学期刊英文论文从广义上讲,应是科技论文。美国生物学编辑协会将科技论文定义为:一篇能被接受的原始科学出版物必须是首次披露,并提供足够的资料,使同行能够评定所观察到资料的价值、重复试验结果、评价整个研究过程的学术水平;此外,它必须易于人们的感官接受、本质上持久、不加限制地为科学界所使用,并成为一种或多种公认的二级情报源(如化学文摘等)所选用。[①]基于此,生物医学期刊英文论文应具有以下两个鲜明特点。

一是学术性。生物医学期刊英文论文的学术性是指论文应具备一定的学术价值。这种价值是针对学科的系统知识和理论体系而言的,既可以是通过严格的逻辑分析和推理对既有知识和操作进行论证和发展;也可以是借助新的理论和研究方法对既有认知进行批判,或推翻重建。所有这些都对作者的学术素养提出了要求,既要具备深厚的专业知识基础,还应具备逻辑分析的思维能力。

二是规范性。规范性具体地体现在两个方面,一是论文呈现的生物医学研究过程的规范性,二是论文写作的规范性。对于前者,生物医学研究的对象是生命体,包括动物和人群,故而研究本身就应该遵循相应的生命规范,比如特定的实验伦理规范等。除此之外,实验室操作以及特定实验试剂的使用也应规范化。对于后者,生物医学期刊英文论文的文字表达首先应规范、准确,语言和技术细节应采用国际法定的名词术语、数字、符号、计量单位等;行文表达要求准确、简明、通顺、条理清楚等,行文结构一般也具有固定的格式。

5.4　生物医学期刊英文论文的写作格式

生物医学期刊英文论文通常都有比较固定的格式。目前学界较重要的期刊,如 *Journal of American Medical Association*, *New England Journal of Medicine*, *British Medical Journal*, *Lancet* 等都遵循国际医学期刊编辑委员会(International Committee of Medical Journal Editor, ICMJE)公布的《生物医学期刊投稿的统一要求》(*Uniform Requirements for Manuscripts Submitted to Biomedical Journals*),即温哥华格式。该要求在 1979 年第一次发布,历经多次修订,2013 年 8 月修订时更名为《学术研究实施与报告和医学期刊编辑与

---

① ［美］金坤林,《如何撰写和发表 SCI 期刊论文》,北京:科学出版社,2016 年,第 29 页。

发 表 的 推 荐 规 范 》 （ *Recommendations for the Conduct，Reporting，Editing，and Publication of Scholarly Work in Medical Journals* ），简称 "ICMJE 推荐规范"①。之后，ICMJE 几乎每年都对规范进行了更新。

"ICMJE 推荐规范"对生物医学期刊英文论文的书写格式、内容和投稿均作了统一规定。根据"ICMJE 推荐规范"，生物医学期刊英文论文主要由文题（Title）、作者（Authorship）、摘要（Abstract）、关键词（Key Words）、引言（Introduction）、材料与方法（Materials and Methods）、结果（Results）、讨论（Discussion）、致谢（Acknowledgements）、参考文献（References）、利益冲突声明（Conflict-of-interest Notification）等部分组成。教材后续章节将对论文的标题、摘要和正文各部分的写作内容和写作方法作详细介绍，因此本章只讲解作者、关键词、致谢、参考文献和利益冲突声明的写作。

5.4.1 作者署名

1. 作者署名的条件

国际医学期刊编辑委员会（ICMJE）在作者身份的标准中明确规定，身为作者须符合以下 4 条标准：（1）对研究的思路或设计有重要贡献，或者为研究获取、分析或解释数据；（2）起草研究论文或者在重要的智力性内容上对论文进行修改；（3）对将要发表的版本作最终定稿；（4）同意对研究工作的各个方面承担责任以确保与论文任何部分的准确性或诚信有关的质疑得到恰当的调查和解决。

论文的通讯作者是在投稿、同行评议及出版过程中主要负责与期刊联系的人。

对论文有贡献但只满足部分而非全部上述 4 条作者署名标准者，如筹得研究资金、参加局部工作或某些试验、参加结果讨论的人员以及译者、审稿者、校对者、提供部分病例和各种资料的单位和人员，经本人同意后，可在致谢或附录中说明。

2. 作者署名的要求

对作者署名的要求如下：

（1）论文的署名排序应由合作者共同确定，根据在研究工作中所负的责任和贡献大小依次排列，而不计资历深浅和学位高低。

（2）一篇医学英文论文的署名人不宜过多。如果研究工作是由众多作者组成的大型团队实施，理想的情况是这个团队在研究开始前就决定谁将成为作者，并且在投稿给期刊发表前确定作者名单。或将作者署名为团队名称，或署以团队名称加上各个作者的姓名。

（3）署名应署真名、全名，不署笔名。中国作者的英文署名，一律按国家规定的汉语拼音书写，姓前名后，姓和名分开写，双姓（如司马、欧阳、诸葛）和双名则不分开写，姓和名的首字母都大写。例如：Wu Xiao（吴晓）、Sima Qian（司马迁）、Ouyang Xiu（欧阳修）、Zhuge Ming（诸葛明）等。若两字拼音连写处出现以元音字母 a，o，e 开头的音节，用隔音符号（ ' ）隔开。如 Chang'an（长安）、Wang Ping'an（王平安）等。外国作者的姓名写法遵从国际惯例。各种医学期刊对拼音书写方法常有不同的要求，论文作者在投稿时应予以

---

① 相关文件材料可登陆官网查看 http://www.icmje.org。

参考。如在《中华医学杂志》中文版的英文摘要中，作者姓的每个字母都大写，名只首字母大写，如：欧阳修为 OUYANG Xiu，王光明为 WANG Guangming；而在英文版，作者姓名除了用英文表示置于标题下之外，还要用括号将姓名以脚注形式再次置于论文首页右下角作者单位之后。对于作者英文署名，姓的首字母大写，名采用缩写形式。如：Sima Qian（司马迁）缩写为 Sima Q，Wang Guangming（王光明）缩写为 Wang GM 等，这种方式便于索引收录。

（4）署名的位置位于文题下方居中书写。作者相互之间用逗号隔开，以利于计算机自动切分。不同工作单位的作者，应在姓名右上角以上标形式加注不同的阿拉伯数字序号。例如：WU Liangjun[1]，LUO Tieyou[2]，HUANG Li[3]。

3. 作者工作单位

文中列出作者单位是为了方便读者、作者及编者间的联系。作者工作单位是指作者从事本文工作时所在的单位。作者单位应采用其公开正式名称，准确完整，不要随便使用简称。

在欧美生物医学期刊的论文中，单位名称的排列顺序大致有 3 种：

（1）小单位在前，大单位在后，这是最常见的一种。其顺序是：组、室、科、院、校、市、州、省、国。

例1

Department of Pathology, College of Basic Medicine, Chongqing Medical University, Chongqing, China

　　译文：重庆医科大学基础医学院病理教研室

（2）大单位在前，小单位在后。

例2

Chongqing Medical University, College of Basic Medicine, Department of Pharmacology

　　译文：重庆医科大学基础医学院药理学教研室

（3）前两种排列顺序的混合型。

例3

Department of Medicine, Division of Digestive Diseases, University of Mississippi Medical Center, Jackson, Mississippi

　　译文：密西西比州杰克逊市密西西比大学医学中心内科消化病组

在国内生物医学期刊英文摘要中，单位名称排列顺序通常采用第一种，即小单位在前、大单位在后的形式。

5.4.2　关键词

关键词是从文稿内容中提炼出来的最能反映论文主要内容，体现文稿种类、目的及实施措施，在论文中出现次数最多，一般在文稿的文题及摘要中出现的关键性用词。

1. 关键词标引要求

（1）标引关键词要从论文的主题分析开始，即对论文的内容和中心思想进行浓缩和提炼，剖析主题结构，确立主题类型。

（2）关键词是文稿论述的核心，应包括：论文标题涉及的主题概念，即核心词；主要论述的课题，即论文论述的重点、研究目的或对象；某种实验研究的目的、手段和结果；某种疾病的预防、诊断和治疗等重要手段、方法的创新；论文中论述篇幅较多的内容。

（3）关键词一般选用专业术语，如 prosthodontics（口腔修复学）；名词短语，如 blood-brain barrier（血脑屏障）；或复合词，如 venous thromboembolism（静脉血栓栓塞），而不选用动词、形容词等。其概念需精确，且有较强的专指性。

2. 关键词的书写要求

生物医学期刊英文论文的关键词，一般 3~5 个左右，以方便索引编辑人员将论文编入互检索引，并因此需要使用规范化词语。

中文关键词英译时，应尽量从美国国立医学图书馆编写的最新版《医学主题词表》（*Medical Subject Headings*, MeSH）中选取。如果《医学主题词表》中的术语不适合新出现的专业术语，则可直接采用新术语。中医药关键词应从中国中医研究院中医药信息研究所编写的《中医药主题词表》中选取。

关键词前冠以 Key words 作为标识，首字母大写，其余小写。Key words 前空两格，后加冒号，其后为关键词内容，每个关键词之间用逗号或分号隔开，最后一个关键词无标点符号。

5.4.3 致谢

如前所述，致谢是作者对为本研究的完成和发表有一定贡献、而又非本文作者的有关人员和单位表示感谢，包括：参加本研究或论文工作讨论或提出过指导性建议者；为本文绘制图表或为实验提供样品者；协助进行某些技术操作或在实验材料、仪器、数据统计处理等方面提供方便的人员和单位以及资金提供者和机构；对论文作全面修改者，等等。

致谢必须实事求是，并应征得被致谢者的书面同意；致谢常置于论文主体之后，参考文献之前；也可将致谢的内容置于论文首页的脚注中，如基金资助常以脚注方式说明。用英语表达致谢时，可开门见山地对本论文研究作出贡献的有关人员和单位表示感谢。

例4

We gratefully acknowledge the financial support of this study from the National Natural Science Foundation of China. We are also greatly indebted to Professor Zhang Ming from the Affiliated Children's Hospital, Chongqing Medical University for his help in data collection, to Wang Ping, MD, from the First Affiliated Hospital, Chongqing Medical University, for technical assistance, and to Huang Qing, MD, from the Second Affiliated Hospital, Chongqing Medical University, for providing the illustrations for this paper.

译文：我们非常感谢国家自然科学基金会给予本课题以资金赞助。同时重庆医科大学附属儿童医院的张明教授为本课题收集数据、重庆医科大学附属第一医院王平博士提供了技术帮助、重庆医科大学附属第二医院黄青博士为本文提供图片资料,在此我们深表谢意。

例5

We thank Dr. Edward V. Prochownik for constructs and compound JKY-2-169, Dr. Shideng Bao for MYC mutant constructs, Dr. Chi V. Dang for P493-6 B cells, and Dr. John M. Sedivy for Rat-1 fibroblast cells. We thank the NUseq and the Robert H. Lurie Comprehensive Cancer Center Flow Cytometry cores of Northwestern University. We thank Dr. Andrew Mazar and Dr. Nicolette Zielinski for helpful discussions on the project design and Lisa Hurley for the technical assistance. This work was supported by grants from the National Cancer Institute：R01CA123484, RO1CA196270, and P50CA180995；and by the New-Cures Biomedical Accelerator of Northwestern University. Part of the work was supported by the H-Foundation Multi-PI Basic Science Synergy Award made possible by a gift from the H Foundation to the Robert H. Lurie Comprehensive Cancer Center. A part of this work was performed by the Northwestern University ChemCore and the Developmental Therapeutics Core，which are funded by Cancer Center Support Grant P30CA060553 from the National Cancer Institute awarded to the Robert H. Lurie Comprehensive Cancer Center，and the Chicago Biomedical Consortium with support from the Searle Funds at the Chicago Community Trust.

译文: 我们感谢 Edward V. Prochownik 博士提供的构建物和化合物 JKY-2-169, Shideng Bao 博士的 MYC 突变构建物,Chi V. Dang 博士的 P493-6 B 细胞,以及 John M. Sedivy 博士的 1 型大鼠成纤维细胞。感谢西北大学 NUseq 和 Robert H. Lurie 综合癌症中心流式细胞术中心。我们感谢 Andrew Mazar 博士和 Nicolette Zie-linski 博士就项目设计进行了有益的讨论,并感谢 Lisa Hurley 提供的技术援助。这项工作得到了国家癌症研究所的资助,资助项目号为 R01CA123484,RO1CA196270 和 P50CA180995;以及西北大学的新治愈生物医学加速器的支持。该研究的部分工作得到了 H 基金会 Multi-PI 基础科学协同奖的支持,这是 H 基金会给罗伯特·H.鲁里综合癌症中心的馈赠。该研究的部分工作由西北大学化学中心和发展治疗学中心完成。中心由国家癌症研究所授予罗伯特·H.鲁里综合癌症中心的癌症中心支持赠款项目(P30CA060553)以及芝加哥社区信托基金的西尔基金支持下的芝加哥生物医学联合会资助。

表示感谢的英文常用表达有:

to thank… for…

to be thankful to… for…

to be grateful to… for…

to be indebted to… for…

to acknowledge… / to be acknowledged

to express… thanks to… for…

to appreciate

to express… appreciation to… for…

5.4.4　参考文献

参考文献是生物医学期刊英文论文的重要组成部分。它表明论文的科学依据和历史背景,体现作者尊重他人研究成果的态度,并提示作者在前人研究基础上的提高、发展与创新。

1. 参考文献的要求

(1) 作者只要可能都应该直接引用原始研究作为参考文献。

(2) 参考文献应是本研究领域内的经典文献,并且参考文献还应该是最新的,以最近一两年以内的为好。

(3) 未公开发表的论文一般不提倡引用。已被期刊接受但尚未发表的文章可引用,但应注明"正在印刷"(in press)或"即将出版"(forthcoming)。

(4) 文献著录时,作者较多时,一般列前 6 位,其余省略,中文省略形式以"等"表示,英文省略形式以"et al"表示。

(5) 医学期刊引用参考文献的数量,少则 10 多条,多达 200 条以上。

(6) 书籍中的出版地为该出版社所在的城市名称,当书籍中印有多个出版地时,仅著录第一出版地。

(7) 参考文献应规范,一般包括期刊、论文集、图书、会议录、国际上的标准化组织或论坛推出的标准、建议、草案等。随着网上资料的增多,网上文章也可以作为参考文献。

2. 参考文献的著录项目

(1) 作者(多个作者之间以","隔开)。主要作者只列姓名,其后不加"著""编""主编"等责任说明。

(2) 文献题名及版本。

(3) 文献类型及载体类型标识。

(4) 出版项(出版社、出版者、出版年)。

(5) 文献出处或电子文献的可获得地址。

(6) 文献起止页码。

(7) 文献标准编号(标准号、专利号等)。

3. 参考文献的著录格式

ICMJE 推荐的参考文献著录格式是基于"国家信息标准组织 NISO Z39.29-2005(R2010)书目参考文献"标准,采用顺序编码制。

参考文献在正文中按引用顺序用 1,2,……上标标注于引文句末;在文末"参考文献"下,按 1,2,……顺序列出。

参考文献的主要著录格式如下[①]:

(1) 专著:

序号. 作者. 书名. 版次. 出版地:出版社;出版年.

---

① 更多著录规范可登陆 http://www.nlm.nih.gov/bsd/uniform-requirements html 查看。

例6

1. Murray PR, Rosenthal KS, Kobayashi GS, Pfaller MA. Medical microbiology. 4th ed. St. Louis：Mosby；2002.

（2）期刊文章：

序号. 作者. 论文名. 刊名. 出版日期；卷号（期号）：起止页码.

例7

1. Halpern SD, Ubel PA, Caplan AL. Solid-organ transplantation in HIV-infected patients. N Engl J Med.2002 Jul 25；347（4）：284-7.

需要注意的是，期刊名称通常不需要著录全名，而是用简称，简称需查阅后著录。

（3）论文集：

序号. 作者或编者. 论文集名. 版次. 出版地：出版者；出版年.

例8

1. Breedlove GK, Schorfheide AM. Adolescent pregnancy.2nd ed. White Plains（NY）：March of Dimes Education Services；2001.

（4）学位论文：

序号. 作者. 论文名. 保存地点：保存单位，授予年份.

例9

1. Borkowski MM. Infant sleep and feeding：a telephone survey of Hispanic Americans [dissertaton]. Mount pleasant（MI）：Central Michigan University，2002.

值得注意的是，不同期刊在参考文献著录格式上也会有差异，所以作者在写作前应参见目标期刊的"投稿须知"。

5.4.5　利益冲突声明

根据"ICMJE 推荐规范"，作者应该报告利益声明，内容包括：（1）作者的利益冲突；（2）研究工作的资助来源，包括资助者名称以及对资助者在以下方面所起作用的解释：研究的设计，数据的收集、分析和解释，报告的撰写，决定将报告投稿发表；或者声明资助者没有参与这些工作；（3）作者是否获得了研究数据，并解释获得途径的性质和获取范围，以及是否可持续获得。对于这些内容，作者可通过填写 ICMJE 的"利益冲突表"①提交。有时，期刊也会要求作者写作声明，置于文后发表。写作形式灵活，具体写作内容需参照目标杂志的要求完成。

例10

Declaration of Interests

We declare no competing interests

---

① 表格可在 ICMJE 的官方网站下载，下载地址：http://www.icmje.org/conflicts-of-interest/。

译文：

利益声明

我们声明没有任何利益冲突。

例11

Conflict of Interest Disclosure

Dr. Koletzko reported being a member of the European Society for Paediatric Gastroenterology, Hepatology and Nutrition guideline group for celiac disease and a member of the PreventCD consortium. No other disclosures were reported.

译文：

利益冲突声明

Koletzko 博士报告说，他是欧洲儿童胃肠病、肝病协会和腹部疾病营养指导小组成员，也是腹部疾病预防联盟的成员。除此之外，没有其他声明。

例12

Competing Interests：All authors have completed the ICMJE uniform disclosure form at www.icmje.org / coi_disclosure.pdf and declare：support from the National Institutes of Health for the submitted work；FBH reports support from grants HL60712, HL118264, and DK112940 from the National Institutes of Health, research support from the California Walnut Commission, honorariums for lectures from Metagenics and Standard Process, and honorariums from, Diet Quality Photo Navigation outside the submitted work；the remaining authors report no other relationships or activities that could appear to have influenced the submitted work.

译文：

利益冲突：所有作者已在 www.ICMJE.org / coi_disclosure.pdf 上填写了 ICMJE 推荐的统一声明表，并声明：国家卫生研究院对提交的工作予以了支持；除所投文稿外，FBH 还报告了国家卫生研究院 HL60712、HL118264 和 DK112940 拨款项目的支持，加州胡桃木委员会提供的研究支持，来自 Metagenics and Standard Process 的讲座酬金，来自 Diet Quality Photo Navigation 的酬金；其余的作者未声明可能影响所投文稿的其他关系或活动。

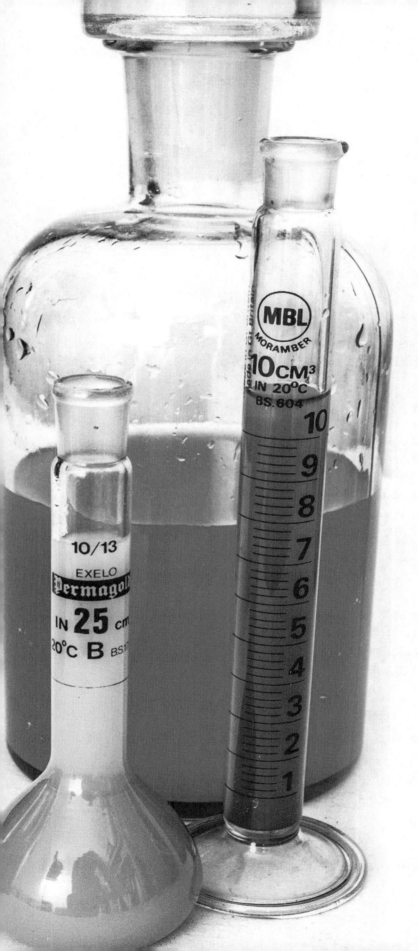

第

6

章

研究论文主体
部分写作指要

6.1 标题

6.1.1 标题的功能

标题对整篇论文进行精炼的描述,它和摘要一起所含有的信息使得对论文的电子检索灵敏而又准确。如读者在美国的 Pub Med(向公众免费开放的医学网站),Amedeo(国际医学文献导引)和我国的《中文科技资料目录 ∗ 医学卷》搜索论文标题,并以此判断文章内容,然后决定是否阅读、收集该文献。因此,研究论文的标题恰当与否是影响医学信息传播的一个重要因素。论文标题必须具备反映论文主题和吸引读者的功能。

6.1.2 标题的内容和结构

6.1.2.1 验证假设型论文标题的内容和结构

1. 反映研究命题

多数情况下,研究论文的标题只反映论文的研究命题,称作为描述性标题(indicative title),通常用短语表达。大部分研究论文属验证假设型论文(hypothesis-testing paper),这类论文完整的命题信息包括:自变量(independent variables)、因变量(dependent variables)和研究对象(subjects)或实验动物(animals)。

有些标题中既有自变量又有因变量,其典型写法如下:

例1

Effect of β Endorphin on Breathing Movements in Fetal Sheep

说明:研究对象为动物时,必须标明动物名称,置于标题最后。

译文:β 内啡肽对胎羊呼吸运动的影响

例2

Effect of Roflumilast on Exacerbations in Patients with Severe Chronic Obstructive Pulmonary Disease Uncontrolled by Combination Therapy(REACT):a Multicentre Randomised Controlled Trial

说明:如果研究对象为特殊人群,则必须标注特殊人群的具体状况。

译文:罗氟司特对联合治疗未能控制的重症 COPD 患者急性加重的疗效(REACT):一项多中心随机对照试验

例3

Association between Maternal Gluten Intake and Type 1 Diabetes in Offspring:National Prospective Cohort Study in Denmark

译文：母体麸质摄入与后代 1 型糖尿病的关系：一项丹麦国家前瞻性队列研究

例4

Semaglutide and Cardiovascular Outcomes in Patients with Type 2 Diabetes

说明：除 effect 这一典型用词外，association，and 也常用于表述自变量与因变量之间的关系。

译文：司美鲁肽与 2 型糖尿病患者心血管转归关系的研究

某些标题只含有因变量或自变量，其写法如下：

例5

Tranexamic Acid in Patients Undergoing Coronary-Artery Surgery

译文：氨甲环酸在行冠状动脉手术患者中的应用

例6

Assessing the Risks Associated with MRI in Patients with a Pacemaker or Defibrillator

译文：植入起搏器或除颤器的患者行 MRI 检查的相关风险评估

2. 揭示研究答案

验证假设型论文的标题除描述研究命题之外，还可揭示研究的结论，称作为结论性标题（declarative title）。使用结论性标题的前提是研究证据充分有力，研究结论明确肯定。因此，相比于描述性题目，结论性标题使用较少，因为不是所有的科学研究都可以得出很确定的结论，而且作者认为很明确的结论，也要接受读者和时间的检验。结论性标题可以用短语或句子表示。

例7

Reduced leaflet motion after transcatheter aortic-valve replacement

说明：在标题最前面，研究的因变量之前加上形容词或起修饰作用的分词，揭示研究答案。

译文：经导管主动脉瓣置换术后小叶运动减少

例8

Restriction of HIV-1 Escape by a Highly Broad and Potent Neutralizing Antibody

说明：也可以在研究因变量之前，用动词的名词化形式叙述研究结论。

译文：高度广泛有效的中和抗体对 HIV-1 逃逸的抑制

例9

Atrial fibrillation is associated with lean body mass in postmenopausal women

说明：结论性标题还可以用一般现在时态的句子。因为表达肯定有力，故句子形式的结论性标题应更谨慎使用。

译文：绝经后妇女房颤与去脂体重相关

6.1.2.2　方法学论文标题的内容和结构

方法学论文（methods paper）的标题应反映该研究论文中研究的方法、仪器或材料，表明其应用目的和应用对象。下面是方法学论文的典型标题：

例10

New pharmacological strategies for protecting kidney function in type 2 diabetes

说明：用介词结构 for + doing... 表示应用目的。

译文：2 型糖尿病患者肾功能保护的新型药物治疗策略

例11

Extracorporeal Photopheresis for Colitis Induced by Checkpoint-Inhibitor Therapy

译文：体外光分离置换法治疗由检查点抑制剂治疗引起的结肠炎

例12

Oil-Based or Water-Based Contrast for Hysterosalpingography in Infertile Women

说明：介词 for 之后也可用名词性词组来表达应用目的。

译文：油性或水溶性造影剂用于不孕妇女子宫输卵管造影

例13

Highly Parallel Genome-wide Expression Profiling of Individual Cells Using Nanoliter Droplets

说明：分词 using 结构也可以用来描写方法或材料。

译文：使用纳升液滴对单个细胞进行高度并行的全基因组表达谱分析

6.1.2.3　描述性论文标题的内容和结构

描述性论文（descriptive paper）的标题常反映研究中的新发现，如一个基因、分子或结构，并阐明其功能。写作时，描述的对象置于标题之首，以同位语、副标题，或句子方式阐明其功能。

例14

Von Willebrand factor, a rapid sensor of paravalvular regurgitation during TRVR

译文：血管性血友病因子，经导管主动脉瓣膜置换术中一种快速检测瓣膜旁返流的传感器

例15

YTH Domain：A Family of N6-methyladenosine（m6A）Readers

译文：YTH 结构域：N6-甲基腺苷（m6A）阅读器家族

例16

ADT-OH, a hydrogen sulfide-releasing donor, induces apoptosis and inhibits the development of melanoma in vivo by upregulating FADD

译文：ADT-OH，一种释放硫化氢的供体，可通过上调 FADD 诱导凋亡并抑制体内黑色素瘤的发展

例17

Astrocytic trans-Differentiation Completes a Multicellular Paracrine Feedback Loop Required for Medulloblastoma Tumor Growth

译文：星形细胞的转分化完成髓母细胞瘤肿瘤生长所需的多细胞旁分泌反馈回路

6.1.3 标题的写作要点

"ICMJE 推荐规范"对论文标题写作的要求只有两点:简练(concise)但信息丰富(informative)。各期刊在征稿启事中对研究论文的标题做了更为明确的写作要求。著名医学杂志 *Cell* 要求标题的字数不超过 10~12 个单词,应阐明论文的整体意义而不提供具体内容,并且特别指明标题应避免使用行话、非标准的缩略语、和标点符号。*JAMA* 规定标题应该简练、具体和信息完整,且不超过 150 个字符,并建议避免写作信息过于宽泛的标题、结论性标题;对于临床试验报告、荟萃分析、系统性回顾,应在题目中用小标题写明研究类型。*Nature* 要求包括空格在内标题应控制在 75 个字符,且通常不建议使用数字、缩略语、或标点符号,但应包含检索需要的足够信息。

具体来讲,撰写研究论文标题时,应注意三个原则:信息准确完整、语义具体清晰、表达简练醒目。

6.1.3.1 信息准确完整

论文标题的准确性是指能准确反映论文内容,恰如其分地描述,不能夸大或缩小事实,更不能名不符实。此外,标题应该足以反映论文的关键信息,如研究对象、研究方法等。

例18

原标题:Experimental study on transplantation of mesenchymal stem cells from human fetal livers for treating myocardial infarction

说明:原标题未描述本研究的研究对象,应予明确。明确研究对象后,原标题中的实验研究就不言而喻,应予省略,达到用词简练的目的。

修改后:Transplantation of mesenchymal stem cells from human fetal livers for treating myocardial infarction in rats

译文:人胎儿肝脏间质干细胞移植治疗大鼠的心肌梗死

例19

原标题:Secretory protein study of Bifidobacterium Longum XY01

说明:原标题只反映了研究内容,但未反映研究方法。

修改后:Two dimensional electrophoresis combined with mass spectrometry for analyzing secretory protein profile in Bifidobacterium Longum XY01

译文:双向电泳-质谱技术分析长双歧杆菌 XY01 分泌蛋白谱

6.1.3.2 语义具体清晰

论文标题所传达的信息是否准确,表达是否具体清晰,直接关系到论文能否被国际读者接受,并且会影响国际检索机构的收录。写作时应注意措辞具体。

例20

原标题:Related research progress of long non-coding RNAs in tumor

说明：原标题未能准确传递研究的命题，且未具体说明研究方法。

修改后：Interaction between lncRNA and microRNA in tumor：a systematic review

译文：肿瘤中 lncRNA 和 microRNA 间的相互作用：一项系统性回顾

例21

原标题：Posttranslational modification of autophagy

说明：原标题表达信息不准确。自噬是一种现象，而研究中真正的命题是自噬相关蛋白。

修改后：Posttranslational modification of autophagy-related protein

译文：自噬相关蛋白的翻译后修饰

6.1.3.3 表达简练醒目

在保证准确、完整和清楚的前提下，论文标题要做到文字简练、易懂。题目越短，给人印象越深。在写作英语标题或将中文标题翻译成英语时应注意以下四个方面：

1. 删除冗词

冗词是指空洞无用之词。冗词因为对论文标题的正确表述并无任何帮助而显得多余，应当删除。常见的冗词有 study of ...，experiment of ...，experience of ...，report of ...，discussion on ...，analysis on ... 等。此外，题目起始处的 the 通常省略，而题目中间的 the 则需保留。

2. 避免赘述

累赘的叙述使得标题重点不突出，不能吸引读者。这时就需要运用技巧简化必要用词，以使标题短小精悍。其中一个重要的简化方法就是用能描述其共同特性的种类名替代不必要的细述。

例22

中文标题：血管内皮生长因子和透明质酸等肿瘤标志物在膀胱癌诊断中的应用价值

原标题：Clinical evaluation of VEGF, HA, BTA stat, NMP22, CD 44v6, surviving and VUC in bladder carcinoma diagnosis

说明：原译的标题含有大量缩略语，理解起来颇费周折，并且显得特别冗长。根据文章内容，发现肿瘤标志物包括英文标题中所提及的 7 项指标，且其重要性相当。如果将 7 项指标全部细述出来，无法让读者抓住重点，一目了然。然而，用肿瘤标志物这一名称来囊括所有的指标则能起到言简意赅的作用。

修改后：Clinical evaluation of tumor markers in bladder carcinoma diagnosis

3. 前置重要内容

写作英文论文标题时应注意将研究中心内容的关键词，即"中心名词"置于首位，然后选择正确的用词顺序清楚表达论文的主题。effect，influence，inhibition，treatment，evaluation，characterization，reduction，expression，association，protection，prevention 等都是研究论文中常用的中心名词。

4. 写作副标题

为了进一步突出论文的某一方面,如病例数、样本、研究方法、意义等,或有系列论文连载,则应使用副标题。或按杂志要求,如 *JAMA* 要求对于临床试验报告、荟萃分析、系统性回顾论文,标题应用小标题写明其研究类型。以下标题都包含副标题。

（1）突出样本

例23

Body-mass index, blood pressure, and cause-specific mortality in India：a prospective cohort study of 500, 810 adults

译文：500810 例印度成年人身体质量指数、血压和特定病因死亡率的前瞻性队列研究

例24

Global trends in insufficient physical activity asmong adolescents：a pooled analysis of 298 population-based surveys with 1.6 million participants

译文：青少年缺乏体育活动的全球趋势：一项纳入 160 万参与者基于 298 项人口调查的汇总分析

（2）突出方法

例25

Antithrombotic treatment after coronary artery bypass graft surgery：systematic review and network meta-analysis

译文：冠状动脉搭桥手术后的抗栓治疗：系统综述和网络荟萃分析

（3）突出意义

例26

Production of functional, stable, unmutated recombinant human papillomavirus E6 oncoprotein：implications for HPV-tumor diagnosis and therapy

译文：功能性、稳定、未突变的重组人乳头瘤病毒 E6 致癌蛋白的产生：对 HPV-肿瘤诊断和治疗的意义

例27

Clinicopathologic features and outcomes of anterior-dominant prostate cancer：implications for diagnosis and treatment

译文：前叶累及为主的前列腺癌的临床病理特征及结局：对诊断及治疗的意义

6.1.4　标题示例

1. 名词词组型标题

Neural Control and Modulation of Thirst, Sodium Appetite, and Hunger（*Cell*, 9 January, 2020）

译文：口渴、钠食欲和饥饿的神经控制和调节

Landscape and Dynamics of Single Immune Cells in Hepatocellular Carcinoma（*Cell*,

31 October, 2019)

译文：肝细胞癌中单个免疫细胞的图谱和动力学

2. 含介词短语结构的标题

IN

Accuracy of pre-hospital trauma triage and field triage decision rules in children (P2-T2 study)：an observational study (*Lancet*, January 31, 2020)

译文：儿童院前创伤类选的准确性和现场类选规则（P2-T2 研究）：一项观察性研究

Widespread Transcriptional Scanning in the Testis Modulates Gene Evolution Rates (*Cell*, 23 January, 2020)

译文：睾丸中的广泛转录扫描调节基因进化速率

WITH

Systemic chemotherapy with or without cetuximab in patients with resectable colorectal liver metastasis (New EPOC)：long-term results of a multicentre, randomised, controlled, phase 3 trial (*Lancet*, January 31, 2020)

译文：可切除结直肠肝转移患者中单用或联用西妥昔单抗的全身化疗（新型 EPOC 研究）：一项多中心、随机、对照、3 期试验的长期结果

A Therapy for Most with Cystic Fibrosis (*Cell*, 23 January, 2020)

译文：一种适用于多数囊性纤维化患者的疗法

FOR

Ropeginterferon alfa-2b versus standard therapy for polycythaemia vera (PROUD-PV and CONTINUATION-PV)：a randomised, non-inferiority, phase 3 trial and its extension study (*Lancet*, January 31, 2020)

译文：新型长效型单修饰脯氨酸干扰素（Ropeginterferon alfa-2b）与标准疗法治疗真性红细胞增多症（PROUD-PV 和 CONTINUATION-PV）：一项随机、非劣效性、3 期临床试验及其扩展研究

Establishing or Exaggerating Causality for the Gut Microbiome：Lessons from Human Microbiota-Associated Rodents (*Cell*, 23 January, 2020)

译文：建立或夸大人类疾病与肠道微生物组的因果关系：一项对人类微生物群相关啮齿动物研究的反思

OF

Impact of Feed the Future initiative on nutrition in children aged less than 5 years in sub-Saharan Africa (*BMJ*, December 11, 2019)

译文：撒哈拉以南非洲地区"未来粮食保障行动计划"对 5 岁以下儿童营养的影响

Population-level impact of human papillomavirus vaccination (*Lancet*, January 20, 2020)

译文：人乳头瘤病毒疫苗接种对人群的影响

BY

Chemosensitization of prostate cancer stem cells in mice by angiogenin and plexin-B2 inhibitors

译文：血管生成素和神经丛蛋白 B2 抑制剂对小鼠前列腺癌干细胞具有化学增敏作用（*Communications Biology*，15 January，2020）

Cysteine Toxicity Drives Age-Related Mitochondrial Decline by Altering Iron Homeostasis（*Cell*，23 January，2020）

译文：半胱氨酸毒性通过改变铁稳态加速年龄相关性线粒体衰老

FROM

Gastrointestinal Bleeding from Metastatic Melanoma（*NEJM*，January 30，2020）

译文：转移性黑素瘤引起的胃肠道出血

Statins for Familial Hypercholesterolemia from Childhood（*Lancet*，January 31，2020）

译文：他汀类药物治疗儿童期家族性高胆固醇血症

BETWEEN

"Asset exchange"—interactions between patient groups and pharmaceutical industry：Australian qualitative study（*BMJ*，December 12，2019）

译文："资产交换"——患者群体与制药行业之间的相互作用：澳大利亚定性研究

Major cardiac events for adult survivors of childhood cancer diagnosed between 1970 and 1999（*BMJ*，January 15，2020）

译文：1970 年至 1999 年诊断为癌症的儿童成年后发生的主要心脏事件

DURING

Maternal smoking during pregnancy and fractures in offspring：national register based sibling comparison study（*BMJ*，29 January，2020）

译文：孕期孕妇吸烟和后代骨折之间的关系：基于国家登记数据的兄弟姐妹比较研究

Local Fatty Acid Channeling into Phospholipid Synthesis Drives Phagophore Expansion during Autophagy（*Cell*，9 January，2020）

译文：自噬过程中磷脂合成产生的局部脂肪酸驱动吞噬泡的扩张

AFTER

Risk of herpes zoster after exposure to varicella to explore the exogenous boosting hypothesis（*BMJ*，January 22，2020）

译文：以水痘暴露后的带状疱疹风险探讨外源性推动假说

Antithrombotic treatment after coronary artery bypass graft surgery：systematic review and network meta-analysis（*Cell*，10 October，2019）

译文：冠状动脉搭桥手术后的抗栓治疗：系统评价和网络荟萃分析

THROUGH

Charting the Complexity of the Marine Microbiome through Single-Cell Genomics（*Cell*，12 December，2019）

译文：通过单细胞基因组图绘制复杂海洋微生物组

A New Class of Medicines through DNA Editing（*NEJM*，March 7，2019）

译文：一类通过 DNA 编辑发挥作用的新型药物

3. 含动词非谓语结构的标题

Modeling the Evolution of Human Brain Development Using Organoids（*Cell*，27 November，2019）

译文：类器官用于人类大脑发育进化的建模

Post-discharge acute care and outcomes following readmission reduction initiatives（*BMJ*，January 15，2020）

译文：减少再入院倡议下出院后急诊护理与结局

Reduced-Intensity Rivaroxaban for the Prevention of Recurrent Venous Thromboembolism

译文：减量利伐沙班用于预防复发性静脉血栓栓塞（*NEJM*，March 30，2017）

4. 句子型标题

FAMIN Is a Multifunctional Purine Enzyme Enabling the Purine Nucleotide Cycle（*Cell*，23 January，2020）

译文：FAMIN 是一种可促进嘌呤核苷酸循环的多功能嘌呤酶

A Single Transcription Factor Drives Toxoplasma gondii Differentiation（*Cell*，23 January，2020）

译文：单一转录因子驱动弓形虫分化

A Successful Trial for Lupus—How Good Is Good Enough?（*NEJM*，January 16，2020）

译文：一项成功的狼疮试验——怎样才算够好？

Exercise

Translate the following "Titles" into English.

1. 体内外环境（environment in vivo and in vitro）对骨髓间充质干细胞（bone mesenchymal stem cell）向神经细胞分化（differentiation）的影响

2. 血管紧张素受体（angiotensin-receptor）拮抗剂（antagonist）伊贝沙坦（irbesartan）在 2 型糖尿病（type 2 diabetes）所致肾病（nephropathy）病人中的肾脏保护作用

3. 接受血液透析（hemodialysis）的病人中金葡菌结合疫苗（staphylococcus aureus conjugate vaccine）的使用

4. 放射免疫法（radioimmunoassay）测定血清 17-羟孕酮（serum 17-OH-progesterone）以诊断与治疗先天性肾上腺增生（congenital adrenal hyperplasia）

5. 人双特异性抗体（bi-specific antibody）FIT-1 具有治疗寨卡（Zika）病毒感染的潜力

6. 甲硝唑（metronidazole）不能防止无症状（asymptomatic）阴道滴虫感染（tricho-

moniasis vaginalis infection）妊娠妇女的早产（preterm delivery）

7. 甲状腺功能低下（hypothyroidism）的妇女在雌激素（estrogen）治疗期对甲状腺素（thyroxine）的需要增加

8. 一氧化氮（nitric oxide）伴或不伴继续降压治疗在急性卒中患者高血压管理中的效应（ENOS）：一项部分析因的（partial-factorial）随机对照试验

9. 度拉糖肽（dulaglutide）每周 1 次与睡前甘精胰岛素（bedtime insulin glargine）均结合用餐时赖脯胰岛素（prandial insulin lispro）治疗 2 型糖尿病的比较（AWARD-4）：一项随机、开放标记、Ⅲ 期、非劣效性研究

10. 用维奈托克靶向 BCL2 治疗复发性慢性淋巴细胞白血病（lymphocytic leukemia）

11. 术前化疗后乳腺癌的卡培他滨（Capecitabine）辅助治疗

12. 富马酸替诺福韦二吡呋酯（Tenofovir Disoproxil Fumarate）与恩替卡韦（Entecavir）治疗慢性 HBV 感染者的远期肾脏效应比较

13. 印度尼西亚初级医疗中尿浸渍检查法（urinary dipstick test）用于管理尿道感染（urinary tract infection）相关症状患者的预测价值：一项横断面研究

14. 高强度聚焦超声（high intensity focused ultrasound）消融激活癌症患者的抗肿瘤免疫力

15. 白介素-13（interleukin-13）和白介素-18 调节支气管哮喘大鼠神经生长因子 mRNA 表达的实验研究

6.2　摘要

6.2.1　摘要的功能

摘要，英语称为 abstract 或 summary，是位于论文正文前面的一段概括性文字，具有独立性（independent）和自含性（self-contained）的特点，即不阅读或参考全文，读者就能通过摘要获得论文的主要信息。因此，摘要具有方便阅读、信息采集和计算机检索的功能。

6.2.2　摘要的内容与结构

研究论文摘要是电子数据库所收录论文的独立成篇部分，犹如论文的微型版本，完整报道论文引言、方法、结果和结论部分的重要内容，因此也被称为资料性摘要。

验证假设型论文摘要概括论文四个部分的内容，即研究问题、研究方法、研究发现和研究答案。此外，还可以在段首描述研究背景，段尾阐述研究价值和意义，作出推测或建议等。[①]

---

① Mimi Zeiger, Essentials of Writing Biomedical Research Papers. U. S. A：The McGraw-Hill companies, Inc., 2000, second edition, p. 269.

与验证假设型论文摘要不同,描述性论文摘要只包括三个部分的内容:论文表达的信息、支持该信息的结果,以及信息的含义。此外,如需阐明研究的原因或信息的重要性,也可以在摘要开始部分添加背景介绍。描述性论文没有假说,因此,摘要一开始就陈述研究信息(message),支持结果紧跟其后,信息的含义写于最后。值得一提的是,研究方法一般不单独成句,而是包含在描述结果的句子中[①]。

方法学论文是描述新型或改良的方法、材料或仪器的一类论文。其摘要包括以下内容:方法、材料、或仪器的名称;使用目的;研究动物或研究人群;材料或仪器的关键特征;方法或仪器的工作原理;具备的优点;检验的方法;以及应用的价值。[②]

写作结构上,资料性摘要分为结构式摘要和非结构式摘要两种。

6.2.3 非结构式摘要的写作要点

非结构式摘要(non-structured abstract)采用传统的一段式,每部分内容无标题及分段。国外一些著名的期刊,如 *Nature*、*Cell*、*Journal of Cerebral Blood Flow & Metabolism*,都采用了非结构式摘要,但使用了不同的标题。*Nature* 使用了小标题 Abstract,而 *Cell* 使用小标题 Summary。

写作时,为帮助读者迅速、有效地理解摘要中的信息,最好使用信息标记语(signal marker)。如在验证假设型论文摘要中,表达研究问题时常用不定式,研究问题和实验内容可以用一个句子表达,例如 To determine whether…, we…, To test the hypothesis that …, we…;也可以分开说明,如 We asked whether…, To answer this question, we…, We hypothesized that…, To test this hypothesis, we…等。叙述结果时,常用 We found…作为标记语。结论开始则常用 We conclude that 或 Our results indicate that 等标记语。如果是根据研究结果预示或推测的结论,则要用 These results suggest that …来加以提示。

6.2.4 非结构式摘要示例

1. 验证假设型论文摘要

例1

Title:Oral administration of a novel lipophilic PPARδ agonist is not neuroprotective after rodent cerebral ischemia

Abstract

Peroxisome proliferator-activated receptors are regulators of inflammatory signaling. This has fostered hope that PPAR agonists might have neuroprotective potential. We hypothesized that PPARδ activation by the novel orally administered lipophilic PPARδ agonist SAR145 may improve short-and long-term outcome after focal brain ischemia. We

---

① Ibid, p. 275

② Ibid, p. 286

induced ischemia by transient filamentous middle cerebral artery occlusion (MCAo) in 227 C57BL/6 mice and administered SAR145 in varying doses and time windows post-injury. Outcome was assessed by three functional tests and histologically determining ischemic lesion sizes. In a second experiment, we tested SAR145 treatment in 40 PPARδ-knockout mice using the same procedures. Three independent groups treated with 10 mg/kg bodyweight SAR145 directly after filament removal showed a mean reduction in lesion sizes of 18 ± 10% compared to vehicle-treated groups. We did not observe a consistent improvement in the long-term functional outcome by SAR145-treatment. PPARδ-knockout mice showed a significantly higher mortality after MCAo. We did not find a reduction of lesion size by SAR145-treatment in PPARδ-knockout mice. In summary, we found no evidence of a long-term neuroprotective effect of post-injury SAR145 treatment in cerebral ischemia. However, PPARδ appears to play a pathophysiologic role in acute infarct development and overall mortality after brain ischemia. (*J Cereb Blood Flow Metab.*, 2018 Jan, 38 (1))

译文:

标题:口服新型亲脂性 PPARδ 激动剂对啮齿小鼠脑缺血后无神经保护作用

摘要

过氧化物酶体增殖物激活受体是炎症信号的调节剂。因此 PPAR 激动剂有望发挥神经保护的潜能。我们的假设是新型口服亲脂性 PPAR 性激动剂 SAR145 可激活 PPARδ 以改善局灶性脑缺血后的短期和长期结局。我们对 227 只 C57BL/6 小鼠进行短暂的丝状大脑中动脉闭塞(MCAo)诱导缺血,并在损伤后不同时间窗给予小鼠不同剂量 SAR145。用三种功能测试和组织学检测的缺血病变大小评估结局。在第二个实验中,我们用相同的程序测试了 SAR145 对 40 只 PPARδ 敲除小鼠的治疗效果。与溶酶对照组相比,三个不同治疗组在去除细丝后按 10 μmg/kg 体重给与 SAR145 治疗,其病变大小平均减少了 18±10%。我们未观察到 SAR145 治疗对长期功能结局的持续改善。PPARδ 敲除小鼠在 MCAo 后死亡率明显升高。我们未发现 SAR145 治疗可减少 PPARδ 敲除小鼠的病变大小。总之,我们并未发现证据表明脑缺血时受伤后 SAR145 治疗具有长期的神经保护作用。但是,PPARδ 似乎在急性脑梗死发展和脑缺血后的总体死亡率中发挥病理生理作用。

研究论文写作中,如果描述的医学术语过长、过难或者出现次数过多时,可以使用缩略语形式简化表达。缩略语具有专业性强、信息量大、简明便捷的优点,但如果作者缩略语使用不当,反而影响学术论文的规范性、可读性、简洁性,所以一定要注意缩略语的使用原则。

英文缩略语通常分为公认缩略语和非公认缩略语两种。

公认缩略语是指被医学界甚至公众普遍熟悉,缩略形式甚至比全称更常见,例如:DNA(脱氧核糖核酸),RNA(核糖核酸),AIDS(艾滋病),MRI(核磁共振成像),ECG(心电图),RBC(红细胞计数),PCR(聚合酶链式反应)等。研究论文中可能用到的公认缩略语还包括化学名和国际通用计量单位,如 CO_2,N_2,mg,kg,min,ml 等。这类缩略语可以在论文中自由使用而无需给出全称。但有时候，很多缩略语只在特定领域中被专业人士熟知，如 COPD（chronic obstructive pulmonary diseases 慢性阻塞性肺疾病），ARDS（acute respiratory distress syndrome 急性呼吸窘迫综合征）等；以及同一个缩略语在不同领域会有多种解释，如 PT 的全称可以理解为：physical therapy（物理治疗），posterior tibial（胫后的）和 paroxysmal tachycardia（阵发性心动过速）等。因此，对于此类非公认缩略语，即作者在论文（正文）写作中为了简化表达而采用的缩略语，一定要在首次出现时给出完整形式（在标题中除外），然后在其后加括号标注缩略形式，通常为每个词的首字母大写。再次使用时，用其缩略形式即可。例如：OSAS（obstructive sleep apnea syndrome）阻塞性睡眠呼吸暂停综合症，HIFU（high intensity focused ultrasound）高强度聚焦超声，PCA（passive cutaneous allergy）被动皮肤过敏反应等。

值得注意的是，缩略语的使用前提是使论文简洁、易懂。一篇论文中不应充斥过多的缩略语；非公认或未审定公布的缩略语要慎用；无需缩略出现次数少于 3～5 次的短语（不同期刊，要求有所不同）；无需缩略较短的单词或短语（如 lung cancer 在论文中即使多次出现，也不建议缩写为 LC）；对仅出现 2～3 次的术语，也不宜缩略，否则反而增加阅读，特别是跨专业阅读的难度。

很多杂志在投稿须知中也提到了常用的缩略语清单，如 the Journal of Clinical Investigation（美国）在官网上列出了标准的缩略语表供投稿者参考（https：// www.jci.org/ kiosk/ publish/ abbreviations）。此外，在写作的时候也可以适当参考缩略词典，如 Dictionary of Medical Acronyms & Abbreviations、AD（Abbreviations Dictionary）等。

2. 描述性论文摘要

例2

Title：Reducing Pericyte-Derived Scarring Promotes Recovery after Spinal Cord Injury

Summary

CNS injury often severs axons. Scar tissue that forms locally at the lesion site is thought to block axonal regeneration, resulting in permanent functional deficits. We report that inhibiting the generation of progeny by a subclass of pericytes led to decreased fibrosis and extracellular matrix deposition after spinal cord injury in mice. Regeneration of raphespinal and corticospinal tract axons was enhanced and sensorimotor function recovery improved following spinal cord injury in animals with attenuated pericyte-derived scarring. Using optogenetic stimulation, we demonstrate that regenerated corticospinal tract axons integrated into the local spinal cord circuitry below the lesion site. The number of regenerated axons correlated with improved sensorimotor function recovery. In conclusion, attenuation of pericyte-derived fibrosis represents a promising therapeutic approach to facilitate recovery following CNS injury. (*Cell*, 2018 Mar 22, 173（1））

译文：

题目：减少周细胞源性瘢痕形成促进脊髓损伤后康复

摘要

中枢神经系统损伤常使轴突断裂。在病变部位形成的局部瘢痕组织往往会阻碍轴突再生，导致永久性的功能缺陷。本文报道了通过周细胞亚群抑制子代产生可以减少小鼠脊髓损伤后纤维化及细胞外基质沉积。周细胞源性瘢痕形成减轻的动物中，脊髓损伤后中脊束轴突和皮质脊髓束轴突的再生得到增强，感觉运动功能恢复得到改善。使用光遗传学刺激，我们证明了再生的皮质脊髓束轴突整合到病变部位下方的局部脊髓回路中。再生轴突的数量与感觉运动功能的改善相关。总之，减轻周细胞源性纤维化可促进中枢神经系统损伤后的恢复，是一种前景良好的治疗方法。

3. 方法学论文摘要

例3

Title： A Method for the Acute and Rapid Degradation of Endogenous Proteins

Summary

Methods for the targeted disruption of protein function have revolutionized science and greatly expedited the systematic characterization of genes. Two main approaches are currently used to disrupt protein function：DNA knockout and RNA interference, which act at the genome and mRNA level, respectively. A method that directly alters endogenous protein levels is currently not available. Here, we present Trim-Away, a technique to degrade endogenous proteins acutely in mammalian cells without prior modification of the genome or mRNA. Trim-Away harnesses the cellular protein degradation machinery to remove unmodified native proteins within minutes of application. This rapidity minimizes the risk that phenotypes are compensated and that secondary, non-specific defects accumulate over time. Because Trim-Away utilizes antibodies, it can be applied to a wide range of target proteins using off-the-shelf reagents. Trim-Away allows the study of protein function in diverse cell types, including non-dividing primary cells where genome-and RNA-targeting methods are limited. (*Cell*, 2017 Dec 14, 171 (7))

译文：

标题：内源性蛋白质急速降解的一种方法

摘要

靶向破坏蛋白质功能的方法彻底改变了科学，加速了基因的系统表征。目前主要有两种方法可用于破坏蛋白质功能：DNA 敲除和 RNA 干扰，分别作用于基因组和 mRNA 水平。当前尚无直接改变内源性蛋白水平的方法。本文中，我们描述了 Trim-Away 技术，该技术在不预先修饰基因组或 mRNA 的情况下，迅速降解哺乳动物细胞中的内源性蛋白质。Trim-Away 技术利用细胞蛋白质降解机制，应用后几分钟内去除未修饰的天然蛋白质。这种快速性可以最大程度地减少表型补偿以及继发、非特异性缺陷随时间累积的风险。由于 Trim-Away 技术使用抗体，因此可以利用现成的试剂将 Trim-Away 技术应用于多种靶蛋白。Trim-Away 技术可用于研究多种细胞类型中的蛋白质功能，包括基因组靶向和 RNA 靶向方法受限的非分裂原代细胞。

6.2.5　结构式摘要的写作要点

结构式摘要（structured abstract），由美国麦克马斯特大学（McMaster University）的海恩斯（R. Brian Haynes）最初提出。完整的结构式摘要包括九个层次，而且每个层次均有特定内容。

背景（background / context）：引出一般研究命题，陈述国内外同类研究的现状。

目的（objective / purpose / aim / goal）：说明研究设想、目的，提出问题的缘由，表明研究的范围及重要性。

设计（design）或**材料和方法**（materials and methods）：说明研究课题的基本设计，及研究分类，使用的材料和方法，如何分组、对照，研究范围及精确程度，数据获得的方法。

研究地点（setting）：写明社区，医疗机构名称。

对象（subjects / participants）：说明研究对象的选取标准，是否遵循随机化原则。如设有对照组，应说明其匹配特征。如果研究对象是患者，应说明临床表现、诊断标准、筛选分组及随访情况。

干预方法（intervention）：说明干预方法的基本特征，使用什么方法及持续时间，是否原创或改进的方法。

主要结局指标（main outcome measures）：说明主要结局的测定方法，及其特异性、灵敏性、准确性。

结果（results）：列出研究的主要结果。主要结果须附有医学统计数据，包括标准差、可信区间、统计学显著检验的确切值。

结论（conclusions）：总结全文，简要说明经验证、论证取得的准确观点，即阐述结果说明什么问题，说明其理论价值或应用价值，是否可以推荐、推广或需进一步研究。

目前，根据"ICMJE 推荐规范"要求，原创性研究、系统综述和荟萃分析摘要应提供研究背景，阐明研究目的、基本过程（受试者的选择、场所、测量方法、分析方法）、主要发现（如果可能，给出具体效应值及其统计学意义和临床意义）及主要结论。临床试验的摘要应包含 CONSORT（试验报告统一标准）小组要求的基本项目。基金来源应单独列于摘要之后，以便突出显示，且便于 MEDLINE 编制供检索之用的索引。

因此，不同的医学刊物对以上结构进行了适当的调整、简化或补充。例如：

Lancet 的摘要结构：Background / Methods / Findings / Interpretation / Funding

背景 / 方法 / 研究发现 / 讨论 / 基金

JAMA 的摘要结构：Context / Objective / Design / Setting and Participants / Main Outcome Measures / Results / Conclusions

背景 / 目的 / 设计 / 研究地点和对象 / 主要结局指标 / 结果 / 结论

BMJ 的摘要结构：Objectives / Design / Setting / Participants / Interventions / Main

Outcome Measures / Results / Conclusions

目的／设计／地点／对象／干预方法／主要结局指标／结果／结论

另外一种较常见的结构式摘要是按温哥华 IMRAD 格式的范畴写作的四层次结构,包括目的／方法／结果／结论。我国医学期刊的摘要基本都采取这种格式。也有期刊使用 Background／Methods／Results／Conclusions(背景／方法／结果／结论)命名的四层次结构式摘要,如 *N Engl J Med*。

结构式摘要易于写作,作者可按层次填入内容,语言表达、结构及时态都比较固定。下面分别予以阐述:

1. 背景

引出一般研究命题或介绍同类研究现状,用现在时或现在完成时。

例4

Background　Recently, increasing evidence has suggested the association between gut dysbiosis and Alzheimer's disease (AD) progression, yet the role of gut microbiota in AD pathogenesis remains obscure.

译文:

背景　近年来,越来越多的证据表明肠道失调与阿尔茨海默病(AD)的进展有关,然而肠道微生物在 AD 发病中的作用尚不清楚。

2. 目的

结构式摘要中叙述研究目的时,多采用不定式,常用动词有 determine, evaluate, investigate, discuss, compare, examine, identify, study, develop, detect 等。

例5

Objective　To evaluate the efficacy and adverse events of a 5-day oral lefamulin regimen in patients with CABP.

译文:

目的　评价口服 lefamulin 5 天方案治疗 CABP 的疗效及不良事件。

用句子表达研究目的时,常用含中心名词 aim, goal, purpose, objective 的系表结构的过去时。

例6

The objective of this study was to determine if there is an increased survival benefit from immediate versus delayed coronary angiography in patients who were successfully resuscitated after out of hospital cardiac arrest without any evidence of STEMI.

译文:本研究的目的是明确与延迟冠状动脉造影相比,即刻冠状动脉造影是否可以提高无任何 STEMI 证据的院外心脏骤停后成功复苏患者的生存获益。

3. 设计、地点、对象、干预方法、主要结局指标

按摘要包括的层次不同,设计、地点、对象、干预方法、主要结局指标的表达结构有所不同。该部分内容多用简单句或短语结构简化表达,动词时态为过去时。

例7

用简单句表达

Design，Setting，and Participants This multicenter diagnostic study enrolled 136 premature infants (gestational age，<37 weeks) in 2 hospitals in Louisiana and 1 hospital in Missouri. Data were collected and analyzed from May 2015 to November 2018.

Interventions Infant stool samples were collected between 24 and 40 or more weeks of postconceptual age. Enrolled infants underwent abdominal radiography at physician and hospital site discretion.

Main Outcomes and Measures Enzyme activity and relative abundance of IAP were measured using fluorometric detection and immunoassays，respectively. After measurements were performed，biochemical data were evaluated against clinical entries from infants' hospital stay.

译文：

设计、地点、对象 这项多中心诊断研究纳入了路易斯安那州 2 所医院和密苏里州 1 所医院的 136 名早产婴儿（胎龄<37 周）。从 2015 年 5 月至 2018 年 11 月收集并分析数据。

干预 受孕后 24 至 40 周或更晚孕周内收集婴儿粪便样本。入选的婴儿由医师和医院地点决定接受腹部 X 线摄片。

主要结局和指标 分别使用荧光检测和免疫测定法测量 LAP 酶活性和相对丰度。在完成测量之后，基于婴儿住院期间的临床数据进行生化数据评估。

例8

用名词性短语表达

Design Population based cohort study.

Setting National Health Service in England between 2005 and 2013.

Population All people undergoing colonoscopy and subsequently diagnosed as having colorectal cancer up to three years after their investigation (PCCRC-3yr).

Main outcome measures National trends in incidence of PCCRC (within 6-36 months of colonoscopy)，univariable and multivariable analyses to explore factors associated with occurrence，and funnel plots to measure variation among providers.

译文：

设计 基于人群的队列研究。

地点 2005 年至 2013 年期间，英国国家卫生局。

对象 所有接受结肠镜检查并随后被诊断为患有结肠直肠癌超过三年的患者（PCCRC-3yr）。

主要结局指标 全国 PCCRC 发病率趋势（结肠镜检查 6~36 个月内），用单变量和多变量分析疾病发生的相关因素，漏斗图用于检测提供者之间的差异。

如果是四个层次的摘要，以上信息则合并为方法部分的内容，叙述时用句子，动词时态为过去时。

4. 结果

结果是摘要中最重要，也是最详尽的内容。叙述时一般用一个句子表达一个结局指标的一个或一组结果，用过去时表述。

例9

Results

Because the mean follow-up was only 3.75 years, our interim analysis had limited statistical power to detect treatment differences. A total of 217 patients in the rosiglitazone group and 202 patients in the control group had the adjudicated primary end point (hazard ratio, 1.08; 95% confidence interval [CI], 0.89 to 1.31). After the inclusion of end points pending adjudication, the hazard ratio was 1.11 (95% CI, 0.93 to 1.32). There were no statistically significant differences between the rosiglitazone group and the control group regarding myocardial infarction and death from cardiovascular causes or any cause. There were more patients with heart failure in the rosiglitazone group than in the control group (hazard ratio, 2.15; 95% CI, 1.30 to 3.57).

译文：

结果

由于平均随访时间只有 3.75 年，因此我们的中期分析对确定治疗差异的统计学效能有限。罗格列酮组中有 217 例患者而对照组中有 202 例患者具有裁定后的主要终点［风险比为 1.08，95% 可信区间（CI）为 0.89～1.31］。纳入待裁定的终点后，风险比为 1.11（95% CI：0.9～1.32）。罗格列酮组和对照组在心肌梗死和心血管原因或任何原因引起的死亡方面无统计学差异。罗格列酮组的心衰患者比对照组多（风险比为 2.15；95% CI：1.30～3.57）。

5. 结论

在阐述结论中最重要的内容，即研究命题的答案时用现在时，表示结论的普遍性。

例10

Conclusions

These comprehensive data show the capacity of countries (including low income countries) to provide optimal care for patients with end stage kidney disease. They demonstrate substantial variability in the burden of such disease and capacity for kidney replacement therapy and conservative kidney management, which have implications for policy.

译文：

结论

这些综合数据显示了各国（包括低收入国家）为终末期肾病患者提供最佳护理的能力。同时还表明这种疾病负担以及肾脏替代疗法和肾脏保守治疗能力在各国之间存在巨大差异，这一发现对政策制定具有启示作用。

写作结论时，作者经常在谓语动词前加情态动词来准确反映结论的肯定程度，其可能性由大到小排列为 will, can, could, would, may, might。

例11

In women with hypothyroidism treated with thyroxine, estrogen therapy may increase the need for thyroxine.

译文：接受甲状腺素治疗的甲低妇女，雌激素治疗可能增加对甲状腺素的需求。

例12

In patients receiving hemodialysis, a conjugate vaccine can offer partial immunity against staphylococcus aureus bacteremia for approximately 40 weeks, after which protection wanes as antibody levels decrease.

译文：在接受血液透析的患者中，结合疫苗可提供抗金黄色葡萄球菌的部分免疫力，持续时间约为40周，此后随着抗体水平下降，保护作用逐渐减弱。

值得一提的是，在少数文章的结论部分，作者只是总结了局限于本研究的主要发现，需用过去时表述。

例13

In the Swedish population, stress related disorders were associated with a subsequent risk of life threatening infections, after controlling for familial background and physical or psychiatric comorbidities.

译文：在瑞典人群中，控制家族背景和身体或精神疾病合并症后，压力相关性疾病与随后威胁生命的感染风险相关。

例14

Among patients with CABP, 5-day oral lefamulin was noninferior to 7-day oral moxifloxacin with respect to early clinical response at 96 hours after first dose.

译文：在CABP患者中，在首剂后96小时的早期临床效果方面，口服lefamulin 5天不劣于口服莫西沙星7天。

如果必要，研究答案之后，应该用一两句话说明其理论价值或应用价值，是否可以推荐、推广或需进一步研究。表述时常用 provide（theoretical, clinical, or pharmacological）evidence for…，provide/offer insights into…，… is important, apply, recommend, speculate, imply, implicate, suggest 等词语作为信息标记语。

例15

Both genes and environment contribute to the correlation between metabolic syndrome and eGFR-defined CKD. The genetic contribution is particularly important to the correlation between abdominal obesity and eGFR.

译文：基因和环境导致了代谢综合征和eGFR定义的CKD之间的相关性，而在腹部肥胖与eGFR的相关性中遗传贡献尤为重要。

例16

These findings implicate regulation of RAB11-dependent vesicular trafficking by TBC1D8B as a novel pathogenetic pathway in nephrotic syndrome.

译文：这些发现提示了TBC1D8B调控RAB11依赖的囊泡转运是肾病综合征的一种新

的致病途径。

例17

Our results identify amphiregulin as a key player in injury-induced kidney fibrosis and suggest therapeutic or diagnostic applications of soluble amphiregulin in kidney disease.

译文:研究结果证实双调蛋白是损伤性肾纤维化的关键因素,提示可溶性双调蛋白可用于治疗或诊断肾脏疾病。

例18

Elevated lipid peroxyl radical levels were associated with ferroptosis onset, whereas radical scavenging by the drugs suppressed ferroptosis-related pathologic changes in different renal cell types and ameliorated organ injuries in mice, suggesting therapeutic potential for such repurposed drugs.

译文:脂质过氧化自由基水平升高与细胞铁死亡发生有关,而药物清除自由基则抑制了不同肾细胞类型中铁死亡相关的病理变化,并减轻了小鼠的器官损伤,提示这种再利用药物具有治疗潜力。

6.2.6　结构式摘要示例

例19

Abstract

Background

Blinatumomab, a bispecific monoclonal antibody construct that enables CD3-positive T cells to recognize and eliminate CD19-positive acute lymphoblastic leukemia (ALL) blasts, was approved for use in patients with relapsed or refractory B-cell precursor ALL on the basis of single-group trials that showed efficacy and manageable toxic effects.

Methods

In this multi-institutional phase 3 trial, we randomly assigned adults with heavily pretreated B-cell precursor ALL, in a 2∶1 ratio, to receive either blinatumomab or standard-of-care chemotherapy. The primary end point was overall survival.

Results

Of the 405 patients who were randomly assigned to receive blinatumomab (271 patients) or chemotherapy (134 patients), 376 patients received at least one dose. Overall survival was significantly longer in the blinatumomab group than in the chemotherapy group. The median overall survival was 7.7 months in the blinatumomab group and 4.0 months in the chemotherapy group (hazard ratio for death with blinatumomab vs. chemotherapy, 0.71; 95% confidence interval [CI], 0.55 to 0.93; P = 0.01). Remission rates within 12 weeks after treatment initiation were significantly higher in the blinatumomab group than in the chemotherapy group, both with respect to complete remission with full hematologic recovery (34% vs.16%, P<0.001) and with respect to complete remission with full, partial, or incomplete hematologic recovery (44% vs.25%, P<0.001). Treatment with blinatumomab resulted in a higher rate of event-free survival than that with chemotherapy (6-month estimates, 31% vs.12%; hazard ratio for an event of relapse after achieving a complete remission with full, partial, or incomplete hematologic recovery, or death, 0.55; 95% CI, 0.43 to 0.71; P<0.001), as well as a longer median duration of remission (7.3 vs. 4.6 months). A total of 24% of the patients in each treatment group underwent allogeneic stem-cell transplantation. Adverse events of grade 3 or higher were reported in 87% of the patients in the blinatumomab group and in 92% of the patients in the chemotherapy group.

Conclusions

Treatment with blinatumomab resulted in significantly longer overall survival than chemotherapy among adult patients with relapsed or refractory B-cell precursor ALL. (Funded by Amgen; TOWER ClinicalTrials.gov number, NCT02013167.)

(Blinatumomab versus Chemotherapy for Advanced Acute Lymphoblastic Leukemia, *N Engl J Med*, 2017 Mar 2,376 (9))

译文:

摘要

背景

博纳吐单抗是一种能使 CD3+ T 细胞识别和清除 CD19+急性淋巴细胞白血病（ALL）原始细胞的双特异性单抗构建体。基于其在单组试验中显示出的疗效和可控的毒性作用，博纳吐单抗获得批准用于复发性或难治性前体 B 细胞 ALL 的治疗。

方法

在本项多机构 3 期临床试验中，我们将接受过大量预处理的前体 B 细胞 ALL 成人患者按照 2∶1 的比例随机分组进行博纳吐单抗或标准化疗。主要终点是总生存期。

结果

在被随机分配接受博纳吐单抗（271 例患者）或化疗（134 例患者）的 405 例患者中，376 例患者接受了至少一剂药治疗。博纳吐单抗组的总生存期显著长于化疗组。博纳吐单抗组的中位总生存期为 7.7 个月而化疗组为 4.0 个月［博纳吐单抗组与化疗组相比的死亡风险比为 0.71；95%可信区间（CI）为 0.55～0.93；P=0.01］。不论是具有完全血液学恢复的完全缓解（34%对 16%，P<0.001），还是具有完全、部分或不完全血液学恢复的完全缓解（44%对 25%，P<0.001）。博纳吐单抗组的治疗开始后 12 周内的缓解率显著高于化疗组，与化疗相比，博纳吐单抗治疗可提高无事件生存率（6 个月估计值，31%对 12%；达到具有完全、部分或不完全血液学恢复的完全缓解后发生复发事件或者死亡的风险比为 0.55；95%可信区间，0.43～0.71；P<0.001），同时可延长中位缓解持续时间（7.3 对 4.6 个月）。各组中共计 24%的患者接受了异体干细胞移植。博纳吐单抗组 87%的患者和化疗组 92%的患者报道发生了≥3 级的不良事件。

结论

与化疗相比，博纳吐单抗治疗可显著延长复发性或难治性前体 B 细胞 ALL 成人患者的总生存期［由安进（Amgen）公司资助；TOWER 在 ClinicalTrials. gov 注册号为 NCT02013167］。（博纳吐单抗和化疗在晚期急性淋巴细胞白血病治疗中的比较研究）①

Exercise

1. Read the samples of "Abstract" and analyze their contents and structures. Recognize the signal markers and sentence patterns to realize these contents. Note the use of tenses for different contents in the writing.

2. Translate the following "Abstracts" into English.

1）俯卧位对急性呼吸衰竭病人生存的影响

背景

虽然将有呼吸衰竭（acute respiratory failure）的病人置于俯卧位（prone position），可使他们当时的氧合作用（oxygenation）提高 60%～70%，但尚不知道对病人生存的作用。

方法

在一项多中心随机化的临床试验（multicenter, randomized clinical trial）中，我们对患急性肺损伤（acute lung injury）或急性呼吸窘迫症（acute respiratory distress syndrome）的病人，进行了常规治疗（仰卧位）与预先规定将病人置于俯卧位连续 10 天、每天 ≥6 小时策略的比较。我们纳入 304 例病人，分为两组，每组 152 例。

结果

10 天研究期间的死亡率为 23.0%，离开加强监护病房（intensive care unit）时的死亡率为 49.3%，6 个月时的死亡率为 60.5%。与仰卧（supine position）组相比，俯卧组的死亡相对危险在研究期结束时为 0.84（95% 可信区间为 0.56～1.27）；在离开加强监护病房时为 1.05（95% 可信区间为 0.84～1.32）；在 6 个月时为 1.06（95% 可信区间为 0.88～1.28）。研究期间，每天早晨在病人仰卧位时所测定的动脉氧分压（the partial pressure of arterial oxygen）与吸入氧分数（the fraction of inspired oxygen）的比值，俯卧组高于仰卧组（63.0±66.8 对 44.6±68.2，p=0.02）。与体位相关的并发症（例如褥疮和意外脱管）（sores and accidental extubation）的发生率两组相似。

结论

虽然将呼吸衰竭的病人置于俯卧位能提高其氧合作用，但不能提高生存率。

2）胰高血糖素样肽-1（GLP-1）和洋甘菊油（Chamomile Oil）联合使用对间充质干细胞向功能性胰岛素产生细胞分化的影响

目的：研究 GLP-1 和洋甘菊油联合使用对间充质干细胞（MSCs）向功能性胰岛素产生

---

① 译文基于"NEJM 医学前沿"，http://www.nejmqianyan.cn/article/yxqyoa1609783，最后登陆时间：2020 年 6 月 17 日。

细胞（IPCs）分化的影响。

材料和方法：在本实验研究中，提取成年雄性新西兰白兔的脂肪 MSC 并分为四组：对照组（不进行任何处理）；GLP-1 组（每隔一天用 10 nM GLP-1 处理细胞 5 天）；洋甘菊油组（每隔一天用 100 ug/ml 母菊洋甘菊花油（*Matricaria chamomilla* L. floweroil）处理细胞 5 天）；和 GLP-1 +洋甘菊油组（每隔一天用 10 nM GLP-1 和 100μg/ml 母菊洋甘菊花油处理细胞 5 天）。使用流式细胞仪（flow cytometry）、茜素红 S 染色（Alizarin red S staining）和油红 O 染色（Oil red O staining）对分离的 MSC 进行表征。使用逆转录酶-聚合酶链反应（RT-PCR）测定法检测 IPCs 特异性基因的表达。使用 ELISA 试剂盒检测对不同葡萄糖浓度反应的胰岛素和裂解的连接肽（cleaved connecting peptide）（C 肽）（C-peptide）。

结果：我们的结果表明，分离的细胞高度表达 MSC 标记物，并能够分化为骨细胞和脂肪细胞。此外，对不同的葡萄糖浓度反应时，与单独使用 GLP-1 或洋甘菊油相比，联合使用 GLP-1 和洋甘菊油表现出更高水平的 IPCs 基因标记物，包括 NK 同源盒基因 2.2（NK homeobox gene 2.2）（*NKX*-2.2），配对盒基因 4（paired box gene 4）（*PAX*4），胰岛素（*INS*）和胰十二指肠同源盒 1（pancreatic duodenal homeobox-1）（*PDX*1），以及胰岛素和 C 肽（$p < 0.05$）。

结论：总之，研究结果为联合使用肽与天然产物以提高在再生医学和肽治疗的效率奠定了坚实的基础。

6.3 引言

6.3.1 引言的功能

引言（Introduction）是研究论文留给读者的第一印象，具有两大功能：引起读者对论文的兴趣和为读者理解全文提供必要的背景知识。为了引起读者兴趣，一篇论文的引言必须简明扼要、直截了当、抓住要点。清晰性（clarity），可读性（readability）和信息性（informativeness）是引言的写作标准。一般来讲，引言应完成以下三方面任务：引出研究主题（introducing the topic），即研究的宏观命题（general topic）；限定研究范畴（limiting the research scope），即研究的具体命题（specific topic）；和陈述研究目的（stating the specific purpose），即研究的具体内容和目标。

6.3.2 引言的内容

不同期刊对引言内容有不同的表述。比如，*Cell* 要求仅提供读者理解研究动机和结果所需的背景信息，在陈述时不使用小标题。*Lancet* 也要求引言提供研究背景信息，同时还强调了学术规范，要求提供相关数据和研究的参考文献；并且引言的结尾需要陈述研究目的的。

引言的内容根据研究类型不同也有所不同。本节重点讲解验证假设型论文的引言内容，而描述性论文和方法学论文的引言只作简要介绍。

6.3.2.1　已知信息，未知信息，研究问题

在验证假设型论文中，引言需首先告知研究的宏观命题，并提供这一命题的相关背景知识，然后再限定研究范围，即具体命题，并围绕这一命题阐述国内外的研究现状以揭示目前研究中的未知信息，最后根据未知信息提出本研究的问题。问题的提出是引言部分最重要的内容，可以是以问题（question），也可以是以假设（hypothesis）的方式提出。

6.3.2.2　研究对象

引言还需明确研究对象。研究对象包括生物材料，如分子（molecule）、细胞系（cell line）、组织（tissue）、器官（organ）及材料来源的生物（organism）；或是动物（animal）及人群（human population）等。

6.3.2.3　参考文献

在阐述研究主题的背景知识和相关研究的现状时必须包括参考文献（references）。选取的参考文献应该反映国内外对同类课题最新、最重要的研究现状、进展及尚待解决的问题以充分反映本论文研究问题的来源。

6.3.2.4　创新性和重要性

一篇论文的价值在于创新性（newness）、可靠性（reliability）或重要性（importance）。论文的引言部分应说明本研究跟以往研究相比的创新之处，如有必要还应阐述研究的重要性。除引言部分外，论文的讨论或结论部分也可以阐述研究的重要性及价值。

6.3.3　引言的结构

验证假设型论文引言的结构呈漏斗模式（funnel model），由三部分构成：宏观命题和具体命题的已知信息（known），具体命题的未知信息（unknown），由已知和未知信息之间的差异产生的问题，以及研究方案。[①]

6.3.3.1　引入已知信息

为了引导读者理解整个研究，引言开头应该简明扼要地介绍本研究的相关背景知识。引言通常以引入宏观命题开始，介绍该命题的性质及意义，然后转入具体命题。宏观命题和具体命题通常也出现在论文的标题中。写作时，突出研究命题已知信息的表达有：…is an important public health issue；… have attracted significant attention thanks to…；There is significant current attention towards…。

---

① Mimi Zeiger, *Essentials of Writing Biomedical Research Papers*. U.S.A.: The McGraw-Hill companies, Inc., second edition, 2000, p. 108

例1

Obstetric hemorrhage accounts for 27% of all maternal deaths.[1] In high-resource settings, maternal death due to postpartum hemorrhage (PPH) has become uncommon, but PPH remains an important cause of severe maternal morbidity.[2-7] Women with persistent PPH are at risk of developing coagulopathy due to depletion of coagulation factors and platelets.[8-12] Coagulopathy can eventually lead to worse maternal outcomes. Timely transfusion of plasma may prevent coagulopathy and thereby improve maternal outcomes.

译文：产科出血占产妇死亡原因的27%。在资源丰富的医疗机构中，产后出血（PPH）导致产妇死亡已不常见，但PPH仍然是严重产妇疾病的重要原因。由于凝血因子和血小板的耗竭，持续性PPH的妇女容易出现凝血病。凝血病最终会恶化产妇结局。及时输注血浆可以预防凝血障碍，从而改善产妇结局。

例2

Cell death is prevalent during development in multicellular organisms and is important for the removal of unnecessary cells and tissues as well as for the correction of developmental error.[1] During vertebrate embryogenesis, dying cells are present during neural tube closure and spinal cord development.[2] Therefore, a rapid and efficient phagocyte response is crucial for the clearance of this debris. In mouse, chicken, and zebrafish, a group of primitive macrophages derived from the yolk sac migrate into the developing brain, differentiate into microglia, and contribute to ongoing neurogenesis by clearing apoptotic debris. York-sac-derived macrophages, however, do not infiltrate the trunk of developing embryos until the formation of the circulatory system at embryonic day 10.5 (E10.5) in mice and 35 h post fertilization (hpf) in zebrafish. However, neural tube closure and motor axon pathfinding start at E9 and 16 hpf in mice and fish, respectively, prior to the colonization of macrophages in the trunk region. Although cell death during neural tube closure has been extensively studied, very little is known about the clearance of debris in the trunk during the earliest stages of neural development.

译文：细胞死亡在多细胞生物的发育过程中普遍存在，对于去除非必需的细胞和组织以及纠正发育错误至关重要。在脊椎动物胚胎形成中，垂死细胞出现在神经管闭合和脊髓发育过程中。因此，快速有效的吞噬细胞反应对于清除这些残骸至关重要。在小鼠、鸡和斑马鱼中，一组由卵黄囊发育形成的原始巨噬细胞迁移到正在发育的大脑中，分化为小胶质细胞，并通过清除凋亡残骸促进神经发育。然而，在小鼠胚胎发育第10.5天（E10.5）和斑马鱼受精后35小时（hpf）形成循环系统之后，卵黄囊发育形成的巨噬细胞才浸润到发育胚胎的躯干。小鼠和鱼类的神经管闭合和运动轴突寻路分别开始于E9和16hpf，均早于巨噬细胞在躯干区域的定植。尽管神经管闭合过程中的细胞死亡已经被广泛研究，但关于在神经发育最早期躯干内残骸的清除却知之甚少。

6.3.3.2 转入未知信息

引言的第二步是提供本研究的研究背景和研究动机，旨在明确具体命题的未知信息。

通常来说,一个研究项目的产生有两个原因。一是目前研究需要深入,二是目前研究存在不足。写作时应首先确定本研究的动机。如果是第一个原因,应选择重要文献突出以往研究取得的成就,及还需深入的部分。如果是第二个原因,应选择重要文献明确指出以往研究的不足之处,包括研究的方法、材料、结果等。这样一来,读者自然会判断出该研究的必然性或者创新性。在引用参考文献时,可以选择综述类文章,为读者提供有关研究的丰富资源。除此之外,选择参考文献时注意引用研究是否经典,是否重要或相关。一般来讲,参考文献应少而精。写作时,常用标记语突出未知信息:There have been few studies of…; There are conflicting data on the…; It also remains unclear whether…; Studies have differed in their conclusion on / about / regarding…; Surprisingly, there is little evidence that…等。

例3

MicroRNAs (miRNAs) are short, regulatory RNAs that act as negative regulators of gene expression by inhibiting mRNA translation or by promoting mRNA degradation [13, 14]. Growing evidence shows that miRNAs are extensively involved in the pathogenesis of heart diseases, including cardiac hypertrophy, dilated cardiomyopathy, and arrhythmia [15, 16, 17, 18, 19]. Although the miRNA expression profiles in both animals and humans with heart diseases have been revealed in several studies [17, 20, 21, 22], the in situ expression patterns of miRNAs in failed hearts have not been fully determined. Whether these miRNAs are synthesized in cardiomyocytes, cardiac fibroblasts, or endothelial cells during the progression of cardiac remodeling is still not fully clear, and needs to be clarified. Recently, exosomal miRNAs have been demonstrated as another functional signaling messenger between adjacent cells [23, 24, 25]. Previous studies have found that miR143 / 145 released from shear-stress-treated endothelial cells could be transferred into adjacent smooth muscle cells (SMC) and regulate the proliferation and contraction of SMC [26]. Meanwhile, exosomal transfer of miR-320 from cardiomyocytes of type 2 diabetic rats also regulates angiogenic activity of surrounding endothelial cells [25].

译文: MicroRNAs (miRNAs) 是一段短 RNAs 序列,通过抑制 mRNA 翻译或促进 mRNA 降解来实现基因表达的负调控。越来越多的证据表明 miRNAs 广泛参与心脏疾病的发病机制,包括心肌肥大、扩张性心肌病和心律失常。尽管几项研究揭示了 miRNA 在患有心脏疾病的动物和人群中的表达图谱,miRNA 在衰竭心脏中的原位表达模式尚未完全清晰。在心脏重塑过程中,这些 miRNAs 是否在心肌细胞、心肌成纤维细胞或内皮细胞中合成也尚未完全清楚,需要厘清。近年来,外泌体 miRNAs 已被证明是相邻细胞间的另一种功能性信号信使。先前的研究发现,剪应力处理后的内皮细胞释放的 miR143 / 145 可以转移到邻近的平滑肌细胞 (SMC) 中,并调节平滑肌细胞的增殖和收缩。同时,外泌体可以将 miR-320 从 2 型糖尿病大鼠心肌细胞经转运至周围的内皮细胞中,以调节其血管生成活性。

例4

In many countries it is recommended that acute hospitals offer influenza vaccine to healthcare workers annually. Employers in the United Kingdom are advised to consider providing vaccination for care home staff, but most do not. Evidence shows that vaccination of healthcare workers can reduce serologically confirmed influenza by nearly 90% in those vaccinated. An indirect effect may also exist whereby immune staffs do not infect patients. Two previous cluster randomised controlled trials showed that influenza vaccination of healthcare workers on wards for the care of elderly people in Scotland led to a decrease in mortality among patients. Results have been questioned owing to the relatively small number of wards randomised (which led to unbalanced randomisation) and because it was not possible to show that the reductions in mortality were related temporally to influenza activity on the wards or in the community.

译文:许多国家建议急性病医院每年为医疗工作者接种流感疫苗。英国也建议资方为疗养院人员接种疫苗,但多数未落实。证据表明,医疗人员接种疫苗可使经血清学证实的流感发病率降低近 90%。还可能存在间接的作用,即接种的医疗人员不会感染患者。两项早期的群体随机对照研究表明,在苏格兰,为病房内老年患者的医疗人员接种流感疫苗降低了患者的死亡率。(然而)这些结果受到了质疑。一是因为随机选取的病房数目相对较小(造成随机分组不平衡),二是因为无法说明死亡率减少是否与病房或整个疗养院内的流感活动程度短时相关。

6.3.3.3 突出本项研究

引言第三步应明确本项研究的问题和/或研究的目的。另外,还应简单描述研究路径。论文的读者都会期望在引言的最后部分找到引言中这些最重要的内容。缺乏清晰明确的研究问题是医学杂志拒绝论文发表的重要原因。写作时,常用标记语突出研究问题:"We designed a prospective trial to test whether…; In this study we asked whether…; We hypothesized that…; We aimed to determine… and to investigate the possible underlying mechanism of…等。

例5

It is reasonable to suggest that exosomal miRNA may play roles to mediate the protective effects of conditioned medium on ameliorating myocardial injury after acute myocardial infarction. In the present study, we analyzed the expression profile of myocardial-disease-associated miRNAs in cardiomyocytes, cardiac fibroblasts, ventricular myocardium, and conditioned medium derived from cardiomyocytes, and then examined the effect of ischemic stress on the expression levels of the miRNAs. An in vitro cultured cell model and an in vivo animal model with myocardial infarction were applied to further determine the role of miRNAs in regulating cardiomyocyte apoptosis, fibroblast activation, immune cell infiltration, and myocardial infarction.

译文:研究合理推论,外泌体 miRNA 可能参与调节条件培养液对改善急性心肌梗死后心肌损伤的保护作用。在本研究中,我们分析了心肌细胞、心肌成纤维细胞、心室肌和心肌细胞条件培养液中与心肌疾病相关的 miRNAs 的表达谱,并研究了缺血应激对 miRNAs 表达水平的影响。应用体外培养的细胞模型和体内心肌梗死动物模型,我们进一步研究了 miRNAs 对心肌细胞凋亡、成纤维细胞活化、免疫细胞浸润和心肌梗死的调节作用。

例6

We studied the effect of vaccinating care home staff against influenza on mortality, health service use, and influenza-like illness among residents. To overcome some of the methodological limitations of previous studies we randomised a large number of units and balanced these on baseline characteristics. We used cluster randomisation to look for indirect effects of vaccination and because the intervention was best applied at the level of the care home. We compared the effectiveness of the intervention during periods with differing levels of influenza activity in the community as this is likely to influence the effect size. The study is reported according to the guidelines of the consolidated standards of reporting trials for cluster randomised controlled trials.

译文:我们研究了为疗养院工作人员接种流感疫苗对疗养人员死亡、就医和流感类疾病患病的影响。为了克服以往研究中的某些方法学上的不足,我们随机选取了大量的病房并且平衡了基线特征。因为干预最好在整个疗养院实施,我们采用群体随机抽样法研究接种的间接作用。另外,我们比较了整个疗养院不同流感活动水平期间的干预效果,因为活动水平可能影响干预效果。本研究的报道符合群体随机对照试验报道的整体标准。

6.3.4 引言的写作要点

6.3.4.1 引言部分的时态

介绍宏观命题和具体命题及其相关背景知识时,用一般现在时。介绍具体命题的研究现状,进展及尚待解决的问题时用一般现在完成时或一般现在时。如具体涉及某一项或几项研究的内容,用过去时表述。陈述本研究问题、研究目的和研究方案时,用过去时。

6.3.4.2 引言部分的综述语

研究论文引言中的文献综述部分,即作者引用其他相关研究者的发现、观点、理论等的引用话语称为综述语,使用的动词称为综述性动词(reporting verbs)。常见的综述性动词有 find, identify, show, suggest, report, think, propose, consider, demonstrate, prove, establish 等,这些词是引言中参考文献引用时的信号词,在引言中起着重要的作用。下面就综述语表达的结构作一简要说明。

1. 以研究名为主语的综述语

例7

Earlier ecologic studies reported a positive correlation between overall animal protein intake and mortality due to cardiovascular disease and cancer. However, only a few epidemiologic studies have evaluated the association between protein intake and mortality outcomes.

译文:早期的生态学研究表明,动物蛋白的总摄入量与心血管疾病和癌症的死亡率呈正相关关系。然而,只有少数流行病学研究评估了蛋白摄入与死亡率结果之间的关系。

例8

Several primary prevention aspirin trials, mostly done before 2010, suggested reduction in myocardial infarction and stroke, although not mortality, and at a cost of increased bleeding events.

译文:几项主要在 2010 年前进行的试验提示,阿司匹林初级预防减少心肌梗死和卒中发病率,不降低死亡率,但会增加出血事件。

例9

Observational cohort studies have shown increasing risks of both macrovascular and microvascular events with increasing average blood glucose levels.

译文:观察队列研究显示,随着平均血糖水平的升高,大血管和微血管事件的风险增加。

例10

Two systematic reviews showed that published trials of fixed-dose combination therapies for atherosclerotic cardiovascular disease had small to moderate sample sizes and short follow-up durations.

译文:两篇系统综述显示,已发表的动脉粥样硬化性心血管疾病固定剂量联合治疗的试验纳入的样本量为小到中等,随访时间短。

这几句参考文献引用话语是以研究名为主语,研究发现为宾语,句子以主动语态表述。这是引言中最常见的一类综述语。

2. 以研究发现为主语的综述语

例11

Caffeine ingestion has been shown to acutely increase insulin resistance.

译文:咖啡因摄入已被证明会急剧增强胰岛素抵抗。

例12

In the context of gliomas, Cx43 has been traditionally considered a tumor suppressor protein because it is downregulated in malignant glioma cell.

译文:在胶质瘤中,Cx43 被认为是一种肿瘤抑制蛋白,因为在恶性胶质瘤细胞中它的表达下调。

例13

It was initially reported that early or late introduction of gluten to infants increased the risk of celiac disease.

译文:最初有报道称,较早或较晚给婴儿添加谷蛋白会增加患小肠吸收不良症的风险。

以上几句综述语以研究发现为主语,用被动语态表达,突出引用的重要信息。研究发现的表达较长时,也可使用形式主语的句型。

引言中一般应避免使用如"Anderson, Lee, and Wilson report in their 2017 study that…"

（Anderson, Lee, and Wilson 在 2017 的研究中报道……）这种影响信息连贯性的综述句式。相反,应直截了当地表述研究信息,而在句末加注参考文献标号。

6.3.4.3　引言部分的常用表达

1. 表达已知信息

It has been reported / observed demonstrated that...

... is widely used in...

... was found / reported / mentioned by...

... is known to...

... has long been successfully applied for...

There is significant current attention towards...

Findings from numerous epidemiological studies have linked... to...

... is an important public health issue, as... is highly prevalent in this age group and has implications for...

... have attracted significant attention thanks to...

Evidence supporting... has emerged in more recent years, with...

This case highlights the potentially remarkable benefit that..., particularly...

2. 表达未知信息

The beneficial effects of... is a topic of much controversy.

Results from studies investigating... have been inconclusive.

Unfortunately, there is limited intervention research on the effects of... on...

The animal experimental studies have been carried out for years. However, to our knowledge, only a few cases with clinical application have been reported.

There is insufficient evidence from randomized studies...

There have been few studies of...

There are conflicting data on the... It also remains unclear whether...

Studies have differed in their conclusion on / about / regarding...

Surprisingly, there is little evidence that...

There have been different / conflicting reports regarding / on...

Little research has been done on...

Relatively little knowledge is available related to...

Little attention has been paid / given to...

It is unclear / uncertain / unknown whether...

... is / remains controversial / unexplored / unclear

... remains an important unsolved problem

However, we have a limited understanding of...

However, ... still remains greatly challenging / a major challenge.

However, … is a barrier to…

However, a key improvement is still needed for…

However, there have been few reports of… owing to…

However, … remains not fully deciphered.

However, while… are known to be associated with…, … has so far been lacking.

Whereas… is known, there is no knowledge whether…

Unfortunately, there is limited research on…

… is a topic of much controversy.

3. 表达未知信息和研究问题之间的连接语

For this purpose, we…

To test the hypothesis, we…

To determine whether…, we…

To answer the question, we…

In an attempt / in an effort / in order to investigate / determine / clarify / assess…, we…

In this study, an attempt was made to…

This study seeks to fill these gaps, provide clarity to…, and…

Using these data, we identified whether…

Therefore, … are highly desirable.

There is thus a clear need for… to….

To address these limitations, we set out to develop…

To further…, a deeper understanding of… is essential to gain valuable insights.

On the basis of published results with… and our previous experience with…, we hypothesized that…

4. 表达研究问题

We designed a prospective trial to test whether…

In this study we asked whether…

We hypothesized that…

We aimed to determine… and to investigate the possible underlying mechanism of…

In this study, we tested the hypothesis that…

The present study aimed to demonstrate…

We conducted this study to determine whether…

We investigated the association between… and…

We undertook this trial to clarify…

We undertook a pilot study to assess…

We conducted an interventional study with the aim of…

The purpose / objective / aim of this study / research / investigation was to…

This study was designed to…

The present study was undertaken to…

The study here reported was undertaken to…

Our aim was to investigate…

Therefore, we designed this protocol to evaluate…

As such, the objectives of this study were to…

Herein, we investigate/present…, which elucidate…

6.3.5　引言示例

1. 验证假设型论文引言

例14

Excessive bleeding and blood transfusions are common in patients undergoing cardiac surgery, [1] and in some of these patients, there is a need for reoperation because of life-threatening bleeding. [2] Both blood transfusion and reoperation are strongly associated with poor outcomes after cardiac surgery. [2,3] Antifibrinolytic therapy reduces the risk of blood loss and transfusion among patients undergoing cardiac surgery, [4,5] but it is unclear whether such therapy reduces the risk of reoperation for bleeding. [4]

译文：

失血过多和输血常见于接受心脏手术的患者,并且这些患者中的一部分因为危及生命的出血需要再次手术。输血和再次手术都与心脏手术后的不良结局密切相关。抗纤维蛋白溶解疗法能降低接受心脏手术患者的失血和输血危险,但是目前尚不清楚这种疗法是否能降低出血导致的再次手术的危险。

Antifibrinolytic agents that have been used in patients undergoing cardiac surgery include aprotinin[6,7] and the lysine analogues tranexamic acid and aminocaproic acid. [8-11] These agents may have prothrombotic effects, and their use may potentially increase the risk of myocardial infarction, stroke, and other thrombotic complications after cardiac surgery. Tranexamic acid in particular seems to be associated with an increased risk of postoperative neurologic events, [12] including seizures. [13] Some studies have shown that tranexamic acid reduces cerebral blood flow[14] and increases the risk of cerebral infarction. [15] This raises the possibility that seisures induced by tranexamic acid may have a thromboembolic basis. We investigated whether tranexamic acid increases the risk of death and thrombotic complications among at risk patients undergoing coronary artery surgery. (Tranexamic Acid in Patients Undergoing Coronary-Artery Surgery, *N Eng J Med.*, 2017 Jan 12, 376 (2))

已经用于行心脏手术患者的抗纤维蛋白溶解剂包括抑肽酶以及赖氨酸类似物氨甲环酸和氨基乙酸。这些药物可能具有促血栓形成作用,并且它们的使用有可能增加心脏手术后心肌梗死、卒中和其他血栓形成性并发症的危险。尤其氨甲环酸似乎与术后神经学事件

（包括惊厥）的危险增加相关。一些研究表明，氨甲环酸减少脑血流量并且增加脑梗死的危险。这提示氨甲环酸诱发的惊厥可能是源于血栓栓塞。我们研究了在行冠状动脉手术的高危患者中，氨甲环酸是否增加死亡和血栓形成并发症的发生危险。（氨甲环酸在行冠状动脉手术患者中的应用）①

说明：这是一篇二段式引言，充分体现了漏斗型的写作模式。命题的已知信息从宏观到具体，分步阐述，逻辑清楚。第一段以宏观命题"失血过多和输血"开始，阐述其重要性，然后缩小命题范畴为"抗纤维蛋白溶解疗法"，并提供已知和未知信息。第二段描述了具体命题"氨甲环酸"作为抗纤维蛋白溶解剂的已知和未知信息，并基于未知信息提出研究的问题。在引言中，whether 引导的句型应引起重视，既可以表达未知信息，如 but it is unclear whether such therapy reduces the risk of reoperation for bleeding，也可以提出研究问题，如 We investigated whether tranexamic acid increases the risk of death and thrombotic complications among at risk patients undergoing coronary artery surgery.

例15

The acute respiratory distress syndrome（ARDS）is caused by an inflammatory injury to the lung that is characterized clinically by acute hypoxemic respiratory failure.[1] Pathologically complex changes in the lung are manifested by an early, exudative phase followed by proliferative and fibrotic phases.[2,3] Persistent ARDS is characterized by ongoing inflammation,[4,5] parenchymal-cell proliferation,[3] and disordered deposition of collagen,[3,6,7,8] all of which may be responsive to corticosteroid therapy.

译文：

急性呼吸窘迫综合征（ARDS）起因于肺的炎症性损伤，临床特征为急性低氧血症性呼吸衰竭。肺脏的病理性改变早期为渗出期，随后是增殖期和纤维化期。持续性 ARDS 的特点是炎症不断发展，肺实质细胞增殖，胶原异常沉着，所有这些改变都可能对皮质类固醇治疗产生疗效反应。

Four trials of high-dose, short-course corticosteroids for early-phase ARDS failed to show improvements in survival.[9,10,11,12] Several reports from small case series suggested a benefit of moderate-dose corticosteroids in patients with persistent ARDS.[8,13,14,15,16,17] A single-center, randomized trial involving 24 patients who had had ARDS for seven or more days reported that moderate-dose corticosteroids improved lung function and survival.[18]

4 项使用大剂量、短疗程皮质类固醇治疗早期 ARDS 的试验，都没有发现该疗法可改善患者生存率。数项小样本病例研究提示，中等剂量皮质类固醇对持续性患者有益。一项单中心随机试验纳入 24 例病程 7 天的 ARDS 病人，结果显示，中等剂量皮质类固醇可改善病人的肺功能和生存率。

The risks associated with corticosteroids in these patients are unclear. Several studies

---

① 本译文基于"NEJM 医学前沿"，http:// www.nejmqianyan.cn/ article/ yxqyoa1606424，最后登陆时间表：2020 年 6 月 17 日。

involving patients with sepsis and ARDS have suggested that high-dose corticosteroids increase the risk of secondary infections,[11,12,19,20,21] yet a meta-analysis of moderate-dose corticosteroids for sepsis did not substantiate this observation.[22] Additional potential risks of corticosteroids include hyperglycemia, poor wound healing, psychosis, pancreatitis, and prolonged muscle weakness with impaired functional status.[23]

目前还不清楚 ARDS 病人中与使用皮质类固醇相关的危险。数项纳入脓毒症和 ARDS 病人的研究提示，大剂量皮质类固醇增加继发性感染的危险。一项关于使用中等剂量皮质类固醇治疗脓毒症的荟萃分析没有证实上述观察结果。皮质类固醇的其他潜在危险包括高血糖、伤口愈合不良、精神病、胰腺炎和长期肌肉无力伴功能障碍。

We conducted a multicenter randomized, controlled trial to determine the efficacy and safety of this therapy. Our hypothesis was that the administration of moderate-dose methylprednisolone to patients with persistent ARDS would improve clinical outcomes without significantly increasing complications. (Efficacy and Safety of Corticosteroids for Persistent Acute Respiratory Distress Syndrome, *N Eng J Med.*, 2006 Apr 20, 354 (16))

我们进行了一项多中心随机对照试验，以确定该疗法的疗效和安全性。我们的假设是：使用中等剂量的甲泼尼龙可改善持续性 ARDS 病人的临床转归，而不显著增加并发症。(皮质类固醇治疗持续性急性呼吸窘迫综合症的疗效和安全性)

说明：这是一篇四段式引言，包括宏观命题已知信息—具体命题已知信息—具体命题未知信息—研究路径—研究假设五个层次。问题是以假设方式提出：Our hypothesis was that the administration of moderate-dose methylprednisolone to patients with persistent ARDS would improve clinical outcomes without significantly increasing complications.

在验证假设型论文中，最科学的问题写作方式是假设。以假设方式提出问题可以使问题更加准确，而读者在阅读时可以更加容易地预测答案。下面是同一个问题的两种提出方式：(1) Our question was whether the administration of moderate-dose methylprednisolone to patients with persistent ARDS would improve clinical outcomes without significantly increasing complications. 我们的问题是：使用中等剂量的甲泼尼龙是否会改善持续性 ARDS 病人的临床转归，而不显著增加并发症。(2) Our hypothesis was that the administration of moderate-dose methylprednisolone to patients with persistent ARDS would improve clinical outcomes without significantly increasing complications. 我们的假设是：使用中等剂量的甲泼尼龙可改善持续性 ARDS 病人的临床转归，而不显著增加并发症。如果问题是以第一种方式，即"问题"的方式提出，读者无法估计研究答案；而第二种方式，即假设的方式，更为准确和具体，读者可以预测确切的影响，并在论文的结论部分应证预期的答案。

虽然"假设"或"问题"这两种问题提出的方式没有绝对的好坏之分，但是以"假设"方式提出的问题能让读者阅读起来更有目的性。

2. 方法学论文引言

方法学论文引言在写作时，开篇需直接陈述使用的方法、仪器设备或材料，并描述理由；接着陈述现有方法、仪器设备或材料存在的问题或局限性；进而再提出新方法、仪器设备或材料,以及它们的优势所在。优势需针对现有问题和局限性。[①]

例16

Introduction

Mammalian neurons possess extensive axonal arbors that project over long distances (Anderson et al., 2002; Braitenberg and Schüz, 2013; Kita and Kita, 2012; Kuramoto et al., 2013; Wu et al., 2014). These projections dictate how information flows across brain areas. Interareal connections have been studied using tracers that label populations of neurons (Gerfen and Sawchenko; Hunnicutt et al., 2014; Luppi et al., 1990; Markov et al., 2014; Oh et al., 2014; Veenman et al., 1992; Zingg et al., 2014) or with functional mapping methods at various spatial scales (Greicius et al., 2009; Petreanu et al., 2007). However, these methods average across large groups of neurons, including multiple cell types, and obscure fine-scale spatial organization. Mapping brain-wide connectivity at the single neuron level is crucial for delineating cell types and understanding the routing of information flow across brain areas, but very few complete morphological reconstructions of individual neurons are available, especially for long-range projection neurons (Ascoli and Wheeler, 2016; Svoboda, 2011).

译文：

引言

哺乳动物的神经元具有广泛的轴突树状结构,可以远距离投射。这些投射指挥信息在大脑区域传递。学界常使用标记神经元种群的示踪剂或用不同空间尺度的函数映射方法研究区域间的联系。然而,这些方法通常描绘神经元群组,包括多种细胞类型,并且会模糊精细的空间组织。在单个神经元层面绘制全脑连接图对于描绘细胞类型和理解跨脑区信息传达的通路至关重要,但目前单个神经元,特别是长程投射神经元的完整形态学重建极少。

Morphological reconstruction is technically challenging because thin axons (diameter, ~100 nm; Anderson et al., 2002; De Paola et al., 2006; Shepherd and Harris, 1998) travel over long distances (centimeters) and across multiple brain regions (Economo et al., 2018; Kita and Kita, 2012; Oh et al., 2014). High-contrast, high-resolution, brain-wide imaging is therefore required to detect and trace axons in their entirety. Earlier studies using imaging in serial sections have reconstructed only small numbers of cells and mostly only partially, because of the difficulty of manual tracing across sections (Blasdel and Lund, 1983; Cowan and Wilson, 1994; Ghosh et al., 2011, 2011; Igarashi et al., 2012; Kawaguchi et al., 1990; Kisvárday et al., 1994; Kita and Kita, 2012; Kuramoto et al., 2009, 2015; Oberlaender et al., 2011; Ohno et al., 2012; Parent and Parent, 2006; Ropireddy et al., 2011; Wittner et al., 2007; Wu et al., 2014). Methods in which a

---

[①] Mimi Zeiger, *Essentials of Writing Biomedical Research Papers.* U.S.A.: The McGraw-Hill companies, Inc., second edition, 2000, p. 120.

precisely assembled volume is generated, for example based on block-face imaging, are more efficient for tracing (Economo et al., 2016; Gong et al., 2016; Han et al., 2018; Lin et al., 2018; Portera-Cailliau et al., 2005), but manual reconstruction has remained a limiting factor. An RNA sequencing-based method (MAPSeq; Han et al., 2018; Kebschull et al., 2016) has provided a complementary, higher throughput approach to examine single neuron projections. However, this method has two significant limitations: the inherent sensitivity of MAPSeq is unknown and the spatial resolution is lower by orders of magnitude—limited by the volume of tissue that can be micro-dissected for sequencing. Microscopy-based neuronal reconstructions therefore remain the 'Gold Standard' for analysis of connectivity and spatial organization of axonal projections.

形态学重建在技术上具有挑战性,因为薄轴突(直径约 100 纳米)跨越长距离(厘米)和多个大脑区域。因此,需要高比对度、高分辨率的全脑成像来检测和追踪轴突的整体。因为很难在整个脑区域进行全层追踪,早期连续多层成像的研究只重建了少量的细胞,并且主要是部分重建。生成精确度量容积量的方法,比如基于块状成像的技术,对于追踪更有效,但手动重建仍然是限制因素。基于 RNA 测序的方法提供了一种互补的、高通量的方法来检测单个神经元的投射。然而,这种方法有两个显著的局限性,一是 MAPSeq 的固有灵敏度未知,二是受到可显微解剖进行测序的组织的体积限制,空间分辨率会低几个数量级。因此,基于显微技术的神经元重建仍然是分析轴突投射连通性和空间组织的"金标准"。

We previously described a serial 2-photon tomography system for imaging the entire brain at sub-micrometer resolution, and manually tracing fine-scale axonal processes across the entire brain (Economo et al., 2016). Here, we improved this method and developed a semi-automated, high-throughput reconstruction pipeline to efficiently trace many neurons per brain. We completely reconstructed more than 1,000 neurons in the neocortex, hippocampus, thalamus and hypothalamus. Reconstructions were made available in an online database with extensive visualization and query capabilities (www.mouselight.janelia. org). We uncovered new cell types and found novel organizational principles governing the connections between brain regions. (Reconstruction of 1,000 projection neurons reveals new cell types and organization of long-range connectivity in the mouse brain, *Cell*, 2019 Sept.19, 179 (1))

我们之前描述了一套连续双光子断层成像系统,用于以亚微米分辨率成像整个大脑,并手动追踪整个大脑的精细化轴突过程。在本研究中,我们改进了这种方法,开发了一个半自动、高通量的重建管道,以有效地追踪每个大脑中的多个神经元。我们在大脑皮层、海马、丘脑和下丘脑完整重建了 1000 多个神经元。重建工作在一个具有广泛可视化和查询功能的在线数据库中进行(www.mouselight.janelia.org)。我们发现了新的细胞类型,并发现了控制大脑区域之间联系的新组织原则。(1000 个投射神经元的重建揭示了小鼠脑中新的细胞类型和长程连接的组织结构)

3. 描述性论文引言

描述性论文没有研究问题和研究假设。因此,描述性论文引言的漏斗状结构与验证假设型论文的漏斗状结构截然不同,不包含已知信息、未知信息和研究问题三部分,而是已知信息和信息描述两部分。①

例17

Introduction

Motor cortex plays critical roles in planning and executing voluntary movements. Activity in motor cortex anticipates specific future movements, often seconds before movement onset. This dynamic neural process, referred to as preparatory activity, is thought to move the state of the motor cortex to an initial condition appropriate for eliciting rapid, accurate movements. In addition, motor cortex activity is highly modulated during movement onset, consistent with commands that control the timing and direction of movements.

译文:

引言

运动皮层在计划和执行随意运动中起着至关重要的作用。运动皮层的活动通常在运动开始前几秒能预测特定的未来运动。这一被称为准备活动的动态神经过程被认为是将运动皮层的状态调整到适宜于激发快速、准确运动的初始状态。此外,在运动开始时,运动皮层的活动受到高度调制,与控制运动时间和方向的指令保持一致。

Reconciling the dual roles of motor cortex requires an understanding of the cell types that make up the cortical circuit, and how these cell types integrate into the multi-regional circuits that maintain short-term memories and produce voluntary movements. Motor cortex comprises distinct cell types that differ in their location, gene expression pattern, electrophysiology, and connectivity. Intratelencephalic (IT) neurons in layers (L) 2-6 receive diverse input from other cortical areas and excite pyramidal tract (PT) neurons. PT neurons, whose somata define neocortical L5b, are of particular significance as they make the only long-range connections linking the motor cortex with premotor centers in the brainstem and spinal cord. PT neurons thus coordinate cortical and subcortical brain regions to produce behavior. Lesioning PT axons cause persistent motor deficits. PT neurons also constitute a major component of the cortical projection to the thalamus. Previous studies have shown that preparatory activity is not maintained by motor cortex in isolation, instead requiring reverberations in a thalamocortical loop. Consistent with roles in both movement planning and initiation, PT neurons show diverse activity patterns, including preparatory activity and movement commands. PT neurons are also structurally heterogenerous, with complex

---

① Mimi Zeiger, *Essentials of Writing Biomedical Research Papers*. U.S.A.: The McGraw-Hill companies, Inc., second edition, 2000, p. 119.

projection patterns in the midbrain and hindbrain.

协调运动皮层的两项功能需要了解构成皮层回路的细胞类型,以及这些细胞类型如何整合到维持短期记忆和产生随意运动的多区域回路中。运动皮层由不同类型细胞组成,这些不同类型的细胞在位置、基因表达模式、电生理学和连接性方面均不同。第 2~6 层的端脑内(IT)神经元接收来自其他皮质区域的不同输入信号,并引发锥体束(PT)神经元兴奋。PT 神经元是连接运动皮层与脑干和脊髓运动前中枢的唯一长距离连接,其神经元体定义新皮质 L5b,具有特殊意义。因而,PT 神经元协调大脑皮层和皮层下区域产生行为。受损的 PT 轴突导致持续性运动障碍。PT 神经元也是皮质投射到丘脑的主要组成内容。之前的研究表明,运动皮层并不是孤立地维持准备活动,而是需要在丘脑皮层回路中产生回响。与运动计划和运动启动中的角色一致,PT 神经元表现出不同的活动模式,包括准备活动和运动指令。PT 神经元在结构上也是异质的,在中脑和后脑有复杂的投射模式。

Here we show that PT neurons in mouse motor cortex comprise two cell types with distinct gene expression profiles and projection patterns. We refer to these cell types as PT Upper and PT Lower neurons, reflecting their distributions in different sublaminae in L5b. PT Upper project to the thalamus, which forms a feedback loop with motor cortex. PT lower neurons project to premotor centers in the medulla. Cell type specific extracellular recordings in the anterior lateral motor cortex (ALM) during a delayed-response task suggest that PT Upper neurons are involved in motor planning, whereas PT Lower neurons play roles in movement execution. Thus, motor cortex coordinates its two complementary roles at the level of distinct cell types. (Distinct Descending Motor Cortex Pathways and Their Roles in Movement, *Nature*, 2018 Nov. 563(7729))

本研究中我们发现小鼠运动皮层中的 PT 神经元由两种细胞类型组成,它们具有不同的基因表达谱和投射模式。我们将这些细胞类型分别命名为 PT 上和 PT 下神经元,以反应它们在 L5b 不同亚层中的分布。PT 上神经元投射到丘脑,形成与运动皮层的反馈环。PT 下神经元投射到延髓运动前中枢。在延迟反应任务中,前侧运动皮质(ALM)的细胞类型特异性细胞外记录表明,PT 上神经元参与运动规划,而 PT 下神经元则参与运动执行。因此,运动皮层在不同细胞类型水平上协调其两种互补作用。(不同的运动皮层下行通路及其在运动中的作用)

Exercise

1. Read the samples of "Introduction" and analyze their contents and structures. Recognize the signal markers and sentence patterns to realize these contents. Note the use of tenses for different contents in the writing.

2. Translate the following sentences in the "Introduction" into English.

1) 长期以来,有心血管植入型电子器械(implantable electronic device)都是进行磁共振成像的禁忌症(contraindication)。

2）人类微生物群（microbiome）含有数千种细菌，在人体不同部位和不同个体之间有不同的组成，并与几种疾病有关。

3）观察研究和荟萃分析（meta-analyses）很好地证实了代谢综合征（metabolic syndrome）患者的心血管疾病风险增加，风险增加部分归因于伴随的动脉粥样硬化性血脂异常（atherogenic dyslipidaemia），这种异常的特征是甘油三酯（triglyceride）与小而密低密度脂蛋白胆固醇（small dense low density lipoprotein cholesterol）水平升高。

4）化疗引起的周围神经病变（peripheral neuropathy）仍然是肿瘤临床的主要局限性之一，其原因是肿瘤患者的数量增加，缺乏有效的治疗策略和疾病复发。

5）在多中心研究（multicenter studies）中，以达到正常血糖水平（blood glucose level）为目标的严格血糖控制未能改善心脏手术后危重（critically ill）成年或儿童患者的结局。而有关未接受心脏手术的危重患儿的研究尚缺乏。

6）目前对这些病毒在其各自宿主物种（host species）中引起的发病机制还不完全了解，这主要是由于无法获得这些蝙蝠物种并将其喂养在适当的环境和生物安全条件下。

7）确定一种新的治疗策略来抵抗这种代谢紊乱的炎性和氧化应激（oxidative stress）成分仍然是非常重要的。

8）我们假设，这一易于临床识别的患者队列（cohort）将是最有可能在治疗效果和安全性之间取得良好平衡的人群，并且三氯格雷（tricagrelor）能满足他们尚未满足的临床需要。

9）因此，在本研究中，我们探讨了 TAT-Cx43 在神经元和星形胶质细胞中的作用，并将其与目前临床试验评估中的其他 c-Src 抑制剂进行了比较。

10）为了评价体内羊膜悬液移植（amniotic suspension allograft）的作用，我们使用了一种完善的大鼠骨关节炎疼痛模型，以评估疼痛和其他行为改变以及滑液和血清中细胞因子的水平。

6.4　方法

6.4.1　方法的功能

研究论文的方法（Methods）部分应清晰描述如何以及为何以某种特定的方法进行研究。通常具有以下三个功能：一是让读者信服——一项研究结果的可信性（reliability）来源于其研究方法和质量；二是让读者受益——方法部分中关于实验材料（experimental material）、实验设备（experimental instrument）、方法学（methodology）、研究对象（study subjects）和处理方式（treatment）等的详细描述可以为同行读者的研究提供参考依据；三是供读者验证——研究的方法步骤应该具有可重复性（replicability），重复研究步骤应该获得相同的研究结果，以此增强研究结果的可信性。

6.4.2　方法的结构

方法部分信息种类繁多、篇幅较长，因此鉴于版面问题，通常期刊会建议作者将研究的具体方案以链接方式开放给读者,正文则应避免详细描述已经发表的方法,除非本研究中需要描述改进或增加的细节,否则用参考文献加以标注即可。因此,*BMJ*、*Nature* 要求该部分一般不超过 3 000 词。该部分可放在正文中,也可以放在全文最后。本章只介绍验证假设型论文的方法部分。

方法部分通常按照信息类别划分为几个小节,并冠以小标题。一般来说,基础类论文常见小标题有:动物研究设计(或伦理)、材料及准备、动物模型、处理、测定方法、统计学分析等;临床类论文常见小标题有:临床研究设计、研究对象、纳入标准、排除标准、干预、测定方法、统计学分析等。

在实际写作中,某些小节如果没有足够的支撑细节,不足以单独成节,可以合并到其他小节,如"材料"和"动物"这两个小节,可以分别放在"测定方法"和"实验准备"中。如果没有需要特别介绍的准备步骤,这一小节也可以直接省掉。同样,临床研究中,"干预方法"和"研究设计"也可以合二为一,通常以"研究方案"标题出现;"研究对象""纳入标准"和"排除标准"也可以合并成"研究对象"。

以下列举部分世界顶级医学期刊杂志关于小节的划分及选用的小标题。

JAMA

Study design and population

Data collection

Intervention

Outcome

Statistical analysis

Lancet

Study design and participants

Randomization and masking

Procedures

Outcomes

Statistical analysis

Funding source

Neuroscience

Animals and sampling / housing

Modeling

Treatments / performances

Assessments

Statistical analysis

值得一提的是,著名医学期刊 *Cell* 指出,完整的方法应该包含"STAR"要素,即Structured(结构合理)、Transparent(信息公开)、Accessible(易懂可行)、Reporting(报道规范)。因而,为使读者直观明了地获取相关信息,该期刊的方法部分要求一级标题一致。一级标题之下,二级小标题通常以研究材料或研究变量以及具体实验步骤命名。如:

Cell

KEY RESOURCES TABLE

CONTACT FOR REAGENT AND RESOURCE SHARING

EXPERIMENTAL MODELS AND SUBJECT DETAILS

    Mice

    Bone Marrow Chimeras

    Induction of EAE

    Influenza Infection

    Rotavirus Infection

    Tritrichomonas musculis Colonization

    Human study participants and fecal sample collection

METHOD DETAILS

    Tissue Harvesting

    Flow Cytometry

    Immunofluorescence microscopy

    Hematoxylin & Eosin and Luxol Fast Blue staining

    ELISPOT analysis

    Parabiosis: Surgical Attachment of Two Female Mice

    Abdominal Surgery for Intestinal Photoconversion in Kaede mice

    PB and / or PC Transfer

    Adoptive transfer EAE in C57BL6 mice

    Isolation of Fecal Bacteria from human samples

    Bacterial Flow Cytometry

    Quantitative IgA ELISAs (human and mouse)

    Statistical Analysis

DATA AND SOFTWARE AVAILABILITY

除此之外,大部分期刊对方法部分小标题的写作没有明确的统一要求。

Nature immunology

Methods

    Mouse splenocyte processing for OT-I spiked-in experiments

    Mouse splenocyte processing for HPV-E7 experiment

    Human subjects

    Human PBMC processing for allergy samples

    Enrichment of TCR transcripts

    Construction of TCR sequencing libraries

Conditions for TCR sequencing

Assessment of TCR transcript enrichment

Determination of clonotypes from sequencing data

Data analysis for transcriptomic data

Single-cell analysis of T cells from mice immunized with HPV-E7

Single-cell analysis of T cells in peanut allergy

MSigDB signature enrichment analysis

Statistics and reproducibility

6.4.3　方法的内容

验证假设型论文的方法部分多呈菜谱模式（cookbook model），详细描述实验材料、研究对象以及研究方法和步骤。以下分别介绍基础实验和临床试验两类文章方法部分的主要内容。

6.4.3.1　基础实验类

1. 研究材料

研究材料包括药物（drug）、培养基（culture medium）、缓冲液（buffer）、气体（gas）等。药物要写出其通用名（generic name）、生产商（manufacturer）、纯度（purity）和浓度（concentration）、剂量（dosage）等。如果是水剂（solution），还应给出溶剂（solvent）、pH值（pH value）、温度（temperature）、给药速度（rate of infusion）、每千克体重给药量（amount of drug administered per kilogram of body）、给药时间（duration of the injection）等。培养基与缓冲液要写出成分（components）和浓度，如果需要还应写出温度、容积（volume）与pH值等；气体应说明其成分、浓度与／或流率（flow rate）。

例1

Vaccine

The vaccine product was generated according to standard techniques. The seed virus was grown to a high titer in eggs, the virions were purified by means of centrifugation, inactivated with the use of formalin, disrupted with the use of Triton X-100, and filtered to remove bacteria. The vaccine underwent further purification and was formulated at concentrations of 90 μg of hemagglutinin protein per milliliter (lot U10915C) and 30 μg of hemagglutinin protein per milliliter (lot U10914C) in vials containing 0.7 ml without preservative. The content of immunologically active hemagglutinin in the final formulation was determined with the use of single-radial-immunodiffusion. Sheep antiserum to bromelain-cleaved native H5 hemagglutinin was used in the agar. Placebo consisted of normal saline. Both vaccine and placebo were stored at 4 ℃ until use.

译文：

疫苗

采用标准技术制备疫苗。在鸡蛋内培育种子病毒至高滴度,采用离心方法纯化病毒颗粒,用福尔马林灭活,用 Triton X-100 打碎,过滤去除细菌。疫苗进一步纯化,制备成血凝素蛋白浓度达 90 μg/ml（批号 U10915C）和 30 μg/ml（批号 U10914C）的成品,每小瓶含量 0.7 ml,无防腐剂。采用单向辐射状免疫扩散技术,测定最终配方中有免疫活性的血凝素含量。琼脂中使用羊抗菠萝蛋白酶裂解的天然 H5 血凝素的抗血清。安慰剂为生理盐水。疫苗和安慰剂都在 4 ℃储藏备用。

2. 实验动物

描述实验动物时,需注明动物的种系（species）、体重（weight）、年龄（age）、性别（sex）、喂养方式（housing）等情况。还应申明该动物研究是否已得到独立的地方、区域或国家审查机构（如伦理委员会、机构审查委员会）的批准（institutional approval）。

例2

Mice

Specific-pathogen-free female, 6-to 8-week-old, CBA/J and C57BL/6 mice were purchased from Taconic (Germantown, NY), and wild-type FVB mice and MMP-9 null (MMP-9KO) breeder mice were purchased from Jackson Laboratory (Bar Harbor, ME). The MMP-9KO breeders were maintained as a colony at Colorado State University. All mice were maintained under barrier conditions with sterile mouse chow and water ad libitum. The specific-pathogen-free nature of the mouse colonies was demonstrated by testing sentinel animals, which were shown to be negative for 12 known mouse pathogens. All experimental procedures were approved by the Colorado State University Animal Care and Use Committee.

译文：

小鼠

无特异病原体,6~8 周大的 CBA/J 与 C57BL/6 雌性小鼠购自 Taconic（纽约州德国镇）；野生型 FVB 小鼠与无 MMP-9（MMP-9 敲除）育种小鼠购自 Jackson 实验室（缅因州巴港）。MMP-9 敲除育种动物以群体方式饲养于美国科罗拉多州大学。所有小鼠都隔栏喂养并随意喂无菌鼠食和水。检测哨兵动物以证实小鼠群体的无特异病原体特征,结果表明12 种已知的小鼠病原体均呈阴性。所有实验步骤均通过美国科罗拉多州大学实验动物管理委员会批准。

例3

Mice

Adult Mus musculus males, females, and postnatal pups on a C57BL/6J background were obtained from the Jackson Laboratory. B6.Cg-Tg (Gfap-cre) 73.12Mvs/J mice (# 012886, The Jackson Laboratory) used previously were crossed with B6.Cg-Gt (ROSA) 26Sortm9 (CAG-tdTomato) Hze/J mice (#007909, The Jackson Laboratory) to generate

Gfap（Cre/+）；TdTomato（f/+）mice. Both male and female pups were sacrificed between P0-P3 for harvesting and culturing astrocytes and sex was assumed to be balanced and differences were not analyzed. Mice were kept in a pathogen-free facility at the Hale Building for Transformative Medicine at Brigham and Women's Hospital in accordance with the IACUC guidelines, fed ad libitum on a 14/10-hour light/dark cycle. Mice were healthy and checked daily by veterinary staff. 8-10 week old mice were used for stereotactic injection and EAE induction. Mice were both drug and test naive and not involved in previous procedures. All mice were at least doubly housed. All procedures were reviewed and approved under the IACUC guidelines at Brigham and Women's Hospital.

译文：

小鼠

C57BL/6J 成年雄鼠、雌鼠以及幼鼠均来自 Jackson 实验室。将之前使用的 B6.Cg-Tg（Gfap-cre）73.12Mvs/J 小鼠（#012886，Jackson 实验室）与 B6.Cg-Gt（ROSA）26Sortm9（CAG-tdTomato）Hze/J 小鼠（#007909，Jackson 实验室）杂交，繁殖 Gfap（Cre/+）；TdTomato（f/+）小鼠。在雄性和雌性幼鼠出生后 0~3 天时将其处死，以获取和培养星形胶质细胞，假设性别均衡故未分析性别差异。按照 IACUC 指导原则，将小鼠饲养于 Brigham and Women's 医院转化医学 Hale 大楼的无菌环境中，在 14/10 小时的光照/黑暗周期中自由进食。小鼠呈健康状态，每天接受兽医检查。对 8~10 周龄小鼠进行立体定向注射和 EAE 诱导。小鼠均为首次给药和受试，此前未参与其他实验。所有小鼠至少两只一笼喂养。Brigham and Women's 医院按照 IACUC 指导原则审查并批准了所有实验操作。

3. 动物模型

详细描述对动物的分组以及各组动物的镇静（sedation）和麻醉（anesthesia）处理，包括所用试剂（agent）、剂量（amount）、给药途径（route）和给药方式（administration）；说明是否为单次（single）、重复（repeated）、或连续（continuous）用药等。

例4

Animals and Induction of Acute Myocardial Infarction in Rats

All experimental animals in this study were housed in an Association for Assessment and Accreditation of Laboratory Animal Care International（AAALAC）-certified animal facility in our hospital with controlled temperature and light cycles（24 ℃ and 12/12 light cycle）. Experimental procedures were performed in pathogen-free, adult male Sprague-Dawley（SD）rats, weighing 275-300 g（Charles River Technology, BioLASCO Taiwan Co., Ltd., Taiwan）. SD rats were anesthetized by intraperitoneal injections of chloral hydrate（35 mg/kg）. Rats were placed in a supine position on a warming pad at 37 ℃ after being shaved on the chest and then intubated with positive-pressure ventilation（180 ml/min）with room air using a small animal ventilator（SAR-830/A, CWE, Inc., Ardmore, PA, USA）. Under sterile conditions, the heart was exposed via a left thoracotomy at the level of the fifth intercostal space. AMI induction was performed via left coronary artery ligation (LCAL) 2 mm below the left atrium with a 7-0 Prolene suture. Regional myocardial ischemia was observed by a rapid discoloration over the anterior surface of the LV, together with the development of akinesia and dilatation over the at-risk area. After induction of AMI, 75 μl of conditioned medium or normal medium was injected into the anterior wall of left ventricle.

译文：

动物及诱导大鼠急性心肌梗塞

本研究中的所有实验动物均在我院由国际实验动物管理评估与认证协会（AAALAC）认证的动物设施中饲养，控制温度和光照周期（24 ℃，12／12 光照周期）。对无病原体，275～300 克重的成年雄性 Sprague-Dawley（SD）大鼠（Charles River Technology，台湾 BioLASCO 有限公司，台湾）实施实验步骤。腹腔注射水合氯醛（35 mg／kg）麻醉 SD 大鼠。胸部剃毛后，将大鼠于 37 ℃热垫上仰卧位放置，然后使用小型动物呼吸机（SAR-830／A，CWE, Inc., Ardmore, PA, USA）以室内空气正压通气插管（180 ml／min）。无菌条件下，于第五肋间隙处打开左侧胸腔，暴露心脏。用 7-0 Prolene 缝线于左心房下方 2 mm 处结扎左冠状动脉（LCAL）以诱导急性心肌梗塞（AMI）。观察到左室前表面快速变色以及该风险区域肌力减少和室扩张则判定为局部心肌缺血。AMI 诱导后，将 75 μl 条件培养基或正常培养基注入左心室前壁。

例5

Rat Monosodium Iodoacetate (MIA) Model Experimental Setup

All animal procedures were completed at Bolder BioPATH (Boulder, CO) and protocols were approved by the Bolder BioPATH Institutional Animal Care and Use Committee (IACUC). Forty-five male Sprague-Dawley rats (Envigo Harlan, Denver, CO) were obtained and acclimated for 8 days prior to the start of any experiments; animal weights were between 175 and 225 g at the beginning of the study. Animals were housed, 4-5 animals per cage on a 12 h／12 h light／dark cycle; Harlan Teklad diet #8640 was fed ad libitum and unrestricted access to tap water was available throughout the study.

译文：

建立大鼠碘乙酸单钠（MIA）实验模型

所有动物处理程序均在 Bolder BioPATH（美国科罗拉多州博尔德市）完成，实验方案已获 Bolder BioPATH 机构实验动物管理委员会（IACUC）批准。取 45 只雄性 Sprague-Dawley 大鼠（Envigo Harlan，丹佛，科罗拉多州），实验开始之前适应 8 天。研究开始时，动物体重为 175～225 g。大鼠用笼舍饲养，每笼 4～5 只，光照／黑暗周期各 12 小时，以 Harlan Teklad #8640 饲料喂养，整个研究过程自由采食和饮用自来水。

On day 0, the right knees of forty rats were injected with 2 mg of MIA to induce OA in the knee (Fig.1). Five rats did not receive MIA and were reserved as age-matched controls (naive group). Following the 7-day period of hypersensitivity reported for this MIA model, rats were randomly placed into their treatment group based on incapacitance testing to ensure a balance in disease severity measured by weight-bearing differences at baseline between all groups. At day 7, rats received an injection into the right knee with one of the following treatments (50 μl volume and n = 10 for all groups): saline (vehicle control), 25 μl ASA (25 μl ASA [ASA, ReNu®; Organogenesis, Birmingham, AL] + 25 μl saline), 50 μl ASA (no dilution), or 0.06 mg triamcinolone acetonide injectable suspension (Kenalog®-10; Bristol Myers Squib, Princeton, NJ; positive control).

第 0 天,在 40 只大鼠的右膝盖注射 2 mg MIA 诱导膝盖部骨关节炎 (OA) (图 1)。5 只大鼠未注射 MIA,设为年龄相匹配的对照组 (未治疗组)。MIA 模型组连续 7 天超敏测试后,根据功能丧失测试检测各组间基线时的负重差异将大鼠随机分入各治疗组,以确保各组间疾病严重程度的均衡性。第 7 天,各组大鼠右膝注射药物如下 (50 μl 体积,每组 10 只): 生理盐水 (溶剂对照组);25 μl ASA (25 μl ASA [ASA, ReNu®; Organogenesis, Birmingham, AL]+25 μl 生理盐水);50 μl ASA (无稀释液组);0.06 mg 醋酸曲安奈德注射悬液 (Kenalog®-10; Bristol Myers Squib, Princeton, NJ;阳性对照组)。

The volume for dosing was established from a previously reported study with recommendations based on the body weight of rats. Behavioral testing was carried out at baseline and during the period following treatment; this schedule can be found in Table 1. Other datails of the model are shown in Figure 1. Fourteen days after treatment (day 21), rats were sacrificed, and serum, synovial fluid, and knee joints were collected for analysis. (tables and figures are omitted)

按先前报道的研究建议,根据大鼠体重确定给药剂量。在治疗之前和治疗期间均进行了行为测试,具体详情见表 1。建模更多细节见图 1。治疗后第 14 天 (第 21 天) 处死大鼠,并收集血清、滑液和膝关节进行分析。(图表省略)

4. 实验处理

例6

Primary astrocyte cultures

Brains of mice aged P0-P3 were dissected into PBS on ice. Cortices were discarded and the brain parenchyma were pooled, centrifuged at 500xg for 10 minutes at 4 ℃ and resuspended in 0.25% Trypsin-EDTA (#25200-072, Thermo Fisher Scientific) at 37 ℃ for 10 minutes. DNase I (#90083, Thermo Fisher Scientific) was then added to the solution (1 mg/ml), and the brains were digested for 10 more minutes. Trypsin was neutralized by adding DMEM/F12 + GlutaMAX (#10565018, Thermo Fisher Scientific) supplemented with 10% FBS (#10438026, Thermo Fisher Scientific) and 1% penicillin/streptomycin (#15140148, Thermo Fisher Scientific), and cells were passed through a 70 mm cell strainer. Cells were centrifuged at 500xg for 10 minutes at 4 ℃, resuspended in DMEM/F12 + GlutaMAX with 10% FBS/1% penicillin/streptomycin and cultured in T-75 flasks (#353136, Falcon) at 37 ℃ in a humidified incubator with 5% CO_2, for 7-10 days until confluency was reached. Astrocytes were shaken for 30 minutes at 180 rpm, the media was changed, then astrocytes were shaken for at least 2 hours at 220 rpm and media was changed again. Medium was replaced every 2-3 days. For microglial cultures, after the first round of shaking, detached cells were replated into a fresh 10-cm dish and cultured at 37 ℃ in a humidified incubator with 5% CO_2.

译文：

星形胶质细胞原代培养

在冰上分离出生后 0~3 天小鼠脑组织于 PBS 中。弃去皮质,采集脑实质,4 ℃下 500xg 离心 10 分钟;37 ℃下,于 0.25% 胰蛋白酶-EDTA（#25200-072, Thermo Fisher Scientific）中重悬 10 分钟。加入 DNase I（#90083, Thermo Fisher Scientific）（1 mg/ml）,并将脑组织再消化 10 分钟。加入 DMEM/F12 + GlutaMAX（#10565018, Thermo Fisher Scientific）并添加 10% 胎牛血清（#10438026, Thermo Fisher Scientific）和 1% 青霉素/链霉素（#15140148, Thermo Fisher Scientific）以中和胰蛋白酶,并用 70 mm 细胞筛过滤细胞。4 ℃下 500xg 将细胞离心 10 分钟,重悬于含 10% 胎牛血清/1% 青霉素/链霉素的 DMEM/F12+GlutaMAX 中,然后置于 T-75 培养瓶（#353136, Falcon）,于 37 ℃、5% CO_2 加湿培养箱中孵育 7~10 天,直至融合。180 rpm 振摇星形胶质细胞 30 分钟,更换培养基,220 rpm 振摇 2 小时以上,再次更换培养基。此后,每 2~3 天更换一次培养基。为了孵育小胶质细胞,在第一次振摇后,将分离的细胞重新铺板至新的 10 cm 培养皿中,并于 37 ℃、5% CO_2 的加湿培养箱中孵育。

5. 测定方法

测定（measurement）部分包括定义测定变量,介绍测定方法和说明测定仪器等。一般需提到仪器名称（包括生产厂家）、溶液及其浓度、测定指标、详细步骤等。

例7

Western blot

Mouse serum was harvested from tumor bearing Igmi and Balbc mice by cardiac puncture. In addition, serum was obtained from non-tumor bearing mice. Serum protein was quantified using DC Protein Assay（Bio-Rad, Hercules CA）and all samples were diluted to equal concentration using water. Samples were separated by electrophoresis on 4%~15% Tris-Glycine polyacrylamide gels（Bio-Rad）, transferred to Hybondâ PVDF membrane（Millipore Sigma, St. Louis MO）, blocked for 1 h at room temperature in 5% BSA（Millipore Sigma）in TBS with 0.05% Tween-20. The membrane was incubated with either IgG1 HRP-conjugated（OBT1508P）or IgM MU CHAIN HRP-conjugated（5276-2504）antibody（Bio-Rad）for 2 h while rocking at room temperature. The membrane was washed three times in TBS with 0.05% Tween-20 and exposed to Super Signal chemiluminescent substrate（Thermo Scientific, Waltham MA）. The membrane was visualized using the Chemi Doc MP Imaging System（Bio-Rad）.

译文：

蛋白质印迹法

心脏穿刺，采集 Igmi 和 Balbc 荷瘤小鼠的血清。另外，获取非荷瘤小鼠血清。采用 DC 蛋白测定法（Bio-Rad，Hercules 加利福利亚州）定量血清蛋白，并用水稀释所有样品至相等浓度。用 4%～15% Tris-甘氨酸聚丙烯酰胺凝胶（Bio-Rad）电泳法分离样品，转移至 Hybondâ PVDF 膜（Millipore Sigma，圣路易斯），室温下用 5% BSA（Millipore Sigma）封闭液（含 0.05% Tween-20 TBS 缓冲液）封闭 1 小时。将膜与 IgG1 HRP 偶联（OBT1508P）或 IgM MU CHAIN HRP 偶联（5276-2504）抗体（Bio-Rad）孵育 2 小时，同时在室温下摇动。含 0.05% Tween-20 TBS 将膜洗涤 3 次，并用 Super Signal 化学发光底物处理（Thermo Scientific，Waltham 马萨诸塞州）。用 Chemi Doc MP 成像系统（Bio-Rad）将膜可视化。

例8

Immunostaining of frozen MS tissue

Frozen brain tissue from 4 MS patients and 4 healthy control individuals was cut into 7 mm thick sections, air-dried, and fixed in ice-cold acetone for 10 minutes. Sections were delipidised in 70% ethanol for 5 minutes, followed by blocking of non-specific binding with 10% donkey serum (#D9663, Sigma-Aldrich). Rabbit anti-human P-IRE1a (#NB100-2323, Novus Biologicals, 1∶50) was incubated with mouse anti-human GFAP-Cy3 (#C9205, Sigma-Aldrich, 1∶50), mouse anti-human NeuN (#MAB377, Millipore, 1∶50), mouse anti-human CNPase (#MAB326, Millipore, 1∶100) or mouse anti-human CD14 (#555397, BD Biosciences, 1∶10) in blocking buffer overnight at 4 ℃. The next day slides were washed with 0.05% PBS-Tween and incubated with a mixture of donkey anti-rabbit Alexa Fluor 488 (#R37118, Life Technologies, 1∶400) and donkey anti-mouse-Cy3 (#715-165-151, Jackson ImmunoResearch, 1∶200) or donkey anti-rabbit-Rhodamine Red X (#711-295-152, Jackson ImmunoResearch, 1∶400) and donkey anti-mouse-Alexa Fluor 488 (Jackson ImmunoResearch, 1∶400) for 40 minutes at room temperature. Sections were mounted in Mowiol (#81381, Sigma-Aldrich) containing TOPRO-3 (#T3605, Invitrogen). In secondary only controls, primary antibodies were omitted to control for non-specific binding.

译文：

免疫染色冰冻多发性硬化（MS）组织

取 4 例 MS 患者和 4 例健康对照者的冰冻脑组织，制备成 7 mm 的切片，风干，在冰冻丙酮中固定 10 分钟。切片在 70% 乙醇中脱脂 5 分钟，然后用 10% 驴血清（#D9663，Sigma-Aldrich）阻断非特异性结合。将兔抗人 P-IRE1a（#NB100-2323，Novus Biologicals，1∶50）与小鼠抗人 GFAP-Cy3（#C9205，Sigma-Aldrich，1∶50）、NeuN（#MAB377，Millipore，1∶50）、CNPase（#MAB326，Millipore，1∶100）或 CD14（#555397，BD Biosciences，1∶10）在封闭缓冲液中孵育，4 ℃过夜。次日，0.05% PBS-Tween 洗片，并用驴抗兔 Alexa Fluor 488（#R37118，Life Technologies，1∶400）和驴抗小鼠-Cy3（#715-165-151，Jackson

ImmunoResearch，1∶200）或驴抗兔-Rhodamine Red X（# 711-295-152，Jackson ImmunoResearch，1∶400）和驴抗小鼠-Alexa Fluor 488（Jackson ImmunoResearch，1∶400）的混合物室温下孵育 40 分钟。然后，在含 TOPRO-3（#T3605，Invitrogen）的 Mowiol（#81381，Sigma-Aldrich）中固定切片。对照样本中仅加入二抗，省去一抗，以控制非特异性结合。

6. 统计学分析

方法部分的最后一般是统计学分析（statistical analysis）的说明，按数据分析应用的统计检验（statistical tests）逐一阐述，以供同行读者通过原始数据判断研究是否恰当，并核实报告结果。如果一种数据涉及几个问题，统计检验则按实验顺序阐述。通常，从描述研究对象的描述统计学（descriptive statistics）开始，然后阐述实验结果或比较研究对象的特殊统计学检验。比较时，用多重比较（multiple comparison）方法，也就是通用的显著性检验（test of significance），然后进行配对比较（pairwise comparisons）。确定统计学差异时，需定义统计学意义（statistical significance）、统计学术语、缩写和大多数符号；若可能，应对结果量化，用能恰当反映测量误差或不确定性的指标（如可信区间）描述结果。传统上的显著性概率（P value），即 p 值为 0.05，但也可以选择不同水平的 p 值（通常更为保守）。另外，还应介绍处理数据（data processing）使用的统计软件（software）及其版本。

例9

Statistical Analysis

All statistical analyses were performed with SPSS software（version 11.5）. Comparison of the proportions for the three cohorts was performed with the use of the chi-square test（$\alpha = 0.05$）；if the null hypothesis was rejected, then pairwise comparisons were performed（$\alpha' = 0.012\ 5$）. Analysis of variance（by means of the Student-Newman-Keuls test）was used to compare the mean ages among the cohorts. Serum thyroglobulin values were compared among the three cohorts with the use of the Student-Newman-Keuls test after logarithmic transformation, because the data had a log-normal distribution rather than a normal distribution. Risk factors were analyzed with the use of logistic regression. The level of significance was set at 5 percent for the Student-Newman-Keuls test and logistic regression.

译文：

统计学分析

所有统计学分析均使用 SPSS 软件（11.5 版），应用卡方检验比较 3 个队列的比例（$\alpha = 0.05$）。如果无效假设被拒绝，则应用配对比较（$\alpha' = 0.012\ 5$）。用变异性分析（通过 Student-Newman-Keuls 检验的方法）比较队列间的平均年龄。对数转换后，用 Student-Newman-Keuls 检验比较 3 个队列的血清甲状腺球蛋白值，因为这些数值呈对数正态分布，而不是正态分布。使用 logistic 回归分析危险因素。Student-Newman-Keuls 检验和 logistic 回归的显著性水平设为 5%。

6.4.3.2　临床试验类

1. 研究设计

一般来说,生物医学期刊发表的临床类论文的方法部分首先会介绍总体的研究设计（study design）。研究设计部分应该短小精悍,通常包括研究时间和地点、研究人群、研究问题、研究类型、干预方法（interventions）、测定的变量（measured variables）和基线（baseline）、对照系列（control series）等内容。如果是已建立的设计方法,应提供参考文献或获取方式（如在线网址）。此外,临床试验的官方注册编号也需要提供,*JAMA*、*Cell* 和 *Lancet* 杂志就有专门的要求。

例10

Study design

This randomised, double-blind, multicentre, phase 3 trial of a single 75 mg dose of rimegepant as an ODT versus placebo in the acute treatment of migraine was done at 69 study centres in the USA in accordance with the principles of the Guidelines for Good Clinical Practice, the Declaration of Helsinki, and all applicable local regulations. The protocol was approved by Advarra IRB（Columbia, MD, USA）and is available in the appendix.

The study is registered with ClinicalTrials.gov, number NCT03461757.

译文:

试验设计

本研究为在美国的 69 个研究中心开展的一项随机、双盲、多中心、Ⅲ 期临床试验,比较了单服 75 mg 瑞格非特口崩片与安慰剂在偏头痛急性治疗中的作用。该试验严格遵循美国《药物临床试验管理规范》《赫尔辛基宣言》及所有适用的当地法规。试验方案经 Advarra IRB（美国马里兰州哥伦比亚）批准,详见附录。

该试验已在 ClinicalTrials.gov 官网注册,编号为 NCT03461757。

例11

Trial Design

We conducted this investigator-initiated, open-label, blinded-outcome-assessor, pragmatic, multicenter, randomized, controlled trial in 25 intensive care units（ICUs）in France（11 in university hospitals and 14 in community hospitals）. The trial rationale and design have been described previously. The research protocol（available with the full text of this article at NEJM.org）was approved by the appropriate ethics committees and French data-protection authorities.

译文:

试验设计

本研究是一项由研究者发起的、开放标签、对结局评估者设盲、实用性、多中心、随机对照试验,在法国的 25 个重症监护病房（ICUs）（11 个在大学医院,14 个在社区医院）中进行。该试验的原理和设计先前已有报道。研究方案（全文见 NEJM.org）已获得相关伦理委员会和法国数据保护机构的批准。

2. 研究对象及设盲

临床论文研究对象多为人群（population），应给出相关人口学数据（demographic data），如年龄（age）、性别（gender or sex）、种族（race）、身高（height）、体重（weight）、健康状况（state of health or disease），及特殊的内科或外科处理（specific medical or surgical management）等。如果是回顾性研究（retrospective study），研究人群的人口学数据应该在方法部分列出。如果是前瞻性（prospective study）研究，则用纳入及排除标准（inclusion and exclusion criteria）选择有代表性的人群，同时描述纳入方式，研究人群的人口学数据应在结果部分列出。如果有对照组（control group），必须描述对照组受试者的选取情况。说明研究组和对照组是随机选取（randomization）还是某类人群的代表，如果是随机，表明所用的随机方法。通常研究组具有一系列的临床指征（clinical indications），明确病人纳入的指征。随后，设盲（masking or blinding）过程应明确。另外，还应说明该人群研究是否获得受试者的知情同意（written or oral informed consent）和相关机构审查委员会的批准（approval of institutional review board），是否符合社会事业机构或地区性的人体试验委员会制定的伦理道德标准（ethics）等。

例12

Participants

Adult patients presenting to hospital in four countries were eligible for inclusion if they were at risk of a recurrent ischaemic stroke and had either a non-cardioembolic ischaemic stroke with limb weakness, dysphasia, or neuroimaging-positive hemianopia, or a non-cardioembolic TIA with at least 10 min of limb weakness or isolated dysphasia. Participants had to be randomly assigned within 48 h of symptom onset. Participants who received intravenous thrombolysis could be randomly assigned but only after 24 h had elapsed after the end of this treatment, and providing post-treatment neuroimaging excluded secondary cerebral bleeding.

译文：

研究对象

受试者是在四个国家就诊的成年患者,合格的纳入标准包括有缺血性卒中复发风险;伴有肢体无力、失语或经神经影像学证实的偏盲的非心脏栓塞性缺血性卒中,亦或是伴有至少 10 分钟肢体无力或仅出现言语障碍的非心脏栓塞性 TIA。受试者在症状发作后 48 h 内接受随机分组。接受静脉溶栓治疗的受试者需在治疗结束后 24 h,且需神经影像学检查排除继发性脑出血,方可接受随机分组。

Key exclusion criteria were age younger than 50 years; isolated sensory symptoms, facial weakness, or vertigo or dizziness; presumed cardioembolic stroke or TIA; parenchymal haemorrhage or other intracranial haemorrhage; non-ischaemic cause for symptoms; definite need for, or contraindication to, aspirin, clopidogrel, or dipyridamole;

definite need for full-dose anticoagulation; premorbid dependency; or severe hypertension. A full list of the study inclusion and exclusion criteria is provided in the appendix.

主要的排除标准包括年龄小于 50 岁；仅出现感觉症状，面瘫，眩晕或头晕；假定的心脏栓塞性卒中或 TIA；脑实质出血或其他颅内出血；引起症状的非缺血性原因；明确需要或禁忌使用阿司匹林，氯吡格雷或双嘧达莫；明确需要足量抗凝治疗；病前生活不能自理；或严重的高血压。研究纳入和排除标准的具体详情见附录。

Patients gave written consent, or written proxy consent was obtained from a relative or carer if the patient lacked capacity. The study was approved by national or local ethics committees in each participating country and site and was adopted in the UK by the National Institute of Health Research Stroke Research Network.

参与者均签署书面同意，若患者无法签署，则由家属或监护人书面代理同意。该研究由各参与国家和地区的国家或地方伦理委员会批准，并被英国国立卫生研究院卒中研究网络采纳。

例13

Randomisation and masking

Patients were randomly assigned (1∶1∶1), via a computer-generated randomisation sequence with an interactive voice-response system, to receive once-weekly dulaglutide 1.5 mg, dulaglutide 0.75 mg, or daily bedtime glargine. Randomisation was stratified by country and metformin use. Participants and study investigators were not masked to treatment allocation, but were unaware of dulaglutide dose assignment.

译文：

随机化和设盲

采用计算机生成的随机序列，通过交互式语音应答系统，将患者按 1∶1∶1 的比例随机分配，接受每周 1 次度拉糖肽 1.5 mg、0.75 mg 或睡前甘精胰岛素治疗。按照国家以及二甲双胍使用情况进行随机化分层。受试者和研究人员知晓治疗分配情况，但不知晓度拉糖肽剂量分配方案。

3. 研究步骤

研究步骤部分详细描述试验的具体实施步骤，没有固定的内容或小标题。原则上，内容可按时间顺序或依重要程度描述，详略程度取决于读者对该方法的熟悉程度。如果是已建立的通用方法，应给出参考文献，无需详细介绍；如果是已经发表但不为人熟知的方法，应给出参考文献并作简要描述；如果是自创或作了较多改良的方法，则要详细描述，并说明采用此方法的理由，对其局限性作出评价。如果是临床研究（clinical study），应介绍治疗方法（treatment）和评估指标（measure），包括药物类型（form of medication）、剂量（dosage）、用药途径（route of medication）、病程（course），以及有无联合用药（with or without combined use of other medicines）等；如果该研究是一项发明，如实验仪器，则应在不违反保密（confidentiality）原则，不影响专利权（patent right）的前提下，全面介绍该仪器的结构（structure）、功能（function）、原理（principle）、用途（usage）、操作（operation）等。

例14

Procedures

Patients were randomly assigned with the use of permuted blocks to receive either intravenous methylprednisolone sodium succinate (methylprednisolone) diluted in 50 ml of 5 percent dextrose in water or placebo (50 ml of 5 percent dextrose in water), stratified according to hospital. A single dose of 2 mg of methylprednisolone per kilogram of predicted body weight [24] was followed by a dose of 0.5 mg per kilogram of predicted body weight every 6 hours for 14 days, a dose of 0.5 mg per kilogram of predicted body weight every 12 hours for 7 days, and then tapering of the dose. Study drug was tapered over a period of 4 days if 21 days of treatment had been completed and the patient was unable to breathe without assistance for a period of 48 hours. Tapering occurred over a two-day period if disseminated fungal infection or septic shock developed or the patient was able to breathe for a period of 48 hours without assistance.

译文：

步骤

我们采用排列分组方法将病人随机分为 2 组，分别接受静脉输注甲泼尼龙琥珀酸纳（甲泼尼龙，将药物溶于 5%葡萄糖溶液 50 ml）或安慰剂（5%葡萄糖溶液 50 ml）。按照病人所在医院进行分层。甲泼尼龙的剂量是首剂 2 mg/kg（按照病人的预计体重计算），随后 0.5 mg/kg，每 6 小时 1 次，共 14 天，然后改为，每 12 小时 1 次，共 7 天，此后逐渐减量停药。如果病人在完成了 21 天的治疗后仍不能在无辅助通气的情况下自主呼吸 48 小时，则在 4 天内减量停药。如果病人发生播散性真菌感染或败血症性休克，或能够在无辅助通气的情况下自主呼吸 48 小时，则在 2 天内减量停药。

The protocol specified how patients were to be weaned from the ventilator. Patients were assessed daily for weaning readiness and weaned by pressure-support ventilation when acceptable arterial oxygenation could be maintained with the use of an FiO_2 of 0.5 or less.

研究方案规定了病人应如何撤离通气机。医师每天对病人进行评估，确定其是否具备撤机条件，如果在 $FiO_2 \leqslant 0.5$ 的条件下，动脉氧合状态仍保持在可接受水平，则采用压力支持通气方法撤机。

Data on demographic characteristics, physiological characteristics, radiographic features, coexisting conditions, and medication were recorded at study entry and on days 1, 2, 3, 4, 5, 7, 14, 21, and 28. Patients were followed until they died, were discharged home while breathing without assistance, or day 180, whichever came first.

在病人入组研究时和研究开始后 1、2、3、4、5、7、14、21 和 28 天，记录其人口统计学特征、生理学特点、X 线片特征、并存症和所用药物。随访病人直至死亡、在无需辅助通气的情况下出院或随访至 180 天，以最早出现者为准。

Patients were monitored daily for cardiovascular, renal, and hepatic failure and coagulation abnormalities, as defined previously, for 28 days.[24] According to our definition, organs were considered failure-free after patients had been discharged from the hospital.

按照以前的规定,在 28 天内每天监测病人是否有心血管、肾脏或肝脏功能衰竭或凝血功能异常。按照我们的定义,病人出院后就被视为不再有器官衰竭。

Any positive culture of material from a normally sterile site, when clinically available cerebrospinal fluid, blood, pleural fluid, urine ($\geq 10^5$ colonies per milliliter), as well as of bile and abdominal (peritoneal) fluid, was recorded. Data from weekly chart reviews were recorded if evidence of serious infections (e. g., nosocomial pneumonia, disseminated fungal infection, or sepsis) or other infections was present (a complete list of prospectively defined infections is provided in the Supplementary Appendix). Bronchoalveolar-lavage fluid and plasma were obtained at study entry and on day 7 and processed as previously described[25] (details are provided in the Supplementary Appendix). Plasma samples were stored in EDTA-treated tubes.

记录临床无菌采集的标本的阳性培养结果,例如脑脊液、血液、胸腔积液、尿 ($\geq 10^5$ 个菌落 / ml)、胆汁和腹水。如果出现患有严重感染的证据 (例如医院内感染的肺炎、播散性真菌感染或脓毒症) 或存在其他感染 (事先定义的感染的完整目录见补充附录),则记录来自病例复习周记的数据。病人入组研究时和研究开始后第 7 天,收集其支气管肺泡灌洗液和血浆标本,按照文献描述的方法处理 (详情见补充附录)。血浆标本贮存在 EDTA 处理过的试管内。

4. 转归

测定的变量包括自变量和因变量,如主要转归 (primary outcomes) 或主要终点 (primary end points)、次要转归 (secondary outcomes) 或次要终点 (secondary end points)。定义时应明确定义标准 (criteria)。

例15

Outcomes

The primary endpoint was a composite of major complications or death within 6 months after randomisation. Major complications were defined as new-onset organ failure (ie, cardiovascular, pulmonary, or renal), bleeding requiring intervention, perforation of a visceral organ requiring intervention (except for the intentionally made perforation during endopscopic treatment), enterocutaneous fistula requiring intervention, and incisional hernia (including burst abdomen). Predefined secondary endpoints included the individual components of the primary endpoint, pancreatic fistula, exocrine and endocrine pancreatic insufficiency, biliary strictures, wound infections, need for necrosectomy, total number of interventions, length of hospital and ICU stay, costs (eg, costs per patient with poor outcome, costs per quality adjusted life-year [QALY], and total direct and indirect medical costs), quality of life, and the total number of crossovers between groups (for definitions of these primary and secondary endpoints see appendix pp 9-10). An adjudication committee composed of five surgeons, three endoscopists, and one radiologist performed a blinded outcome assessment. They individually evaluated each patient for the occurrence of the primary endpoint. Disagreements were resolved during a plenary consensus meeting before data analysis started.

After enrolment of each consecutive group of 25 patients, an independent data safety and monitoring committee evaluated the progress of inclusion and safety endpoints for each patient with unblinded data. Patient reports and a list of potential adverse events were presented to the data safety and monitoring committee (see appendix p7).

译文：

转归

主要终点是随机化后 6 个月内主要并发症的联合终点或死亡。主要并发症定义为新发生的器官衰竭（即心血管、肺或肾）、需要介入的出血、需要介入的内脏器官穿孔（除在内镜治疗中有意制造的穿孔）、需要介入的肠外瘘和切口疝（包括腹脏内伤）。预先定义的次要终点包括主要终点的各单一终点、胰腺瘘、胰腺外分泌和内分泌功能不全、胆管狭窄、伤口感染、需要坏死清除、介入总次数、住院时间和 ICU 入住时间、费用[如不良转归患者的平均费用，平均生命质量调整年的费用（QALY），总的直接和间接医疗费用]，生活质量和组间的交叉总数（这些主要和次要终点的定义见附录 9~10 页）。由 5 位外科医生，3 位内镜医生和 1 位放射科医生组成的裁判委员会进行盲法结果评估。他们分别评估每位患者主要终点的发生情况。在数据分析开始之前，全体共识会议解决了分歧。

25 名患者的每个连续组别纳入研究后，独立的数据安全和监测委员会利用非盲数据评估每个患者的纳入进展和安全终点的情况。患者报告单和潜在不良事件清单也递交给数据安全和监测委员会（见附录第 7 页）。

5. 统计学分析

例16

Statistical Analysis

All the patients who underwent randomization were included in the intention-to-treat population, which was used for all efficacy analyses. The safety analysis included all the patients in the intention-to-treat population who had received at least one dose of a trial drug and for whom data were available after the administration of the drug.

译文：

统计学分析

所有的有效性分析均基于意向治疗人群；所有接受随机分组的患者均包括在意向治疗人群中。安全性分析包括意向治疗人群中所有接受至少一剂试验药物治疗的患者，而且可以获得这些患者使用药物后的数据。

We used the log-rank test stratified according to Asian or non-Asian race to compare the duration of progression-free survival between the two treatment groups. We used the Breslow approach for handling tied events and the Kaplan-Meier method to summarize the results. Data for patients who had not had a progression event or had not died at the time of the analysis were censored at the time of the last RECIST assessment.

采用按照亚洲人种或非亚洲人种进行分层的时序检验法对两个治疗组间的无进展生存期进行比较。采用 Breslow 法处理关联事件,采用 Kaplan-Meier 法对结果进行总结。对于分析时仍未发生进展事件或死亡的患者,采用最后一次 RECIST(实体瘤疗效评价标准)对其数据进行截尾处理。

We determined that 221 events of progression or death would provide a power of 80% to reject the null hypothesis of no significant difference in the duration of progression-free survival between the two treatment groups, assuming a treatment effect hazard ratio of 0.67 with a P value of 0.05 indicating two-sided statistical significance. (Additional details are provided in the Supplementary Methods section in the Supplementary Appendix.) The data cutoff date was April 15, 2016.

假定治疗效应的风险比为 0.67,双侧统计学显著性的 P 值设为 0.05,我们确定 221 例疾病进展或死亡事件能够提供 80% 的统计学效能,足以否定两个治疗组间无进展生存期无显著差异这一无效假设(更多详情列于补充附录的补充方法部分)。数据收集的截止日期为 2016 年 4 月 15 日。

从以上例子可以发现,基础或临床研究中方法部分的某些细节信息应该置于括号中(information in parenthesis),以使内容更简洁,语言表达更流畅和连贯。常置于括号中的信息为动物的体重、年龄、获取来源;受试者的体重、年龄、身高等人口学资料;溶液的浓度、药物的剂量、药物或仪器的生产商名,以及厂家、型号、批次等。具体参见本节各例。

6.4.4　方法的写作要点

6.4.4.1　方法部分的时态

方法部分属回顾性叙述,多采用过去时态。说明研究或实验之前发生的动作或情况,用过去完成时。说明数据表示方法用现在时;有关解释、说明的信息,事实性的信息也用现在时描述。具体参见本节各例。

6.4.4.2　方法部分的信息标记语

方法部分可以用小标题、主题句和连接语来标记主题。小标题标记每个小节的主题。如果一个小节含有一个以上的段落,可以用主题句标记每一个段落的主题。另外,如本书第 4 章段落写作原则所述,生物医学期刊英文论文中常用动词不定式或介词结构作为连接语,置于段首或段落中,作为陈述实验目的的标记语。

例17

In vivo imaging

Mice were anesthetized using an isofluorane chamber and anesthesia was maintained throughout the course of the experiment with vaporized isofluorane delivered by a nose cone as previously described[52,53]. Image stacks were acquired with a LaVision TriM Scope II (LaVision Biotec, Germany) laser scanning microscope equipped with a tunable Two-photon Chameleon Ultra (Coherent, USA) Ti:Sapphire laser. To acquire serial optical sections, a laser beam (940 nm for H2BGFP, actinGFP and mTmG; 1040 nm for H2BPAmCherry and tdTomato) was focused through a 20X or 40X water immersion lens (N.A.1.0 and 1.1 respectively; Zeiss, USA) and scanned with a field of view of 0.5×0.5 mm^2 or 0.25×0.25 mm^2 respectively at 600 Hz. Z-stacks were acquired in 1-3 μm steps to image a total depth of 200 μm of tissue[52]. To visualize large areas, 3-36 tiles of optical fields were imaged using a motorized stage to automatically acquire sequential fields of view as previously described [54]. For time-lapse imaging, serial optical sections were obtained in a range of 1 to 12 minute intervals depending on the experimental setup. The duration of time-lapse imaging ranged from 4-12 hours.

译文：

体内成像

用异氟烷麻醉舱麻醉小鼠。如前所述,在整个实验过程中用鼻锥吸入异氟烷蒸气以保持麻醉状态。使用现有可调谐双光子 Chameleon Ultra(Coherent,美国)Ti:Sapphire 激光器的激光扫描显微镜 LaVision TriM Scope II(LaVision Biotec,德国)采集图像堆栈。为了获取连续的光学成像,采用不同波长的激光束(H2BGFP,actinGFP 和 mTmG 采用940 nm;H2BPAmCherry 和 tdTomato 采用1 040 nm)通过 20 倍或 40 倍浸没物镜(分别为 NA 1.0 和 1.1;Zeiss,美国)观察成像,并在 600 Hz 时以 0.5×0.5 mm^2 或 0.25×0.25 mm^2 的视场进行扫描。Z 堆栈以 1~3 μm 的步长采集,以形成总深度 200 μm 的组织成像。为了可视化大面积区域,如前所述,使用电动载物台对 3~36 片场进行成像,以自动获取连续的视场。根据实验装置,对 1~12 分钟各间隔获取的连续光学切片进行延时成像。延时成像的持续时间为 4~12 小时。

Topical drug treatment

To inhibit cell proliferation in the epidermis, Mitomycin C (MMC)[55] was delivered topically by applying it to the wound and the surrounding ear skin. MMC was dissolved in a 15 mg/ml stock solution in dimethyl sulfoxide (DMSO) and later the stock solution was diluted 100 times in 100% petroleum jelly (Vaseline; final concentration is 150 μg/ml). 100 mg of the mixture of the MMC and the petroleum jelly was spread evenly on the wounded area at 1 and 2 days PWI. A mixture of 100% DMSO in petroleum jelly (1:100) was used as a vehicle control. Colcemid was used to block microtubule polymerization[56,57]. Colcemid was dissolved to 25 mg/ml stock solution in the DMSO and delivered as described for the MMC treatment.

局部用药

为了抑制表皮细胞增殖,将丝裂霉素 C(MMC)局部涂抹于耳部伤口以及周围皮肤。将 MMC 溶解于含二甲亚砜(DMSO)的储备溶液中(15 mg/ml),然后将储备溶液在

100%凡士林（最终浓度：150 μg／ml）中稀释 100 倍。伤口形成后第 1 天和第 2 天，将 100 mg MMC 和凡士林的混合物均匀涂抹于伤口上。100% DMSO 与凡士林的混合物（1∶100）用于溶剂对照组。秋水仙胺用于阻止微管聚合。将秋水仙胺溶于含 DMSO 的储备溶液中（25 mg／ml），并按照 MMC 治疗中描述的方法使用。

　　说明：本例文在描述实验时，首先采用小标题 In vivo imaging，Topical drug treatment 表明了该段落的实验内容。具体描述时，采用了不定式如 To acquire serial optical sections…，To visualize large areas…，和介词短语 For time-lapse imaging… 等连接语来表明具体某一步骤的目的；而段落主旨句 To inhibit cell proliferation in the epidermis, Mitomycin C（MMC）was delivered topically by applying it to the wound and the surrounding ear skin.概括了本段的中心内容。这些连接语或标记语使得文章逻辑更加严密，可读性更强。

6.4.4.3　方法部分的语态

　　传统医学英文论文的"方法部分"都是用第三人称的被动语态来写，以避免提及有关的执行者，排除主观成分。然而从 20 世纪 60—70 年代开始，不少国际医学写作组织及文体专家明确主张使用主动语态，以使科学论文和著作的文字生动、有活力、信息突出；多用人称代词 we 以显示研究者对研究积极、负责的态度。

　　事实上，主动和被动语态之间并没有绝对的优劣之分，使用主动与被动语态要根据句子表达清晰、流畅的需要。写作时，可以选择整个"方法部分"只用一种语态表达；或者有些小节选择使用主动语态，例如，"研究设计"小节，以强调研究者在研究中的作用；而另一些小节则使用被动语态（例如，阐述实验的方法、测定的变量等小节），将研究的对象和观察指标等作为叙述重点，而行为动作的执行者或实验者则不言而明。还可以选择被动语态作为某个小节的基本语态，但有些句子则有意改用主动语态，以显示研究者勇于承担的态度。被动语态与主动语态的不同使用具体参见本节各例。

6.4.4.4　方法部分的常用表达

1. 表达研究对象的选取

Patients were eligible for inclusion in the… if they had evidence of…

The present study enrolled／enlisted…

Subjects were eligible to participate if…

Patients meeting the following criteria were included in the study…

… subjects were recruited／included／entered on a voluntary basis…

All included subjects were examined with…

Patients were included in our study if they had presented with…

The study population consisted of patients with…

… were excluded from the study／participation／enrollment if they had any of the following…

… were considered ineligible for…

The criteria for exclusion were...

... were excluded on the basis of...

We also recruited a control population including...

... analysis was available for... patients.

The present study consisted of a cross-section analysis of... participants.

... participants were excluded due to a previous history of / their use of a...

We excluded patients with...

2. 表达对象分组情况

Patients were divided into... groups.

... groups were selected at random.

... were randomly assigned by a computerized system.

... were randomly assigned to... groups.

... were randomized into... with...

... was divided into four sub-groups：

... was grouped / categorized as follows：

3. 表达研究的伦理规范和有效性

... were conducted in agreement with...

The research procedure was carried out in accordance with...

All procedures complied with the guiding principles for the care and use of animals approved by...

The experiment / protocol was approved by...

All participants gave written informed consent.

The requirements for written informed consent were waved by...

Verbal consent was obtained from...

Participation in the study was optioned for...

All participants signed / gave the written informed consent form before participation in the study.

All methods were conducted according to the relevant guidelines and regulations of...

All methods were carried out under license in accordance with relevant guidelines and regulations from the appropriate competent authorities and all experimental protocols were approved by... ethics committee.

4. 表达材料来源

... was (were) supplied / provided by...

... was (were) donated by...；... was the / a gift of / from...；... was a donation from...

... were obtained / ordered / purchased / derived from... and certified by... via...

We obtained... from...

The following reagents were purchased from...

... used in this study came from...

5. 表达实验方法

Sections of... were prepared as previously described.

... was (were) prepared according to the method described by...

The procedures were similar to those in previous studies.

The... model was established (set up) by... methods.

... were assayed by... method derived from sb.

... were assayed by... technique adapted from previously published methods.

... were prepared / dissolved to a concentration of...

... was compared between A and B using...

We observed... using / by...

... model was then fitted to estimate the effects of... on... using...

The method used to... was based on...

To reconstitute..., we followed a similar strategy as described before / previously.

To remove variants that..., we excluded...

Using..., we confirmed that... We next used... techniques to confirm that... We further investigated whether...

6. 表达实验步骤

... was (were) pretreated for... minutes.

The blood samples were collected / taken / obtained / withdrawn from...

... was (were) seeded in... and maintained in...

... was (were) harvested with...

... was (were) collected / harvested under... conditions.

... was (were) fixed with...

... was (were) stained with...

... was (were) implanted in...

... was (were) embedded in...

... was (were) grown in... medium.

... was (were) cloned into...

... was (were) incubated / cultured in...

... was (were) injected / administered with...

... was (were) exposed / subjected to...

... was (were) treated with... in the presence or absence of...

... was (were) extracted using...

... was (were) suspended in...

... was (were) dehydrated in...

... was (were) diluted to...

… was (were) purified from… with the use of…

… was (were) amplified by…

… was (were) dissolved in…

… was (were) stored at… until use…

… was (were) synthesized by…

… was (were) multiplied by…

… was (were) anesthetized with…

… was (were) sacrificed with…

… was (were) killed by decapitation / cervical dislocation / exsanguination.

To eliminate…, we filtered… We further filtered… Finally, sth. were inspected using… to confirm…

… were generated by…

7. 表达测定方法

… was(were) measured / determined / detected / evaluated / assessed / by using…

Assessment of experiments was carried out using analysis of…

Analyses were performed with…

… procedures were performed / carried out according to… techniques.

… was (were) histologically analyzed and morphometrically evaluated.

Primary / Secondary outcome measures were…

Information was obtained through…

… was (were) sorted / determined / estimated on the basis of / according to…

To remove / analyse / validate…, we used…

Using…,… were identified…

Using… models, we assessed factors that influenced…

To ensure that…, we visually inspected…

… were applied to identify…

8. 表达统计学分析

… was used to determine the statistical significance of differences between groups.

Data were analyzed with…

All statistical analyses were performed / accomplished with the use of / using…

We used logistic regression analysis to identify…

The level of significance for all outcome was 0.5.

Statistical analysis was performed by… test, and statistical significance was defined as $P<0.05$.

We analyzed data, with a 5% significance level.

P values were judged significant if they were less than 0.05.

The categorical variables were described as…

All the variables with p < … in … analysis were selected for … in the multivariate analysis.

Multiple linear regression (forward) was applied for…

The data were adjusted for…

The continuous variables were described by the means and standard deviations (SDs) or medians and interquartile ranges.

6.4.5 方法示例

例18

Methods

Mice

K14-H2BGFP[21] and *K14-actinGFP*[43] mice were obtained from Elaine Fuchs (Rockefeller University). TetO-Cre[44] mice were obtained from Katerina Politi (Yale). *K14-rtTA*[45], *tetO-Cdkn1b*[46], *Rac1*[-/-28], *Rosa-stop-tdTomato*[47], *Rosa-mTomato-stop-mGFP* (*mTmG*)[48] and *K14-CreER*[49] mice were obtained from Jackson Laboratories. *K14-H2BPAmCherry* mice were generated by the Yale Transgenic Facility[28]. For the photo-activation experiment, *K14-H2BPAmCherry* mice were mated with *K14-actinGFP* mice to visualize the structure of the epidermis (*K14-H2BPAmCherry*; *K14-actinGFP*). For the migration inhibition experiment, *K14-CreER*; *Rac1*[-/-]; *tdTomato*; *K14-H2BGFP* were generated. To block the migration of epithelial cells, three intraperitoneal injections of tamoxifen (100 mg/kg in corn oil) at postnatal day 10, 12 and 14. Inhibition of migration was monitored by time-lapse imaging via two-photon laser scanning microscopy described below. *K14-CreER*; *Rac1*[+/-]; *tdTomato*; *K14-H2BGFP* mice were used as controls.

译文：

方法

小鼠

K14-H2BGFP 和 *K14-actinGFP* 小鼠由洛克菲勒大学的 Elaine Fuchs 教授提供。TetO-Cre 小鼠由耶鲁大学的 Katerina Politi 教授提供。*K14-rtTA*, *tetO-Cdkn1b*, *Rac1*[-/-28], *Rosa-stop-tdTomato*, *Rosa-mTomato-stop-mGFP* (*mTmG*) 和 *K14-CreER* 小鼠均由杰克逊实验室提供。*K14-H2BPAmCherry* 小鼠由耶鲁转基因实验室提供。为了光激活实验，将 *K14-H2BPAmCherry* 小鼠与 *K14-actinGFP* 小鼠交配以可视化上皮结构（*K14-H2BPAmCherry*; *K14-actinGFP*）。制备的 *K14-CreER*; *Rac1*[-/-]; *tdTomato*; *K14-H2BGFP* 用于迁移抑制实验。为了阻止上皮细胞的迁移，小鼠出生后分别于第 10、12 和 14 天腹腔内注射他莫昔芬（100 mg/kg，溶剂为玉米油）为监测细胞迁移的抑制，用双光子激光扫描显微镜（如下文所述）进行延时成像。取 *K14-CreER*; *Rac1*[+/-]; *tdTomato*; *K14-H2BGFP* 小鼠作对照组。

For the proliferation inhibition experiment, *K14-rtTA*; *tetO-Cdkn1b*; *tetO-Cre*; *Rosa-*

stop-tdTomato；*K14-H2BGFP* were generated. To block the proliferation of epithelial cells, these mice were given doxycycicline（1 mg/ml）in potable water with 1% sucrose starting 1 day before the punch biopsy. Doxycycline treatment was sustained until imaging was performed. tdTomato signal was used to monitor Cre activation. Inhibition of proliferation was monitored by time-lapse imaging via two-photon laser scanning microscopy described below. *K14-rtTA*；*tetO-Cre*；*Rosa-stop-tdTomato*；*K14-H2BGFP* mice were used as controls.

制备 *K14-rtTA*；*tetO-Cdkn1b*；*tetO-Cre*；*Rosa-stop-tdTomato*；*K14-H2BGFP* 用于增殖抑制实验。为了阻断上皮细胞的增殖，强力霉素（1 mg/ml）溶于含1%蔗糖的饮用水，灌注小鼠，第二天进行穿刺活检。持续使用强力霉素直至显像。tdTomato 信号用于监测 Cre 的激活。为监测增殖的抑制，用双光子激光扫描显微镜（如下文所述）进行延时成像。选用 *K14-rtTA*；*tetO-Cre*；*Rosa-stop-tdTomato*；*K14-H2BGFP* 小鼠作为对照组。

For cell membrane labeling experiments, Cre expression was induced with a single intraperitoneal injection of tamoxifen（1 mg/kg in corn oil）at postnatal day 21 in *K14-CreER*；*mTmG* mice. Mice from experimental and control groups were randomly selected of either gender for live imaging experiments. No blinding was done. All procedures involving animal subjects were performed under the approval of the Institutional Animal Care and Use Committee（IACUC）of the Yale School of Medicine.

细胞膜标记实验中，*K14-CreER*；*mTmG* 小鼠于出生后第 21 天腹腔内单次注射他莫昔芬（1 mg/kg；溶剂为玉米油）以诱导 Cre 的表达。从实验组和对照组中随机选择任意性别的小鼠进行实时成像。没有设盲。所有动物处理程序均获得耶鲁医学院的研究所实验动物管理委员会（IACUC）的批准。

Antibodies and reagents

Mitomycin C（MMC）was purchased from Research Products International Corp（M92010）, Colcemid from Sigma（D7385-5MG）, rabbit polyclonal anti-keratin 10 from Biolegend/Covance（PRB-159P, used at 1∶1000）, rabbit polyclonal anti-keratin 5 from Biolegend/Covance（PRB-160P, used at 1∶1000）, donkey anti-rabbit Rhodamine Red-X from Jackson Lab（711-295-152, used at 1∶100）and donkey anti-rabbit Alexa 647 from ThermoFisher（A-31573, used at 1∶200）.

抗体和试剂

丝裂霉素 C（MMC）购自 Research Products International Corp 公司（M92010）；秋水仙胺（Colcemid）购自 Sigma 集团（D7385-5MG）；兔抗 KRT10 多克隆抗体购自 Biolegend/Covance 公司（PRB-159P, 1∶1000 使用）；兔抗 KRT5 多克隆抗体购自 Biolegend/Covance 公司（PRB-160P, 1∶1000 使用）；RRX 标记驴抗兔抗体购自 Jackson 实验室（711-295-152, 1∶100 使用）；Alexa 647 标记驴抗兔抗体购自 ThermoFisher 公司（A-31573, 1∶200 使用）。

Wounding

Three-week-old mice were anesthetized by intraperitoneal injection of ketamine and xylazine cocktail mix (100 mg / kg and 10 mg / kg, respectively in phosphate-buffered saline). Once a surgical plane of anesthesia was verified by the absence of a physical and physiologic response to a noxious stimulus, a punch biopsy was performed using a 1 mm diameter punch biopsy tool (Miltex, USA). The punch biopsy tool was used to make a circular full thickness wound on the dorsal side of mouse ear. Wounds did not penetrate the ear and remained above the cartilage. The ear is chosen as a convenient region for imaging and for its similarity with respect to epithelial functions to other regions of mouse skin[50,51]. Dermal components such as cartilage are however different from back skin.

建立伤口

选 3 周龄小鼠,腹腔内注射氯胺酮和甲苯噻嗪混合物(磷酸盐缓冲液中分别含 100 mg / kg 和 10 mg / kg)进行麻醉。若对有害刺激物的物理和生理反应消失则判定动物处于麻醉状态,便可用直径 1 mm 的打孔活检工具(Miltex,美国)进行活检。用该工具在小鼠耳背面形成全层皮肤缺损的圆形伤口。伤口未贯穿耳朵,仅止于软骨层上方。选择耳部进行活检是因为耳部区域不仅方便成像而且其上皮功能与小鼠其他区域皮肤相似;然而,真皮部分(如软骨)不同于背部皮肤。

In vivo imaging

Mice were anesthetized using an isofluorane chamber and anesthesia was maintained throughout the course of the experiment with isofluorane delivered by a nose cone as previously described[52,53]. Image stacks were acquired with a LaVision TriM Scope II (LaVision Biotec, Germany) laser scanning microscope equipped with a tunable Two-photon Chameleon Ultra (Coherent, USA) Ti:Sapphire laser. To acquire serial optical sections, a laser beam (940 nm for H2BGFP, actinGFP and mTmG; 1040 nm for H2BPAmCherry and tdTomato) was focused through a 20X or 40X water immersion lens (N.A.1.0 and 1.1 respectively; Zeiss, USA) and scanned with a field of view of 0.5×0.5 mm^2 or 0.25×0.25 mm^2 respectively at 600 Hz. Z-stacks were acquired in $1 \sim 3$ μm steps to image a total depth of 200 μm of tissue[52]. To visualize large areas, $3 \sim 36$ tiles of optical fields were imaged using a motorized stage to automatically acquire sequential fields of view as previously described[54]. For time-lapse imaging, serial optical sections were obtained in a range of 1 to 12 minute intervals depending on the experimental setup. The duration of time-lapse imaging ranged from 4-12 hours.

体内成像

用异氟烷麻醉舱麻醉小鼠。如之前所述,在整个实验过程中用鼻锥吸入异氟烷蒸气以保持麻醉状态。使用现有可调谐双光子 Chameleon Ultra(Coherent,美国)Ti:Sapphire 激光器的激光扫描显微镜 LaVision TriM Scope II(LaVision Biotec,德国)采集图像堆栈。为了获取连续的光学成像,采用不同波长的激光束(H2BGFP,actinGFP 和 mTmG 采用 940 nm;H2BPAmCherry 和 tdTomato 采用 1040 nm)通过 20 倍或 40 倍浸没物镜(分别为 NA 1.0 和 1.1;Zeiss,美国)观察成像,并在 600 Hz 时以 0.5×0.5 mm^2 或 0.25×0.25 mm^2

的视场进行扫描。Z 堆栈以 1~3 μm 的步长采集,以形成总深度 200 μm 的组织成像。为了可视化大面积区域,如前所述,使用电动载物台对 3~36 片光场进行成像,以自动获取连续的视场。根据实验装置,对 1~12 分钟各间隔获取的连续光学切片进行延时成像。延时成像的持续时间为 4~12 小时。

Photo-activation

Photo-activation in *K14-H2BPAmCherry* mice was carried out with the same optical equipment used for image acquisition. An 810 nm laser beam at 5% laser power was used for 1 minute to scan the target area (100×100 mm^2) and activate the PAmCherry protein.

光激活

K14-H2BPAmCherry 小鼠的光激活与图像采集由同一台光学设备完成。在 5% 激光功率下用 810 nm 激光束扫描目标区域 (100×100 mm^2) 1 分钟并激活 PAmCherry 蛋白。

Topical drug treatment

To inhibit cell proliferation in the epidermis, Mitomycin C (MMC)[55] was delivered topically by applying it to the wound and the surrounding ear skin. MMC was dissolved in a 15 mg / ml stock solution in dimethyl sulfoxide (DMSO) and later the stock solution was diluted 100 times in 100% petroleum jelly (Vaseline; final concentration is 150 μg / ml). 100 mg of the mixture of the MMC and the petroleum jelly was spread evenly on the wounded area at 1 and 2 days PWI (post wound induction). A mixture of 100% DMSO in petroleum jelly (1 : 100) was used as a vehicle control. Colcemid was used to block microtubule polymerization[56,57]. Colcemid was dissolved to 25 mg / ml stock solution in the DMSO and delivered as described for the MMC treatment.

局部用药

为了抑制表皮细胞增殖,将丝裂霉素 C (MMC) 局部涂抹于耳部伤口以及周围皮肤处。将 MMC 溶解于含二甲亚砜 (DMSO) 的储备溶液中 (15 mg / ml),然后将储备溶液在 100% 凡士林 (最终浓度:150 μg / ml) 中稀释 100 倍。伤口形成后第 1 天和第 2 天,将 100 mg MMC 和凡士林的混合物均匀地涂抹在伤口上。100% DMSO 与凡士林的混合物 (1:100) 用于溶剂对照组。秋水仙胺用于阻止微管聚合。将秋水仙胺溶于含 DMSO 的储备溶液中 (25 mg / ml),并按照 MMC 治疗中描述的方法使用。

Image Analysis

Raw image stacks were imported into Fiji (NIH, USA) or Imaris software (Bitplane / Perkin Elmer) for further analysis. Imaris software was used to track cells and obtain xyz coordinates from individual tracked cells over time. All cell tracks were individually examined to confirm that they reported the behavior of a single cell. Only cells that could be tracked for the full duration of a movie were included in the final analysis. For the wound, a surface was manually defined in Imaris by the absence of cells within the wound area at the beginning of each movie. Imaris' distance transformation module from their X Tensions library was then utilized to determine the starting distance of each track from the wound's surface.

图像分析

将原始图像堆栈导入到 Fiji（NIH，美国）或 Imaris 软件（Bitplane/Perkin Elmer）中进一步分析。使用 Imaris 软件持续追踪细胞并获取其 xyz 三维坐标。分别检查所有的细胞轨迹，以确认它们显示了每个细胞的行迹。最终分析仅针对在整个追踪过程中都可拍摄到的细胞。每次拍摄开始时，将缺失细胞的伤口区域在 Imaris 中手动定义为伤口表面。然后，利用 X Tensions 库中的 Imaris 距离转换模块来确定每个轨迹距伤口表面的起始距离。

Prism software（Graphpad）was used to graph the data and to calculate non-linear trend-line（exponential growth equation, weight by $1/Y^2$）for a WT movie（Fig.3a）. To quantify migration in vehicle and drug-treated mice, migrating cells were isolated by track straightness（track length/track displacement）> 0.3 and binned every 100 μm from the wound. The bin calculated means were used to yield trend-lines（Fig.1h and 5b）. For the tracking of photolabeled H2BPAmCherry cells, an artificial surface was created using second-harmonic generation（SHG）from fibrillar collagens and the interface with the K14-actinGFP positive epithelial cells.

Prism 软件（Graphpad 绘图工具）用于绘制数据并计算 WT 视频的非线性趋势线（指数增长方程，权重系数为 $1/Y^2$）（图 3a）。为了定量对照组和药物处理组小鼠中的细胞迁移，依据路径直线度（长度与位移之比）>0.3 分离出迁移细胞，细胞从伤口处每迁移 100 μm 则纳入统计，纳入统计的值取平均值用于生成趋势线。（图 1h 和 5b）。为了跟踪光标记的 H2BPAmCherry 细胞，我们将来自胶原纤维的二次谐波（SHG）与 K14-actinGFP 阳性上皮细胞界面来制备人工表面。

This interface roughly defines the basement membrane. From this basement membrane, H2BPAmCherry signal was identified using Imaris spot analysis, and used to determine the minimum distance from each spot to the basement membrane surface using the distance transformation module in Imaris XTensions. Day 3 labeling（where only basal layer cells are labeled）was then utilized at the later time points to determine cell permanence within the basal layer or their displacement into suprabasal layers. Provided images and supplementary videos are typically presented as a maximal projection of 3 to 6 μm optical sections, unless otherwise specified. For visualizing individual labeled cells expressing the H2BPAmCherry reporter, the brightness and contrast were adjusted accordingly for the green（GFP）and red（H2BPAmCherry）channels and composite serial image sequences were assembled as previously described[58]. The tiled images were stitched by a grid/collection stitching plugin in Fiji. Migrating cell tracking analysis and 3D reconstitution of photo-activated cells were performed in Imaris software.

这一界面可基本界定基底膜。基于该基底膜，用 Imaris 斑点分析识别出该膜中 H2BPAmCherry 信号，并用 Imaris X Tensions 中的距离转换模块确定每个斑点与基底膜表面的最短距离。在后面的时间点用 3 天标记法（仅标记基底层细胞）确定细胞是否停留在基底层内或移入基底上层。除非特殊标明,文中展示的图片和补充材料中的视频均采用最大投射 3~6 μm 的光学成像。为了可视化表达 H2BPAmCherry 报道基因的单个标记细胞,对绿色(GFP)和红色(H2BPAmCherry)通道的亮度和对比度进行了相应的调整,并如先前所述合成了复合系列图像序列。平铺图片由 Fiji 的网格/集合插件拼接而成。在 Imaris 软件中,完成迁移细胞路径跟踪分析和光激活细胞的 3D 重建。

Immunostaining

Frozen skin sections were fixed in 4% paraformaldehyde and used for histological analysis as previously described[59,60]. Immunofluorescence was performed by incubating sections at 4 ℃ overnight with primary antibodies: rabbit anti-keratin 10 (1:1000, Covance) and rabbit anti-keratin 5 (1:1000, Covance). One hour incubation at room temperature was then performed with secondary antibodies: donkey anti-rabbit Rhodamine Red-X (1:100, Jackson Lab) and donkey anti-rabbit Alexa 647 (1:200, Alexa Fluor). Two photon microscope or a Zeiss Axioimager was used to collect images.

免疫染色法

如前所述,将冷冻皮肤切片以 4% 多聚甲醛固定后进行组织学分析。用一抗[兔抗角蛋白 10(1:1000,Covance)和兔抗角蛋白 5(1:1000,Covance)]在 4 ℃孵化切片过夜后进行免疫荧光分析。然后室温下用二抗[驴抗兔罗丹明 Red-X(1:100,Jackson 实验室)和驴抗兔 Alexa 647(1:200,Alexa Fluor)]孵育 1 小时。用双光子显微镜或生物显微镜(Zeiss Axioimager)收集图像。

Quantitative characterization of tissue deformation

The tracking of cell nuclei over time made the measurement of local tissue deformation possible. Based on the profile of the average displacement toward the wound and distance to the basement membrane, we first estimated that nuclei belonging to the most basal layer of cells were in the range of 0-10 μm distance to the basement membrane. For each time point, we therefore selected the "basal nuclei" based on this threshold.

组织变形的定量表征

持续追踪细胞核可以测量局部组织的变形。根据向伤口的平均位移和距基底膜的距离,我们先估测出属于最基础细胞层的细胞核距基底膜距离在 0~10 μm 之间。因此,在每个时间点,我们都基于该阈值选择了"基础核"。

Then we aimed to characterize the deformation of the basal layer of cells based on nuclei displacements. To achieve this, we used a quantitative approach that was recently developed and validated, and which is based on the evolution of links connecting neighboring cell centroids[34]. Therefore, we first determined neighbor relationships between nuclei, which then enabled us to define the pairs of neighbor nuclei that will be connected with a link. To this end, in each image, we used the nuclei positions as generators to build a Voronoi tessellation that established neighbor relationships between nuclei and between their corresponding Voronoi regions. In each image, we defined the links joining the centers of neighboring Voronoi regions. Then, based on the tracking of nuclei, we could record the evolution of those links over time (Supplementary Fig. 6a-c).

　　然后，我们根据核位移来表征细胞基础层的变形。为此，我们使用了一种最近开发和验证的定量方法，该方法是基于相邻细胞中心的连接演变。因此，我们首先确定了细胞核间的相邻关系，以此定义连接的一对相邻细胞核。在每帧图像中，用细胞核的位置生成泰森多边形图（Voronoi tessellation），以确立细胞核之间及其对应的 Voronoi 区之间的相邻关系。在每帧图像中，我们定义相邻 Voronoi 区域中心的连接。然后，根据对细胞核的跟踪，我们可以记录随着时间推移这些连接的演变（见补充图 6a-c）。

To characterize tissue deformation across the tissue surrounding the wound and its spatial variations, we defined sub-regions in the tissue of about 80×80 μm^2 containing approximately 50 to 200 cells. The sub-region size was chosen so that it was large enough to contain many nuclei and links, ensuring accurate statistical measurements, but also small enough so that tissue deformations could be estimated at various locations across the tissue and that deformations within each sub-region remain rather homogeneous. The nuclei initially assigned to each sub-region were kept in the same sub-region deforming over time (Lagrangian approach). Then, we determined the local tissue deformation in each sub-region, the calculation of which was solely based on the change of geometry of links that were conserved in this region between two images[34].

　　为了表征伤口周围组织的变形及其空间变化，我们将 80×80 μm^2 左右大小，包含约 50 到 200 个细胞的组织定义为一个子区域。确定这一子区域面积是因为，一方面一个子区域足以包含诸多细胞核和连接，确保了统计测量的准确性；另一方面一个子区域可以用来评估整个组织各细小部位的变形，确保各子区域内的变形一致。最初分到每个子区域的细胞核在同一子区域中渐渐变形（拉格朗日法）。接下来，我们测定了各个子区域的局部组织形变，形变的计算仅仅依赖于在子区域里守恒的连接在几何上的变化。

Note that, if the contributions of cell behaviors to tissue deformation indeed depends on the actual cell network and requires the knowledge of actual cell geometries and topologies, this is not the case for tissue deformation that only involves the variation of conserved link geometry in the sub-region. Also, it is not sensitive to the type of tessellation chosen, as long as each sub-region contains enough conserved links between two successive images.

　　值得一提的是，如果细胞行为对组织变形的影响取决于实际的细胞网，并且需要有关细胞几何学和拓扑学的知识，那么就不适宜于仅涉及子区域中守恒连接在几何上变化的组织变形。同样，只要各子区域在两帧连续图像之间有足够保守的连接，对所选区面类型也不敏感。

Statistics and reproducibility

Data are expressed either as absolute numbers or percentages ± S. D. An unpaired Student's t-test was used to analyze data sets with two groups and [*] $p < 0.05$ to [****] $p < 0.000\ 1$

indicate a significant difference. Statistical calculations were performed using the Prism software package (GraphPad, USA). No statistical method was used to predetermine sample size. Panels showing representative images are representative of at least two independent experiments and up to five, as indicated in the figure legends. (Tissue-scale coordination of cellular behavior promotes epidermal wound repair in live mice, *Nature Cell Biology.*, 2017 Mar 1, 19 (2))

统计学分析与可重复性

数据表达为绝对数字或百分比±S.D.。用未配对 Student's *t* 检验分析两组数据,*p < 0.05 至 ****p<0.000 1 表明显著差异。用 Prism 软件包(GraphPad,美国)进行统计学计算。样本量没有使用统计学方法来预测。如图注所示,代表性图像的面板数据代表至少两个,最多五个独立实验。(组织水平的细胞行为协调促进活体小鼠的表皮伤口修复)

例19

Methods

Study design and patients

We did a phase 3, randomised, double-blind, placebo-controlled, two-centre trial. From March, 2009, to August, 2012, we recruited patients from Rady Children's Hospital San Diego, CA, USA, and Nationwide Children's Hospital in Columbus, OH, USA. Eligible participants were children aged 4 weeks-17 years with Kawasaki disease who had fever (≥38.0 ℃) for 3-10 days. The full inclusion criteria, as per the American Heart Association case definitions, and exclusion criteria are listed in the appendix. Because many children with Kawasaki disease are anergic to delayed-type hypersensitivity skin tests, all patients also had a chest radiograph within the week before infusion of study drug with no evidence of tuberculosis or other infection. The study protocol was reviewed and approved by the University of California San Diego's and Nationwide Children's Hospital's Institutional Review Boards. Written informed consent was obtained from the parents or legal guardians and assent, when appropriate, was obtained from the patient.

译文:

方法

试验设计与对象

本研究是一项 III 期、随机、双盲、安慰剂对照、双中心试验。2009 年 3 月至 2012 年 8 月,从美国加利福尼亚州圣地亚哥瑞迪儿童医院和美国俄亥俄州哥伦比亚国家儿童医院招募患者。合格的受试者是 4 周至 17 岁发热(≥38.0 ℃)3~10 天的川崎病患者。依据美国心脏病协会制定的纳入标准和排除标准详见附录。由于很多川崎病患儿对皮肤迟发型过敏试验无变应性,因此所有患者在注射研究药物前 1 周内拍胸片以排除患有结核或其他感染灶。研究方案由圣地亚哥加利福尼亚大学和国家儿童医院的审查委员会审核和批准。由患者父母或法定监护人签署书面知情同意书,并在可能的情况下,获得患者的同意。

Randomisation and masking

After validation of eligibility criteria, patients were randomly assigned to either the infliximab or placebo group in a 1 : 1 ratio. Randomisation was based on a randomly permuted block design with block sizes of two and four participants, stratified by age (< 1 year or ≥1 year), sex, and centre. Patients received either infliximab (5 mg / kg at 1 mg / ml intravenously over 2 h) or placebo (normal saline intravenously, 5 ml / kg). Patients, treating physicians and staff, study team members, and the echocardiographer were all masked to assignment. The placebo was similar in colour, volume, and manner of administration to the infliximab.

随机化和盲法

纳入标准确定后,将患者以 1∶1 的比例随机分入英夫利昔单抗组或安慰剂组。随机分组基于随机排列的区组设计,2~4 例参与者组成一个区组,按年龄 (< 1 岁或 ≥ 1 岁)、性别、和治疗中心分层。患者接受英夫利昔单抗 (5 mg / kg,1 mg / ml 静脉注射 2 小时以上) 或安慰剂 (生理盐水 5 ml / kg,静脉注射)。患者、医护人员、研究人员及超声心动图检查者均不知晓治疗分组情况。安慰剂的颜色、容积及给药方式与英夫利昔单抗相似。

Procedures

After randomization, all patients received diphenhydramine (1 mg per kg intravenously, maximum 50 mg) and acetaminophen (15 mg per kg orally, maximum 650 mg) 30 min before receiving study drug. All patients received intravenous immunoglobulin (Gammagard [Baxter Pharmaceuticals, Westlake Village, CA, USA], 2 g per kg over 10-12h) immediately after administration of study drug. Aspirin (80-100 mg / kg per day divided every 6 h) was administered orally until the patient was discharged from the hospital when the dose was reduced to 3-5 mg / kg per day for the duration of the study, or longer if clinically indicated. The primary outcome measure, treatment resistance, was defined as a temperature of 38.0 ℃ or higher between 36 h and 7 days after completion of the intravenous immunoglobulin infusion without another likely source. Treatment-resistant children received a second infusion of intravenous immunoglobulin (2 g per kg). Patients who had persistent fever 24 h after the end of their second intravenous infusion without another likely source were treated at the discretion of the centre investigator.

步骤

随机分组之后,所有患者在接受研究药物 30 分钟之前使用苯海拉明 (1 mg / kg 静脉注射,最大剂量 50 mg) 和对乙酰氨基酚 (15 mg / kg 口服,最大剂量 650 mg)。所有患者在接受研究药物之后即刻接受免疫球蛋白静脉 (IVIG) 输注 [Gammagard (Baxter 制药,西湖村,加利福尼亚州,美国) 2 g / kg,10~12 小时以上]。口服阿司匹林[80~100 mg / (kg·d),每 6 小时一次],出院后减至 3~5 mg / (kg·d),根据临床指标持续应用于研究期间或更长时间。主要的结局指标为治疗抵抗,定义为 IVIG 输注治疗结束后 36 小时到 7 天,患者体温 ≥ 38.0 ℃,并排除其他可能的发热原因。治疗抵抗的儿童接受第二次 IVIG 输注 (2 g / kg)。

在第二次 IVIG 输注后持续发热 24 小时并除外其他可能发热原因的患者由各医疗中心的研究人员酌情治疗。

After completion of the intravenous immunoglobulin infusion, body temperatures were measured every 6 h before the aspirin dose by either the rectal or oral route with a digital thermometer. On discharge, the legal guardian recorded temperatures by the oral, rectal, or axillary route once a day for 3 days. The family was contacted by a study coordinator 3 days and 10 weeks after discharge to monitor the child's recovery.

完成 IVIG 输注后, 阿司匹林给药前用电子温度计每 6 小时测量一次肛温或口腔温度。出院后, 由法定监护人记录口腔温度、肛温或腋温, 每日 1 次, 共记录 3 天。出院后 3 天至 10 周内, 由研究协调员随访患者家人以监测患儿的恢复情况。

Secondary outcome measures were: Z_{max} (largest of the blinded, single-observer, echocardiographic measurements of the internal diameter normalised for body surface area of the proximal right coronary artery and left anterior descending coronary artery at weeks 2 and 5 after treatment) and change in Z score from baseline to weeks 2 and 5; change in concentrations of age-adjusted haemoglobin, C-reactive protein, alanine transaminase, albumin, and γ-glutamyl transferase; change in erythrocyte sedimentation rate, platelet count, white blood cell count, and absolute cell counts; number of fever days (24 h period with a temperature of at least 38.0 ℃) from enrolment; duration of hospital stay; and intravenous immunoglobulin and infliximab infusion reactions.

次要结局指标:Z 最大值(治疗后第 2 周和第 5 周, 校正体表面积后, 由同一超声心动图测量者盲法测得的右冠状动脉近端和左冠状动脉前降支的最大内径值。) 及从基线至第 2 周和第 5 周 Z 值的变化;年龄校正的血红蛋白、C 反应蛋白、丙氨酸氨基转移酶、白蛋白和 γ 谷氨酰转移酶浓度的变化;以及红细胞沉降率 (ESR)、血小板计数、白细胞计数和绝对细胞计数的变化;纳入后的发热天数(24 h 内体温≥38.0 ℃);住院时间;IVIG 输注和英夫利昔单抗输液反应。

We obtained laboratory data at baseline, 24 h after completion of the intravenous immunoglobulin infusion, and at week 2 (study day 14, or within 2 days beforehand or afterwards; Rady Children's Hospital site only) and week 5 (study day 35, or within 2 days beforehand or afterwards) after randomisation. Echocardiograms were obtained during the initial hospitalisation and at the week 2 and 5 visits. Patients younger than 3 years were sedated with chloral hydrate (75 mg/kg per dose orally, maximum 1 g) for the chocardiogram. An echocardiographer (BFP) interpreted all echocardiograms across both centres and reported coronary artery dimensions as Z cores. Patients were classified as having normal (Z score <2.5), dilated (Z score ≥2.5), or aneurysmal (focal dilation of an arterial segment≥1.5 times the diameter of the adjacent segment) coronary arteries based on the maximum internal diameters of the proximal right coronary artery or left anterior descending coronary artery.

基线时、IVIG 输注后 24 h、随机分组后第 2 周（研究的第 14 天或提前及推后 2 天内；仅在瑞迪儿童医院站点）和第 5 周（研究的第 35 天或提前及推后 2 天内）收集实验室检查数据。入院时和第 2 周、第 5 周随访时检查超声心动图。3 岁以下患儿采用水合氯醛镇静 [75 mg／(kg·次)，口服，最大剂量不超过 1 g] 进行超声心动图检查。一名超声心动图测量者（BFP）负责解读两家医疗中心所有超声心动图，并以 Z 值报告冠状动脉内径。根据右冠状动脉近端或左冠状动脉前降支的最大内径将患者划分为冠状动脉正常（Z 值<2.5）、冠状动脉扩张（Z 值≥2.5）或冠状动脉瘤（冠状动脉扩张内径≥1.5 倍相邻段内径）。

An intravenous immunoglobulin infusion reaction was defined as fever with chills or hypotension for age that warranted interruption of the intravenous immunoglobulin infusion. A data and safety monitoring board reviewed safety data after enrolment of 25, 50, and 100 patients.

IVIG 输注反应定义为发热伴寒战；或出现需要及时中断 IVIG 输注的年龄校正的低血压。数据和安全监测委员会分别在纳入 25 例、50 例和 100 例患者后多次评估安全数据。

Statistical analyses

To have 80% power to detect a reduction in treatment resistance from 20% to 5%, with a two-sided α of 0.048 and an attrition rate of 10%, based on a two-sample binomial test for proportions, the study required 196 participants. The data and safety monitoring board did an interim analysis for efficacy (with a threshold of 0.002) after 100 participants were enrolled.

统计学分析

研究纳入 196 例受试者，分析基于双样本二项分布检验，检测出治疗抵抗从 20% 降至 5% 的效能为 80%，双侧 α 值为 0.048，失访率为 10%。数据和安全监测委员会在纳入 100 例受试者后进行了一项中期疗效分析（临界值 0.002）。

The primary outcome was analysed on the basis of a modified intent-to-treat population, which was defined as all the randomised patients who received study drug (98 infliximab and 97 placebo). The primary analysis used a logistic regression model to compare the resistance rates between groups adjusting for illness days (illness day 1 = first day of fever), alanine transaminase, γ-glutamyl transferase, age-adjusted haemoglobin, and percent bands at baseline, previously identified as predictors of intravenous immunoglobulin resistance. For the secondary outcome measure of coronary artery internal dimension, a linear regression model was used to compare Zmax between treatment groups, adjusted for the same covariates as in the primary analysis. Change in Z scores from baseline for the left main coronary artery and proximal right coronary artery and left anterior descending coronary artery at week 2 and week 5 were analysed with mixed model repeated measures. The time point was treated as a categorical variable and an unstructured variance covariance error matrix was applied. The laboratory values that were secondary outcome measures were assessed at several timepoints. If the parameter was measured at more than two timepoints, similar mixed model analysis as described above was done. If the parameter was measured only at two timepoints, an ANCOVA model was used to assess the difference between the treatment groups in change score, with adjustment for the baseline measure. Intravenous immunoglobulin infusion reaction rates were compared between groups with Fisher's exact test. Duration of hospital stay and number of fever days were analysed with the Wilcoxon rank sum test. Safety data were summarised by treatment groups and overall. Fisher's exact test was used to compare the number of patients who experienced any adverse events between the groups. A p value of less than 0.05 was considered statistically significant for secondary measures. No adjustments were made for multiple comparisons. Statistical analyses were done in R, version 2.14.0.

主要结局基于改良的意向治疗人群,定义为所有随机接受研究药物的患者(98 例英夫利昔单抗组患者和 97 例安慰剂组患者)。使用 logistic 回归分析模型完成主要结局分析,按之前定义的 IVIG 抵抗的预测指标比较两组的治疗抵抗率,包括校正的发病时间(发病时间 1 = 发热第 1 天)、丙氨酸氨基转移酶、γ 谷氨酰转移酶、年龄校正的血红蛋白浓度,以及基线中性粒细胞带状百分比。次要结局指标为冠状动脉内径,用线性回归模型比较治疗组间 Z 最大值,校正为与主要结局分析时相同的协变量。用重复测量混合模型分析第 2 周和第 5 周时左冠状动脉主干和右冠状动脉近端及左冠状动脉前降支 Z 值较基线值的改变。时间点作为一个分类变量,应用非结构化的误差协方差矩阵。实验室数据作为次要结局,在不同的时间点进行评估。如果在多于两个时间点检测某参数,则应用上述的类似混合模型分析。如果只在两个时间点衡量某参数,则采用 ANCOVA 分析模型并校正基线指标来评估治疗组间数值变化的差异。两组间 IVIG 药物不良反应率用 Fisher 确切概率法比较。住院时间和发热天数采用 Wilcoxon 秩和检验来分析。对各治疗组和全部参与者的安全数据进行总结。用 Fisher 确切概率法比较两组出现不良事件的患者数量。比较次要结局时,P 值<0.05 被认为具有统计学意义。对于多重比较未进行校正。应用 R 2.14.0 版本进行统计学分析。

This study is registered with ClinicalTrials.gov, number NCT00760435.

本项试验已在 ClinicalTrials.gov 上注册,注册编号 NCT00760435。

Role of the funding source

Grant support was provided by the US Food and Drug Administration and the Robert Wood Johnson Foundation. Janssen Biotech, the manufacturer of infliximab, provided commercial-grade drug for this study. The sponsors of this study had no role in the study design, data collection and analysis, or decision to submit for publication. Janssen Biotech reviewed the manuscript and suggested changes, but the final decision on content was retained exclusively by the authors.

(Infliximab for intensification of primary therapy for Kawasaki disease: a phase 3 randomised, double-blind, placebo-controlled trial, *Lancet.*, 2014 Feb 24, 383)

基金来源

本研究由美国食品药品监督管理局和罗伯特·伍德·约翰逊基金会提供拨款支持。强生生物技术公司作为英夫利昔单抗的生产商,为本研究提供商业用药。研究赞助者未参与试验设计、数据收集和数据分析,或论文提交与发表的决定。强生生物技术公司审核原稿并建议修改,但内容的最终决定权完全由作者保留。

（英夫利昔单抗用于川崎病的初始强化治疗：一项 3 期、随机、双盲、安慰剂对照试验）

Exercise

1. Read the samples of "Methods" and analyze their contents and structures. Recognize the signal markers and sentence patterns to realize these contents. Note the use of tenses for different contents in the writing.

2. Translate the following sentences in the "Methods" into English.

1）在一项多中心、随机对照、开放标签试验中,我们使用了相同的方法和设计来评估同样的干预措施,即使用低分子量肝素进行抗凝剂治疗（anticoagulant therapy with low-molecular-weight heparin）。研究方案（可在线阅读：NEJM.org）和试验设计均得到莱顿大学医学中心（Leiden University Medical Center）医学伦理委员会的批准。试验由荷兰健康研究中心资助。

2）本研究参与者是通过当地报纸刊登广告以及在商场现场招募方式征集。纳入标准为 18 ～ 60 岁,全职工作,未患流感并发症的高危病症,如慢性心肺病（chronic cardiopulmonary disease）、糖尿病或其他严重病症。排除标准包括有鸡蛋和硫柳汞（thimerosal）速发型超敏反应史（immediate hypersensitivity reactions）,或有流感疫苗接种史。本研究获得所有受试者的知情同意。

3）本实验研究中,从伊朗 Razi 研究所获得 20 只,平均体重 2.5 kg 的雄性新西兰白兔。25±1 ℃室内饲养白兔,12 / 12 小时明暗周期。将兔置于兔笼,自由进食和饮水。所有步骤和实验测试均获 Shahid Beheshti 医科大学动物伦理委员会批准。

4）纳入患者以 1：1 的比例随机分组,分别接受标准药物化疗或安慰剂治疗。治疗药物为柔红霉素 daunorubicin（每日 60 mg / m^2,在第 1、2 和 3 日静脉给药）和阿糖胞苷 cytarabine（每日 200 mg / m^2,从第 1 至第 7 日连续静脉给药）。米哚妥林（Mildotolin）或安慰剂在第 8 日至第 21 日以双盲方式给药（50 mg,每日口服 2 次）。

5）使用兔胰岛素 ELISA 试剂盒（rabbit insulin ELISA kit）测量培养基中的胰岛素水平。首先用 Krebs-Ringer 缓冲液在 37 ℃下预孵育（pre-incubate）细胞 2 小时。然后用含有不同剂量葡萄糖（0、15 和 30 mM）的 Krebs-Ringer 缓冲液在 37 ℃孵育细胞 1 小时。最后,收集培养基并进行评估。

6）将雄性 Wistar 大鼠（240～300 g,8 周龄）随机分为两组：对照组（非糖尿病组）以标准食谱喂养（n = 6）;糖尿病组以高热量食谱喂养,包含 20 kcal %蛋白质,25 kcal %碳水化合物和 45 kcal %脂肪（n = 18）。14 天后,将链脲佐菌素（STZ；Sigma-AldrichCo., StLouis, MO, USA）注入糖尿病组大鼠的尾静脉（35 mg / kg）以诱导 2 型糖尿病。非糖尿病组大鼠口服复方溶剂（compound vehicle）,即苄醇（benzylalcohol）、聚山梨酯 80（polysorbate80）、EDTA 二钠（disodium EDTA）、羟乙基纤维素（hydroxyethyl cellulose）和水的混合物。

6.5 结果

6.5.1 结果的功能

结果（Results）部分是研究论文的核心（core），代表着论文的学术科研水平或技术创新的程度。写作时应按照逻辑顺序在正文和图表中合理准确地阐明研究、试验、调查等所获得的客观、真实的结果。该部分不包括作者对结果的评述，写作时应注意结果和结论部分在内容和表达方式上不同。

6.5.2 结果的结构

结果部分没有固定的结构，叙述的顺序取决于实验的目的和设计，可以按时间顺序或从最重要结果到次重要结果的顺序写作。不同期刊的具体要求也有所不同，如 *Cell*，*Nature* 规定采用小标题以更有序地呈现结果，而 *Lancet* 明确规定结果部分不使用小标题。

Cell 对于小标题的使用明确指出：We encourage subtitle like *Factor X requires Factor Y to function in Process Z* rather than *Analysis of Factors X and Y using Approach Q.* 所以小标题要尽量详尽，而不是笼统概括。例如：

Cell

Results

NCCs, but Not Macrophages, Colonize the Trunk during Early Development

NCCs Migrate away from Their Segmental Stream of Origin to Engulf Cellular Debris

Engulfing NCCs Have Distinct Migratory Patterns but Are Not Lineage Restricted

NCCs Form PI (3) P + and Lamp1 + Phagosomes after Engulfment

Cell Ablation Induces NCC Phagocytosis

NCCs and Macrophages Clear Debris during Distinct Developmental Stages

NCCs Migrate into the Spinal Cord and Clear CNS Debris

Il-1β Recruits NCCs to Debris after Damage

Cell

Results

Mutational Dataset and Driver Gene Identification Power

Landscape of Cancer Driver Genes

Approaches to Driver Mutation Discovery

Functionally Validated Mutations Confirm Structure-Based Analysis

Hypermutated Phenotypes and Immune Infiltrates

Therapeutic Implications of Molecular Events

BMJ

Results

Baseline characteristics

Adherence

n-3 LCPUFA supplementation and BMI development during childhood

n-3 LCPUFA supplementation and body composition

Maternal FADS genotype and BMI development during childhood

6.5.3　结果的内容

6.5.3.1　结果和数据

结果部分的主要内容为结果。叙述结果不必面面俱到，而是列出与"引言"中提出的问题相关的结果，即支持或不支持假设的结果。在写作结果部分时，应注意数据、数字和结果的区别。数字，英文为 number 或 figure，是实验时的原始记录，也称为原始数据（raw data）；数字或原始数据经过计算（calculating）或加工处理（processing）后成为"数据"（processed data）；而结果表达的是建立在数字和数据基础上的信息（message）。写作时，要特别注意区分数据和结果，以准确有效地传递信息。

例1

数据而非结果

In the 20 control subjects, the mean resting blood pressure was 85±5（SD）mmHg. In comparison, in the 30 tennis players, the mean resting blood pressure was 94±3（SD）mmHg.

说明：这个句子仅叙述了两个比较组中平均静息血压值，即数据，然而这两个数据传递的信息，即结果（两组间的这两个值相似还是不同）并不一目了然。

译文：20 例对照者的平均静息血压为 85±5（SD）mmHg，而 30 名网球选手的平均静息血压为 94±3（SD）mmHg。

例2

结果

The mean resting blood pressure was higher in the 30 tennis players than in the 20 control subjects［94±3（SD）vs. 85±5（SD）mmHg, P<0.02］.

说明：这个句子中的信息，即结果，表达清楚：30 名网球选手的平均静息血压值高于 20 例对照者。为了强调结果，将结果在正文中阐述，而数据置于括号内。

译文：30 名网球选手的平均静息血压值高于 20 例对照者［94±3（SD）vs. 85±5（SD）mmHg, P<0.02］。

例3

结果及差异的量值

The mean resting blood pressure was 10% higher in the 30 tennis players than in the 20 control subjects [94±3（SD）vs. 85±5（SD）mmHg, P<0.02].

说明：为了进一步准确表达结果，表明两组血压值的准确差异，此句中用百分比表示差异的量值（magnitude）。

译文：30名网球选手的平均静息血压值比20例对照者高10%[94±3（SD）vs. 85±5（SD）mmHg, P<0.02]。

6.5.3.2 示意图、插图、表格等

结果的表达除了使用文字以外，还应尽量按照具体期刊的要求多运用表图叙述的方式。表格与插图（table and illustration）是生物医学论文写作的一种重要表达形式，可以起到形象直观、简明扼要、一目了然的作用，具有用文字叙述难以达到的效果（注意：无需在正文中重复图表中的所有数据，仅需强调或概述最重要的观察结果）。如果表格中的项目很多，可用线图代替；图与表的数据不能重复。

例4

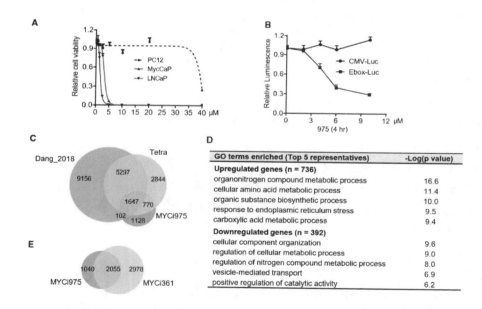

Figure 7. 975 Selectively Inhibits MYC-Dependent Cancer Cell Viability and the MYC Transcriptional Program
(A) Anti-proliferative effects of 975 on prostate cancer cells and PC12 following 5 days of treatment.
(B) Dose-response effect of 975 on MYC transcriptional activity in E-box luciferase reporter assay compared with CMV luciferase reporter.
(C) Venn diagram showing overlap of genes regulated in P493-6 cells by: (1) silencing MYC by Tetra 0.1 μg/mL for 48 h, log fold change >0.5 from Dang (2018); (2) silencing MYC by Tetra, 0.1 μg/mL for 24 h, adj-p <0.05, this study; and (3) 975 treatment at 6 μM for 24 h, adj-p < 0.05, from this study.
(D) GO biological process analysis on 975 uniquely regulated genes (1,128) in P493-6 cells.
(E) Venn diagram showing overlap of genes regulated by 361 (6 μM, 24 h) and 975 (8 μM, 24 h) treatment of PC3 cells from RNA-seq. Genes with adj-p < 0.05, and log fold change >0.5 were included.
Error bars represent mean ± SEM, n = 4 replicates in (A and B), data are representative of 2 to 3 independent experiments with similar results. RNA-seq data were assessed in triplicates (C–E).
See also Tables S3 and S4.

例5

Table 2　Primary and secondary endpoints according to the intention-to-treat analysis

	Endoscopic step-up approach (n=51)	Surgical step-up approach (n=47)	Relative risk (95% CI)	p value
Primary endpoint				
Major complications or death*	22 (43%)	21 (45%)	0·97 (0·62–1·51)	0·88
Secondary endpoints				
New-onset organ failure†				
Pulmonary	4 (8%)	7 (15%)	0·53 (0·16–1·68)	0·27
Persistent pulmonary	4 (8%)	5 (11%)	0·74 (0·21–2·58)	0·63
Cardiovascular	3 (6%)	9 (19%)	0·31 (0·09–1·07)	0·045
Persistent cardiovascular	2 (4%)	8 (17%)	0·23 (0·05–1·03)	0·032
Renal	2 (4%)	6 (13%)	0·31 (0·07–1·45)	0·11
Persistent renal	2 (4%)	6 (13%)	0·31 (0·07–1·45)	0·11
Single organ failure	7 (14%)	13 (28%)	0·50 (0·22–1·14)	0·087
Persistent single organ failure	6 (12%)	11 (23%)	0·50 (0·20–1·25)	0·13
Multiple organ failure	2 (4%)	6 (13%)	0·31 (0·07–1·45)	0·11
Persistent multiple organ failure	2 (4%)	5 (11%)	0·37 (0·08–1·81)	0·20
Bleeding (requiring intervention)	11 (22%)	10 (21%)	1·01 (0·47–2·17)	0·97
Perforation of a visceral organ or enterocutaneous fistula (requiring intervention)	4 (8%)	8 (17%)	0·46 (0·15–1·43)	0·17
Incisional hernia	0	1 (2%)	··	0·30
Death	9 (18%)	6 (13%)	1·38 (0·53–3·59)	0·50
Other endpoints‡				
Pancreatic fistula	2/42 (5%)	13/41 (32%)	0·15 (0·04–0·62)	0·0011
Exocrine insufficiency				
Use of enzymes	16/42 (38%)	13/41 (32%)	1·20 (0·66–2·17)	0·54
Fecal elastase <200 mg/g	22/42 (52%)	19/41 (46%)	1·13 (0·73–1·75)	0·58
Steatorrhoea	6/42 (14%)	7/41 (17%)	0·84 (0·31–2·28)	0·73
Endocrine insufficiency	10/42 (24%)	9/41 (22%)	1·08 (0·49–2·39)	0·84
Biliary strictures	3 (6%)	3 (6%)	0·92 (0·20–4·34)	0·92
Wound infections	2 (4%)	3 (6%)	0·61 (0·11–3·52)	0·58

Continued

	Endoscopic step-up approach (n=51)	Surgical step-up approach (n=47)	Relative risk (95% CI)	p value
Median number of interventions§	3 (2–6)	4 (2–6)	..	0·35
Drainage procedures¶	1 (1–3)	3 (1–5)	..	0·0041
Necrosectomies‖	2 (1–4)	1 (1–1)	..	0·0004
Number of necrosectomies	..	..	..	0·0062
0	22 (43%)	24 (51%)	0·84 (0·55–1·29)	..
1	9 (18%)	18 (38%)	0·46 (0·23–0·92)	..
2	8 (16%)	3 (6%)	2·46 (0·69–8·72)	..
≥3	12 (24%)	2 (4%)	5·53 (1·31–23·42)	..
Additional percutaneous drainage in the endoscopy group	14 (27%)	..	..	..
Additional VARD procedure in the endoscopy group	2 (4%)	..	..	..
Additional endoscopic drainage in the surgical group	..	2 (4%)	..	..
Additional endoscopic necrosectomy in the surgical group	..	0	..	..
Days between first drainage and first necrosectomy				
Median (range)	10 (5–16)	23 (9–62)	..	0·013
Mean (SD)	14 (14)	33 (30)	..	
Days in ICU within 6 months of randomisation**				
Median (IQR)	0 (0–3)	2 (0–11)	..	..
Mean (SD)	13 (31)	13 (21)	..	0·31
Days in hospital within 6 months of randomisation				
Median (IQR)	35 (19–85)	65 (40–90)	..	..
Mean (SD)	53 (47)	69 (38)	..	0·014

Data are n (%), mean (SD), or median (IQR) unless otherwise stated. Relative risk is reported for dichotomous variables for the endoscopic step-up approach as compared with the surgical step-up approach. ICU=intensive care unit. VARD=video-assisted retroperitoneal debridement. *Multiple events in the same patient were considered as one endpoint. †Organ failure occurring after randomisation and not present 24 h before randomisation. ‡Patients were assessed 6 months after randomisation; patient deaths were excluded. §This category included all drainage procedures (endoscopic or percutaneous) and necrosectomies (endoscopic or VARD) as part of the endoscopic or surgical step-up approach. ¶This category included primary drainage procedures (endoscopic or percutaneous) as part of the endoscopic or surgical step-up approach and additional drainage procedures before and after necrosectomy in both treatment groups. ‖This category included all necrosectomies (endoscopic or VARD procedure) as part of the endoscopic or surgical step-up approach. **For patients not present in ICU 24 h before randomisation.

1. 图表标题

图表的标题应简明扼要、清楚正确地总结表的内容。书写英文标题时根据拟投稿杂志的要求，通常有三种形式：一是首词的第一个字母大写，其他首字母小写；二是每个词的第一个字母大写，其中虚词要小写；三是标题中的所有字母均大写。可采用一般现在时的句子（如例 4）或短语（如例 5）形式呈现。若图表中包含多种形式，如饼状图、线型图、曲线图等（如例 4），则还应给出各小图具体的小标题。

2. 栏目

栏目（column）包括表中列举的所有表目（headings），需要时还包括子表目（subheadings）和测量单位（units of measurement）。表目分为横表目和纵表目。横表目位于表的左边，表示研究对象或研究内容，可能还设总表目；纵表目位于表的右边，说明各统计指标的含义。在描述测量单位时，长度、高度、质量和体积的测量值应采用公制单位（米、千克、升）或其十进倍数和分数单位表述。温度的单位应该用摄氏度。血压的单位应该用毫米汞柱，除非期刊特别要求使用其他单位。报告血液学和临床生化指标以及其他一些测量值，须参阅拟投稿期刊的须知，同时用当地单位和国际单位制（International System of Units，SI）单位报告实验室检测信息。

如例 5 中纵表目的总表目：主要终点、次要终点、其他终点和就医情况；纵表目：主要并发症或死亡、新出现的器官衰竭、出血，等等；横表目：内窥镜阶梯式治疗、外科阶梯式手术治疗、相对风险和 P 值。英文栏目名多用名词或介词结构表达，首词的第一个字母或每个词的第一个字母大写，虚词小写。

3. 正文

表内横表目通常应为研究的自变量，纵表目为因变量。如果是以前发表过的图，必须注明出处，并征得版权所有者书面同意（公有领域中的文件除外）。纵表目中数据通常用阿拉伯数字表示，但也可以表达为文字或符号。

4. 图表注

注释文字通常置于图表注中，不放在栏目标题中，对标题、栏目或图表内容予以说明。说明顺序依次涉及实验方法及结果、缩略语或符号，以及统计学信息，但统计学信息中有关数据表示方式的说明往往置于缩略语或符号定义之前。表注通常用符号或字母标注。标准的图表注使用符号依次为：∗,†,‡,§,¶,||,e,∗∗ 等，字母为 a，b，c 等。如图表注只涉及统计学显著性差异，通常使用以下序列的符号：∗ $P < 0.05$，$P^{**} < 0.01$，∗∗∗ $P < 0.001$。

写作英文图表注时应注意结构和时态。说明实验方法及结果时用句子的过去时表达，如例 4 中：RNA-seq data were assessed in triplicates；例 5 中：Patients were assessed 6 months after randomization；patient deaths were excluded.

定义缩略语、说明符号含义或说明数据可用一般现在时态的句子，也可用短语及符号 = 或：表达。如例 4 中 Error bars represent mean±SEM，n = 4 replicates in（A and B），data are representative of 2 to 3 independent experiments with similar results. 例 5 中：ICU = intensive care unit；VARD = video-assisted retroperitoneal debridement.∗∗ For patients not present in ICU 24 h before randomisation.

6.5.3.3　结果的主体内容

1. 所有实验经预先设计的研究

对所有预先设计好实验步骤的研究，即方法部分包括设计内容的研究，结果部分只叙述结果。通常一个段落叙述一个方面的结果,按时间顺序或从最重要结果到次重要结果的顺序。下例是一项验证假设型研究的结果部分,为帮助理解,列出该研究的研究背景。

例6

Background

Infected necrotising pancreatitis is a potentially lethal disease and an indication for invasive intervention. The surgical step-up approach is the standard treatment. A promising alternative is the endoscopic step-up approach. We compared both approaches to see whether the endoscopic step-up approach was superior to the surgical step-up approach in terms of clinical and economic outcomes.

译文:

背景

感染性坏死性胰腺炎是潜在的致死性疾病,也是有创介入治疗的适应症。标准治疗方法是外科阶梯式手术治疗。另一种前景良好的治疗方法是内镜阶梯式治疗。我们对这两种方式进行了比较,以明确内镜阶梯式治疗在临床及经济结局方面是否优于外科阶梯式手术治疗。

Results

Between Sept 20, 2011, and Jan 29, 2015, 418 patients with pancreatic or extrapancreatic necrosis in 19 Dutch hospitals were screened, of which 98 were eligible (figure). 51 patients were randomly assigned to the endoscopic step-up approach and 47 to the surgical step-up approach. In each treatment group, one patient did not undergo any intervention because of spontaneous clinical improvement shortly after randomisation. In two other patients in the endoscopy group, owing to the technical difficulty of the drainage procedure, the endoscopist was not able to successfully puncture the collection. These two patients underwent treatment within the surgical step-up approach and were analysed according to the intention-to-treat principle in the endoscopy group. Baseline characteristics were equally distributed between groups (table 1).

结果

本研究于 2011 年 9 月 20 日至 2015 年 1 月 29 日期间在荷兰的 19 家医院筛选 418 例胰腺或胰腺外坏死的患者,其中 98 例符合纳入标准(见图)。51 例患者被随机分到内镜阶梯式组,47 例患者被分配到外科阶梯式组。两组中均有一名患者在随机分组后不久由于短期内自发好转未接受任何干预。由于引流操作的技术难度,内镜医师无法对内镜组的另外两名患者进行成功刺穿采集标本。这两名患者接受了外科阶梯式治疗,并根据意向治疗原则在内镜组完成分析。两组间基线特征平均分布(表1)。

The primary composite endpoint occurred in 22 (43%) patients in the endoscopy group and in 21 (45%) in the surgery group (relative risk 0.97, 95% CI 0.62-1.51; p = 0.88; table 2). We observed no significant difference in new-onset single organ failure between groups (table 2); however, new-onset cardiovascular organ failure and persistent cardiovascular organ failure occurred more frequently in the surgery group (table 2). We observed no differences in major complications including bleeding, perforation of a visceral organ, enterocutaneous fistula, and incisional hernia. Mortality was similar in both groups

(table 2). The causes of death between both groups did not differ, with most patients dying because of progressive sepsis (two [22%] of nine patients in the endoscopy group, two [33%] of six in the surgery group) and multiple organ failure (four [44%] in the endoscopy group, two [33%] in the surgery group).

内镜组 22 例（43%）和手术组 21 例（45%）（RR 0.97, 95% CI 0.62-1.51; P = 0.88; 表 2）出现了主要复合终点。我们观察到两组之间在新发单器官衰竭方面无显著差异（表 2）；然而，外科手术组中新发心血管器官衰竭和持续性心血管器官衰竭的发生频率更高（表 2）。在主要并发症包括出血、内脏器官穿孔、肠皮瘘、切口疝等方面，两组间未观察到差异。两组死亡率相似（表 2）。两组死亡原因无差异，多数患者因进行性脓毒症［内镜组 9 例中有 2 例（22%），手术组 6 例中有 2 例（33%）］，和多脏器功能衰竭［内镜组 4 例（44%），手术组 2 例（33%）］死亡。

The incidence of pancreatic fistulas was lower in the endoscopy group than in the surgery group (table 2). All patients with pancreatic fistulas required persistent drainage during follow-up and nine (60%) of these patients (one patient in the endoscopy group and eight in the surgery group) underwent an additional endoscopic retrograde cholangiopancreatography with pancreatic sphincterotomy or stent placement. At 6-month follow up, we observed no differences regarding exocrine and endocrine insufficiency, biliary strictures, and wound infections (table 2).

内镜组胰瘘发生率低于手术组（表 2）。所有胰瘘患者在随访期间需要持续引流，其中 9 例（60%）患者（内镜组 1 例，手术组 8 例）另接受在内镜逆行胰胆管造影下行胰胆管括约肌切开术或支架植入。在 6 个月的随访中，两组在外分泌和内分泌功能不全、胆管狭窄和伤口感染方面未见差异（表 2）。

Mean length of hospital stay was 16 days shorter in the endoscopy group compared with the surgery group (table 2).22 (43%) patients in the endoscopy group and 24 (51%) patients in the surgery group were treated with catheter drainage only (table 2). The remaining patients underwent necrosectomy, occurring sooner in the endoscopy group compared with the surgery group (table 2). More necrosectomy procedures were done in the endoscopy group compared with the surgery group. We observed no difference in the median number of interventions (drainage or necrosectomy) between groups (table 2).

内镜组平均住院天数比手术组少 16 天（表 2）。内镜组 22 例（43%），手术组 24 例（51%）仅行导管引流（表 2）。其余患者行坏死组织清除术，且内镜组行手术的时间早于手术组（表 2）。与手术组比较，内镜组行坏死组织切除手术的例数更多。两组之间干预（引流或坏死清除）的中位数未见差异（表 2）。

The most common adverse events were pneumonia (16 [31%] patients in the endoscopy group vs. 9 [19%] in the surgery group), bacteraemia (11 [22%] vs. 6 [13%]), ascites (7[14%] vs. 8[17%]), urinary tract infection (6[12%] vs. 4[9%]), cholecystitis or cholangitis (4 [8%] vs. 3 [6%]), and atrial fibrillation (3 [6%] vs. 2 [4%]). All adverse events are listed in the appendix (pp 21-22).

最常见的不良事件是肺炎［内镜组 16 例（31%）vs. 手术组 9 例（19%）］、菌血症［内镜组 11 例（22%）vs. 手术组 6 例（13%）]、腹水 [内镜组 7 例（14%）vs. 手术组 8 例（17%）]、尿路感染 [内镜组 6 例（12%）vs. 手术组 4 例（9%）]、胆囊炎或胆管炎 [内镜组 4 例（8%）vs. 手术组 3 例（6%）] 以及心房颤动 [内镜组 3 例（6%）vs. 手术组 2 例（4%）]。所有不良事件见附录（21-22 页）。

Correction for trends in baseline characteristics（ie, chronic renal insufficiency, systemic inflammatory response syndrome, and modified multiple organ dysfunction syndrome）with multivariable regression analyses did not affect the results（appendix p 26）. Predefined subgroup analyses for time of randomisation and institution showed no significant differences in the primary endpoint（appendix p 12）. We found no differences in outcome in the subgroup of patients with organ failure at randomisation or after correction for imbalances in baseline in this subgroup. Additional perprotocol analyses did not affect the results, except that persistent cardiovascular organ failure no longer differed between groups（appendix pp 13~14）.

基线特征的趋势（即慢性肾功能不全、全身炎症反应综合征和改善的多器官功能不全综合征）用多变量回归分析校正后对结果并无影响（附录 26 页）。预先定义的亚组分析显示，随机分组的时间和入组机构，在主要终点无显著差异（附录 12 页）。在随机化分组时或校正该组中的基线失衡后，器官衰竭患者亚组的转归没有差异。除了两组间持续心血管器官衰竭不再有差异之外，额外的符合方案分析不影响结果（附录 13-14 页）。

The mean costs of the index interventions（ie, all drainage and necrosectomy procedures）were €3785 in the endoscopy group and €2851 in the surgery group, with a mean difference of €934（BCa 95% CI -€82 to €2097）. The mean total costs per patient from randomisation until 6-month follow-up were €60228 for the endoscopic step-up approach and €73883 for the surgical step-up approach. The resulting mean difference of -€13655（-€35782 to €10836）per patient was not significant.

有干预指征的操作（包括引流和清除坏死组织等），内镜组的平均费用为 3785 欧元，手术组为 2851 欧元，平均差值为 934 欧元（BCa 95% CI-82 到 2097 欧元）。从随机分组到 6 个月随访，内镜阶梯式治疗的病人平均总费用是 60228 欧元，外科阶梯式为 73883 欧元。每个患者的平均差异为-13655 欧元（-35782 到 10836 欧元），不具有显著性。

The number of QALYs gained for the endoscopy group was 0.2788（BCa 95% CI 0.2458 to 0.3110）compared with 0.2988（0.2524 to 0.3398）for the surgery group. The mean difference was -0.0199（-0.0732 to 0.0395）. The savings per loss of a single QALY were €684455. The probability of the endoscopic step-up approach being cost-effective is 0.896 at a societal willingness-to pay level of €50000 per QALY（see appendix pp 15-20 for details of the cost analysis）.（Endoscopic or surgical step-up approach for infected necrotising pancreatitis：a multicentre randomised trial, Lancet., 2017 Nov 3, 391）

内镜组的质量调整寿命年（QALYs）为 0.2788（BCa 95% CI 0.2458-0.3110），而手术组为 0.2988（0.2524-0.3398）。平均差值为-0.0199（-0.0732-0.0395）。每减少一个 QALY 节省 684455 欧元。社会愿意支付每个 QALY 50000 欧元的情况下，内镜阶梯式治疗具有成本效益的可能性为 0.896（费用分析详见附录 15~20 页）。（内窥镜或外科介入治疗坏死性

胰腺炎：一项多中心随机试验）

Table 1 Baseline Characteristics

表 1 基线特征

	Endoscopic step-up approach (n=51)	Surgical step-up approach (n=47)
Age, years	63 (14)	60 (11)
Female	17 (33%)	18 (38%)
Male	34 (67%)	29 (62%)
Cause of pancreatitis		
Gallstones	26 (51%)	30 (64%)
Alcohol abuse	7 (14%)	7 (15%)
Other*	18 (35%)	10 (21%)
Body-mass index†	29 (25–32)	28 (25–30)
Coexisting condition		
Cardiovascular disease	26 (51%)	18 (38%)
Pulmonary disease	8 (16%)	6 (13%)
Chronic renal insufficiency	4 (8%)	0
Diabetes	11 (22%)	7 (15%)
ASA class on admission		
I: healthy status	17 (33%)	18 (38%)
II: mild systemic disease	29 (57%)	27 (57%)
III: severe systemic disease	5 (10%)	2 (4%)
CT severity index‡	6 (6–8)	8 (6–10)
Extent of pancreatic necrosis		
<30%	26 (51%)	22 (47%)
30–50%	15 (29%)	10 (21%)
>50%	10 (20%)	15 (32%)
Necrosis extending >5 cm down the retrocolic gutters	20 (39%)	22 (47%)
Encapsulation of the necrotic collection		
Partial	15 (29%)	14 (30%)
Complete	36 (71%)	33 (70%)
Gas configurations within the necrotic collection	23 (45%)	27 (57%)
Disease severity§		
Admitted to the ICU at randomisation	21 (41%)	25 (53%)
SIRS¶	33 (65%)	38 (81%)
APACHE II score‖	9 (5–13)	10 (6–13)
APACHE II score ≥20‖	3 (6%)	4 (9%)
Modified Glasgow score**	2 (1–3)	2 (1–3)
Modified MODS score††	0 (0–1)	0 (0–2)
SOFA score††	0 (0–4)	1 (0–3)
C-reactive protein mg/L/‡‡	168 (105–258)	189 (136–301)
White cell count ×10⁹ per L§§	14·4 (9·4–18·0)	13·1 (10·5–17·4)
Single organ failure	13 (25%)	14 (30%)
Respiratory	11 (22%)	13 (28%)
Cardiovascular	11 (22%)	7 (15%)
Renal	3 (6%)	1 (2%)
Multiple organ failure	9 (18%)	7 (15%)

Continued

	Endoscopic step-up approach (n=51)	Surgical step-up approach (n=47)
Time since onset of symptoms, days	39 (28–54)	41 (28–52)
Antibiotic treatment at randomisation	10 (20%)	9 (19%)
Tertiary referral	35 (69%)	35 (74%)
Confirmed infected necrosis¶¶	46 (90%)	46 (98%)

Data are mean (SD), median (IQR), or n (%). ASA=American Society of Anesthesiologists. ICU=intensive care unit. SIRS=systemic inflammatory response syndrome. APACHE=Acute Physiology and Chronic Health Evaluation. MODS=multiple organ dysfunction syndrome. SOFA=Sequential Organ Failure Assessment. *Includes, among others, medication, anatomic abnormalities, and unknown aetiology. †Data missing in 34 patients. ‡Data were derived from the CT performed just before randomisation. Scores range from 0 to 10, with higher scores indicating more extensive pancreatic necrosis and extrapancreatic collections. §Data were based on maximum values during the 24 h before randomisation unless stated otherwise. ¶SIRS was defined according to the consensus-conference criteria of the American College of Chest Physicians and the Society of Critical Care Medicine. ||Scores range from 0 to 71, with higher scores indicating more severe disease.**Scores range from 0 to 8, with higher scores indicating more severe disease. ††Scores range from 0 to 24, with higher scores reflecting more severe organ dysfunction. ‡‡Data missing in 10 patients. §§Data missing in two patients. ¶¶Confirmed infected necrosis was defined as a positive culture of pancreatic or extrapancreatic necrotic tissue obtained by fine-needle aspiration or from the first drainage procedure or operation, or the presence of gas in the collection on contrast-enhanced CT.

数据表达为平均值（SD），中位数（IQR），或 n（%）。ASA＝美国麻醉师协会。ICU＝重症监护室。SIRS＝全身炎症反应综合征。APACHE＝急性生理学和慢性健康评价。MODS＝多器官功能障碍综合征。SOFA＝连续器官衰竭评估。* 包括药物、解剖异常以及未知的病因。†34 例患者资料丢失。‡ 数据来源于随机分组前的 CT 检查。得分范围从 0 到 10，分数越高，胰腺坏死和胰腺外坏死越广泛。除非另有说明，数据以随机化前 24 小内的最大值为基础。¶SIRS 根据美国胸科医师学会和重症监护医学会的共识会议标准来定义。|| 评分为 0～71 分，得分越高，病情越严重。** 得分在 0～8 之间，得分越高，病情越严重。†† 评分为 0～24 分，评分越高则脏器功能障碍越严重。‡‡ 缺失 10 例患者数据。§§ 缺失 2 例患者数据。¶¶ 确认感染坏死是依据通过穿刺或第一次引流或手术而获得的胰腺或胰腺外坏死组织的阳性培养物，或在增强 CT 显示坏死腔中有气体。

Table 2　Primary and secondary endpoints according to the intention-to-treat analysis

表 2　根据意向治疗分析的主要和次要终点

	Endoscopic step-up approach (n=51)	Surgical step-up approach (n=47)	Relative risk (95% CI)	p value
Primary endpoint				
Major complications or death*	22 (43%)	21 (45%)	0·97 (0·62–1·51)	0·88
Secondary endpoints				
New-onset organ failure†				
Pulmonary	4 (8%)	7 (15%)	0·53 (0·16–1·68)	0·27
Persistent pulmonary	4 (8%)	5 (11%)	0·74 (0·21–2·58)	0·63
Cardiovascular	3 (6%)	9 (19%)	0·31 (0·09–1·07)	0·045
Persistent cardiovascular	2 (4%)	8 (17%)	0·23 (0·05–1·03)	0·032
Renal	2 (4%)	6 (13%)	0·31 (0·07–1·45)	0·11
Persistent renal	2 (4%)	6 (13%)	0·31 (0·07–1·45)	0·11
Single organ failure	7 (14%)	13 (28%)	0·50 (0·22–1·14)	0·087
Persistent single organ failure	6 (12%)	11 (23%)	0·50 (0·20–1·25)	0·13
Multiple organ failure	2 (4%)	6 (13%)	0·31 (0·07–1·45)	0·11
Persistent multiple organ failure	2 (4%)	5 (11%)	0·37 (0·08–1·81)	0·20
Bleeding (requiring intervention)	11 (22%)	10 (21%)	1·01 (0·47–2·17)	0·97
Perforation of a visceral organ or enterocutaneous fistula (requiring intervention)	4 (8%)	8 (17%)	0·46 (0·15–1·43)	0·17
Incisional hernia	0	1 (2%)	··	0·30
Death	9 (18%)	6 (13%)	1·38 (0·53–3·59)	0·50
Other endpoints‡				
Pancreatic fistula	2/42 (5%)	13/41 (32%)	0·15 (0·04–0·62)	0·0011
Exocrine insufficiency				
Use of enzymes	16/42 (38%)	13/41 (32%)	1·20 (0·66–2·17)	0·54
Fecal elastase <200 mg/g	22/42 (52%)	19/41 (46%)	1·13 (0·73–1·75)	0·58
Steatorrhoea	6/42 (14%)	7/41 (17%)	0·84 (0·31–2·28)	0·73
Endocrine insufficiency	10/42 (24%)	9/41 (22%)	1·08 (0·49–2·39)	0·84
Biliary strictures	3 (6%)	3 (6%)	0·92 (0·20–4·34)	0·92
Wound infections	2 (4%)	3 (6%)	0·61 (0·11–3·52)	0·58

Continued

	Endoscopic step-up approach (n=51)	Surgical step-up approach (n=47)	Relative risk (95% CI)	p value
Health-care use				
Median number of interventions§	3 (2–6)	4 (2–6)	··	0·35
Drainage procedures¶	1 (1–3)	3 (1–5)	··	0·0041
Necrosectomies‖	2 (1–4)	1 (1–1)	··	0·0004
Number of necrosectomies	··	··	··	0·0062
0	22 (43%)	24 (51%)	0·84 (0·55–1·29)	··
1	9 (18%)	18 (38%)	0·46 (0·23–0·92)	··
2	8 (16%)	3 (6%)	2·46 (0·69–8·72)	··
≥3	12 (24%)	2 (4%)	5·53 (1·31–23·42)	··
Additional percutaneous drainage in the endoscopy group	14 (27%)	··	··	··
Additional VARD procedure in the endoscopy group	2 (4%)	··	··	··
Additional endoscopic drainage in the surgical group	··	2 (4%)	··	··
Additional endoscopic necrosectomy in the surgical group	··	0	··	··
Days between first drainage and first necrosectomy				
Median (range)	10 (5–16)	23 (9–62)	··	0·013
Mean (SD)	14 (14)	33 (30)	··	··
Days in ICU within 6 months of randomisation**				
Median (IQR)	0 (0–3)	2 (0–11)	··	··
Mean (SD)	13 (31)	13 (21)	··	0·31
Days in hospital within 6 months of randomisation				
Median (IQR)	35 (19–85)	65 (40–90)	··	··
Mean (SD)	53 (47)	69 (38)	··	0·014

Data are n (%), mean (SD), or median (IQR) unless otherwise stated. Relative risk is reported for dichotomous variables for the endoscopic step-up approach as compared with the surgical step-up approach. ICU=intensive care unit. VARD=video-assisted retroperitoneal debridement. *Multiple events in the same patient were considered as one endpoint. †Organ failure occurring after randomisation and not present 24 h before randomisation. ‡Patients were assessed 6 months after randomisation; patient deaths were excluded. §This category included all drainage procedures (endoscopic or percutaneous) and necrosectomies (endoscopic or VARD) as part of the endoscopic or surgical step-up approach. ¶This category included primary drainage procedures (endoscopic or percutaneous) as part of the endoscopic or surgical step-up approach and additional drainage procedures before and after necrosectomy in both treatment groups. ‖This category included all necrosectomies (endoscopic or VARD procedure) as part of the endoscopic or surgical step-up approach. **For patients not present in ICU 24 h before randomisation.

　　数据为 n（%），平均值（SD）或中位数（IQR）。与外科手术相比,内镜手术二分变量报道的相对风险较高。ICU = 重症监护病房。VARD = 视频辅助腹膜后清创术。* 同一患者的多次事件被视为一个终点。† 器官衰竭发生在随机分组后,而不是在随机分组前 24 小时出现。‡ 随机分配 6 个月后评估患者;排除患者死亡。§此类别包括所有引流程序（内窥镜式或经皮肤）和坏死组织切除术（内窥镜或 VARD），作为内窥镜或外科手术的一部分。¶该类别包括作为内窥镜或外科手术的主要引流程序（内镜或经皮肤），以及两个治疗组在坏死切除术之前和之后的其他引流程序。‖此类别包括所有作为内窥镜或外科手术中的坏死组织切除术（内窥镜或 VARD 手术）。** 对于随机分组前 24 小时未在 ICU 中就诊的患者。

2. 前一个实验步骤结果决定下一个实验步骤的研究

对前一个实验步骤结果决定下一个实验步骤的研究，每一项实验结果的叙述通常包括四个步骤：问题（question）—实验回顾（overview of the experiments）—结果（results）—问题的答案（answer to the question）。四个步骤的内容在一个段落或多个段落完成。如果必要，还可以回顾提出问题的背景及实验步骤的目的或原因。

例7

Question Whether the nematode gene ceh-22 and the vertebrate gene nkx2.5 perform similar functions.

译文：

问题 线虫基因 ceh-22 与脊椎动物的基因 nkx2.5 是否具有相似功能。

Experimental approach Examination of the ability of the zebrafish nkx2.5 gene to substitute for the nematode ceh-22 gene in transgenic caenorhabditis elegans.

实验路径 研究斑马鱼的 nkx2.5 基因是否能替代转基因秀丽隐杆线虫中线虫 ceh-22 基因

Results

结果

Zebrafish nkx2.5 can activate myo-2 expression when expressed in C. elegans body wall muscle. To determine whether zebrafish nkx2.5 can function similarly to ceh-22, we expressed nkx2.5 in C. elegans body wall muscle and examined expression of the endogenous myo-2 gene by antibody staining. The rationale for this approach was as follows. In wild type C. elegans, ceh-22 is expressed exclusively in pharyngeal muscle, where it activates expression of the pharyngeal muscle specific myosin heavy chain gene myo-2 (14). However, ectopic expression of ceh-22 in body wall muscle can activate expression of myo-2 (15). Because myo-2 is normally never expressed in body wall muscle, this ectopic expression assay provides a sensitive test for ceh-22 function. We generated two transgenic lines expressing an nkx2.5 cDNA under the control of the unc-54 body wall muscle specific promoter. In both lines, we detected myo-2 expression in the body wall muscles (Fig.1A and 1B). These results show that nkx.2.5 can function ceh-22 to induce myo-2 expression.

斑马鱼 *nkx2.5 在秀丽隐杆线虫的体壁肌肉中表达时能够激活 myo-2 的表达*。为了确定斑马鱼 nkx2.5 是否和 ceh-22 的功能相似，我们在秀丽隐杆线虫的体壁肌肉中表达了 nkx2.5，用抗体染色法检测了内源性 myo-2 基因的表达。这一方法的原理如下：在野生型秀丽隐杆线虫中，ceh-22 只在咽部肌肉表达，并激活咽部肌肉特异性肌球蛋白重链基因 myo-2。

然而,体壁肌肉中 ceh-22 的异位表达能够激活 myo-2 的表达。因为正常情况下 myo-2 从不在体壁肌肉表达,异位表达检测可以作为 ceh-22 功能的敏感性测试。我们生成了两条转基因链表达在 unc-54 体壁肌肉特异性启动子控制下的 nkx2.5 cDNA。在两条基因链中,检测到了 myo-2 在体壁肌肉的表达（图 1A 和 1B）。这些结果表明 nkx2.5 与 ceh-22 功能相似,能够诱导 myo-2 的表达。

We next asked whether nkx2.5 directly interacts with the same sequences recognized by ceh-22. To answer this question, we examined expression of a reporter gene under the control of multimerized ceh-22 binding sites. Ceh-22 binds a region within the myo-2 enhancer termed the β sub-element (14). In wild type animals, a lacZ reporter under control of a synthetic enhancer consisting of four copies of a 28 bp β sub element oligonucleotide is expressed specifically in pharyngeal muscle; only occasional expression is observed outside the pharynx (Table 1; ref.14). In a transgenic strain bearing the unc-54 :: nkx2.5 expression construct, we found a significant increase in the number of animals expressing β galactosidase in body wall muscle (from 2.5 to 16.5%) (Table 1; Fig.1C). To rule out the possibility that nkx2.5 was indirectly increasing expression of myo-2 or the β sub-element reported by activating ectopic expression of the ceh-22 gene, we examined expression of a ceh-22 :: lacZ fusion in animals bearing the unc-54 :: nkx2.5 transgene. Expression of β galactosidase was limited to pharyngeal muscle (Table1), a pattern identical to that observed in wild type animals. Thus, nkx2.5, like ceh-22, activates transcription by interacting directly with the β sub-element of the myo-2 enhancer.

接下来,我们提出 nkx2.5 是否与 ceh-22 识别的同样序列直接相互作用。为了回答这一问题,我们检测了多聚化 ceh-22 结合位点控制下的一个报告基因的表达。Ceh-22 与 myo-2 增强子,β 亚基内的一个部位结合。在野生型动物中,在含有 4 个拷贝的 28-bp β 亚基低聚核苷酸的合成增强子控制下,lacZ 报告基因只在咽部肌肉表达;咽部外只是偶尔有表达（表 1;参考文献 14）。在一条含有 unc-54 :: nkx2.5 表达的转基因链中,我们发现表达 β 单奶糖苷酶的动物数显著增加（从 2.5% 增至 16.5%）（表 1;图 1C）。为了排除 nkx2.5 通过激活 ceh-22 基因异位表达而间接增加 myo-2 或 β 亚基的表达这一可能性,我们检测了含有 unc-54 :: nkx2.5 转基因结构的动物中 ceh-22 :: lacZ 融合的表达,发现 β 单奶糖苷酶只在咽部肌肉表达（表 1）,与野生型动物中观察到的方式一样。因此,跟 ceh-22 一样,nkx2.5 也是与 myo-2 增强子的 β 亚基直接作用从而激活转录。

In addition to its role in myo-2activation, ceh-22 likely regulates other genes required for pharyngeal development. Indeed, a ceh-22 mutant exhibits profound contractile and morphological defects in the pharynx, despite expressing myo-2 nearly as well as wild type. To examine the extent to which nkx2.5 and ceh-22 are functionally equivalent, we asked if expression of nkx2.5 in pharyngeal muscle can rescue a ceh-22 mutant. ①

---

① Mimi Zeiger, *Essentials of Writing Biomedical Research Papers*. U.S.A.: The McGraw-Hill companies, Inc.. second edition, 2000, P.159.

除了激活 myo-2 的作用,ceh-22 可能调节咽部发育的其他基因。实际上,尽管几乎跟野生型一样能表达 myo-2,ceh-22 突变基因在咽部中造成严重的收缩和结构上的缺陷。为了检测 nkx2.5 和 ceh-22 究竟在多大程度上功能相当,我们提出咽部肌肉中 nkx2.5 的表达是否能拯救 ceh-22 突变体。

6.5.4 结果的写作要点

6.5.4.1 重要内容前置

如前所述,结果部分应突出结果。可以运用多种技巧突出结果,如省略、浓缩次重要信息或将重要信息置于重要位置。例如,将重要结果置于醒目位置,如段首,然后再叙述次重要的结果。

例8

The duration of ARDS before study entry and procollagen peptide type III levels at baseline were found to interact with treatment and mortality. Treatment with methylprednisolone was associated with a significantly increased mortality rate among patients who had had ARDS for more than 13 days before enrollment and a significantly decreased mortality rate among those with higher-than-median levels of procollagen peptide type III in bronchoalveolar-lavage fluid at baseline (Table 2 and Table 3). None of the other interactions, including tidal volume (P = 0.63) and date of enrollment (P = 0.34), were significant. There were no significant differences between the group enrolled 7 to 13 days after the onset of ARDS and the group enrolled at least 14 days after the onset of ARDS, other than in the percentage of men and the positive end-expiratory pressure at baseline (13.3 + 5.0 and 10.8 + 5.1 cm of water, respectively; P = 0.004) (Table 4 of the Supplementary Appendix).

译文:分析发现,纳入研究前的 ARDS 病程及基线 III 型前胶原肽水平,与甲泼尼龙治疗及病死率存在相互作用。甲泼尼龙治疗显著增加纳入研究前 ARDS 病程>13 天病人的病死率,显著降低基线高于中位数值病人的病死率(表 2 和表 3)。其他相互影响均无显著性,包括潮气量(P = 0.63)和纳入研究日期(P = 0.34)。ARDS 发病后 7~13 天纳入研究组与 ARDS 发病后≥14 天纳入研究组之间无显著差异,但男性病人的百分比和基线呼气末正压[分别为(13.3±5.0)cm 水柱和(10.8±5.1)cm 水柱,P = 0.004]除外(补充附录表 4)。

也可以将结果作为主题句开启段落,然后叙述支撑数据等相关内容。值得注意的是,数据应该主要罗列在图表中,正文中出现过多的数据会扰乱结果的表达。如果需要,正文中只列举几个最重要的数据,在陈述结果之后用括号加注图表名。列举结果时,如果有组间对照,应先列举实验组、干预组,然后才是空白组或对照组。

例9

The mean serum glucose level was not significantly different between groups at baseline but was significantly higher in the methylprednisolone group than the placebo group on days 1（Figure 3），2，and 4. The difference in means decreased from 77.1 mg per deciliter（4.3 mmol per liter）on day 1（95 percent confidence interval，52.1 to 102.1 mg per deciliter [2.9 to 5.7 mmol per liter]）to 20.2 mg per deciliter（1.1 mmol per liter）on day 4（95 percent confidence interval，2.4 to 37.9 mg per deciliter [0.1 to 2.1 mmol per liter]）（Figure 5 of the Supplementary Appendix）

译文：基线时两组病人的平均血清葡萄糖水平无显著差异，但第 1 天（图3）、2 天和 4 天时，甲泼尼龙组病人的平均血糖水平显著高于安慰剂组。两组病人的平均血糖水平之差，从第 1 天时的 77.1 mg / dl（4.3 mmol / l）[95% CI 为 52.1 mg / dl～102.1 mg / dl（2.9 mmol / l～5.7 mmol / l）]，降至第 4 天时的 20.2 mg / dl（1.1mmol / l）[95% CI 为 2.4 mg / dl～37.9 mg / dl（0.1 mmol / l～2.1 mmol / l）]（补充附录图5）。

6.5.4.2 结果部分的时态

结果部分的时态为一般过去时；陈述研究实验结果时，有时追述结果之前的情况，则用过去完成时。具体参见本节各例。

6.5.4.3 结果部分的比较句型

研究论文的结果部分经常涉及对比较内容的描述。比较句型是本部分写作的重要内容。

1. 自身对照的描述

自身对照的描述表示"经过某种处理"或"一段时间后"，某项（些）指标的变化。句中常含有表示时间变化的形容词、副词或介词词组，如 previously，after，during，with time，over time 等。另外，也常含有表示变化的动词，如 become，reach，increase，rise，elevate，decrease，decline，fall，diminish，drop 等。

例10

The use of elagolix at two doses（150 mg once daily and 200 mg twice daily）resulted in reductions in the pain symptoms of endometriosis，dysmenorrhea and nonmenstrual pelvic pain，after both 3 months and 6 months of treatment.

译文：在治疗 3 个月和 6 个月后，以两种剂量使用 elagolix（150 mg，q.d.；200 mg，b.i.d.）可减轻子宫内膜异位症、痛经和非经期盆腔痛引起的疼痛症状。

例11

Using the FPG（fever practice guideline）resulted in a 78% reduction in the time to treatment and a cost reduction in fever work-ups of more than 60%.

译文：使用 FPG（发热治疗指南）使治疗时间减少了 78%，发烧检查费用降低了 60% 以上。

例12

After treatment with PHM（polysaccharide hemostatic microsphere），hemostatic time shortened from 210 s (negative group) to 45 s. Amount of bleeding decreased from 155 mg (negative group) to 33 mg.

译文：用 PHM（多糖止血微球）治疗后，止血时间从 210 秒（阴性组）缩短到 45 秒。出血量从 155 mg（阴性组）降至 33 mg。

2. 组间对照的描述

组间对照的描述用于实验组与对照组的比较，或实验组之间的比较。比较时，根据结果有无统计学差异及差异大小分为以下几种情况。

（1）结果无统计学差异

结果无统计学差异时，常用 was similar to, did not differ, there was no significant difference between…, … was not different from…, no significant difference was found…等表示。

例13

Data in Table 2 did not show a significant difference in body weight between the groups of rats.

译文：表 2 中的数据显示两组之间大鼠的体重无显著差异。

例14

The mean serum levels in the oral group were similar to those in the topical group.

译文：口服组的平均血清水平与局部用药组相似。

例15

The range of motion of the affected extremity also did not differ significantly between the two groups.

译文：两组间患肢的活动范围也无显著差异。

例16

There were no significant between-group differences in either trial in any other neurocognitive or pregnancy outcomes or in the incidence of adverse events, which was low in both groups.

译文：在任一试验中，在其他神经认知或妊娠结局或者在不良事件发生率方面，无显著的组间差异，两组的不良事件发生率均较低。

（2）结果有差异但无比较

表达结果的差异时，不直接说明孰高孰低，而是客观地交代数值。句中常含有表示转折或比较的标记语，如 but, however, whereas, versus 等。

例17

In the matched cohort, we observed an average of 24 adverse maternal outcomes (21.2%) in women with plasma transfusion within 60 minutes vs. 23 adverse maternal outcomes (19.9%) in women with no or later plasma transfusion.

译文：在配对队列中，我们观察到 60 分钟内输血浆的女性平均有 24 例产妇不良结局（21.2%），而没有或之后输血浆的女性平均有 23 例产妇不良结局（19.9%）。

例18

The mean total costs per patient from randomisation until 6-month follow-up were € 60228 for the endoscopic step-up approach and € 73883 for the surgical step-up approach.

译文:从随机分组到 6 个月随访,内镜阶梯式治疗的病人平均总费用是 60228 欧元,外科阶梯式为 73883 欧元。

例19

The cumulative incidence of metastatic prostate cancer at 12 years was 14.5% in the bicalutamide group, as compared with 23.0% in the placebo group (P = 0.005).

译文:在第 12 年时,比卡鲁胺组中前列腺癌转移的累计发生率为 14.5%,而安慰剂组为 23.0% (P = 0.005)。

（3）结果有差异且有比较

为了清楚地展示不同结果间的差异,用 more, higher, greater, lower, less 等形容词比较级,或 elevate, increase, decrease, rise, decline 等表示变化的动词,或由这些动词演变的分词或名词来表达组间的比较结果,比较句结构用 than 或 compared with。

例20

Mice from the tMCAO + teriflunomide group had lower brain water content than those from the tMCAO + vehicle group.

译文:tMCAO +特氟醚胺组的小鼠脑水含量低于 tMCAO +载体组的小鼠。

例21

The incidence risk was significantly lower in both treatment groups than in the placebo group, for which the incidence risk was 48.73%.

译文:两个治疗组的发生风险均显著低于安慰剂组,安慰剂组的发生风险为 48.73%。

例22

The efficacy of an unsupervised 14-day primaquine regimen was significantly lower than that of a daily observed 14-day regimen.

译文:14 天无监督的伯氨喹治疗方案的疗效显著低于 14 天持续观察的方案。

例23

The expressions of mesenchymal stem cell (MSC) markers such as CD73-PE and CD 105 PE, were higher than those of the hematopoietic progenitor marker CD34 and the pan-leukocyte marker CD45.

译文:间质干细胞(MSC)标记物(如 CD73-PE 和 CD 105 PE)的表达高于造血祖细胞标记物 CD34 和泛白细胞标记物 CD45 的表达。

例24

The decrease in mean nocturnal plasma glucose was significantly greater with glargine than with the dulaglutide 1.5 mg or 0.75 mg doses.

译文:甘精胰岛素组夜间平均血糖降低显著大于度拉糖肽 1.5 mg 剂量组或 0.75 mg 剂量组。

例25

The mean dose of total daily insulin was roughly 30% lower in patients receiving dulaglutide than in those receiving glargine (table 2).

译文：度拉糖肽组患者的胰岛素平均总日剂量比甘精胰岛素组患者约低30%（表2）。

需要注意的是，在比较句型中描述"增加"或"减少"的具体量值时，要慎用 compared with，否则可能引起歧义，影响结果的正确表达，如：

例26

Experimental rabbits had a 28% decrease in alveolar phospholipids as compared with control rabbits during normal ventilation.

这一句子可以有三种理解：

① Experimental rabbits had a 28% greater decrease in alveolar phospholipids than did control rabbits during normal ventilation. 正常通气时，实验兔比对照兔肺泡磷脂的降低程度大28%。

② Experimental rabbits had a 28% decrease in alveolar phospholipids but control rabbits had no decrease during normal ventilation. 正常通气时，实验兔中肺泡磷脂降低28%，而对照兔没有降低。

③ Experimental rabbits had 28% less alveolar phospholipids than did control rabbits during normal ventilation. 正常通气时，实验兔的肺泡磷脂比对照兔的肺泡磷脂少28%。

另外，写作比较句时一定要分清比较内容和比较对象，确保比较的对应性。比较对象不一致是比较句写作中的常见错误。如：

例27

原句：The incidences of our study were higher than the report in Taiwan.

修改句：The incidences in our study were higher than those in the report of Taiwan.

译文：我们研究中的发病率高于台湾的相关报告。

6.5.4.4　结果部分的常用表达

1. 描述研究结果

After… treatment, a significant increase in… was observed in…

… increased markedly in… but not in…

… was highly associated with…

There was a direct relationship between… and…

Positive / negative co-relationship was found between…

There was a clear direct dose-dependent relationship between…

… correlated well with…

We found a marked difference / clear relationship between… and…

There was no evidence of association for use of… and…

This model provided the estimated probability of… as follows.

... was strongly associated with / inversely correlated with / in direct proportion to...

The study results revealed that patients (with...) presented elevated / reduced...

There were no distinct differences in...

... verified that all included studies presented no evident impacts on...

2. 图表相关表达

Figure 1 shows / displays / indicates / demonstrates that...

Clinical characteristics and laboratory data of the patients are summarized in table 1.

General clinical characteristics of patients...are summarized in Table 1.

Comparisons between... and... are presented in table 2 according to extent of disease.

3. 描述结果的统计学意义

By contrast with... there was no significant correlation between... and...

The difference was not statistically significant.

There was a significant / weak / negative / positive correlation between... and...

As shown in table 1, no statistically significant differences were found between... and...

We did not find any statistical difference in... levels between... and...

... had no significant effect on...

These phenomena were observed in a dose-dependent manner and were statistically significant.

We found no statistical difference in... levels between... and...

Statistical analysis or test showed difference / no difference / significant difference in sth. between groups.

... was significantly associated with...

... did not differ significantly between the treatment and the control groups.

4. 表达结果的比较

Rats of group A and B had few differences from those of control group.

The mean value of... was statistically increased in patients with... (disease) compared with the control group.

The composition of... was significantly different in the two groups, but... was similar.

... were larger in Group 1 than in Group 2, while... were similar in both groups.

In control experiments, similar experiments revealed no detectable interaction.

No significant differences were found / observed / identified between... and...

... were significantly increased while... did not change...

Group A, compared to B, showed statistically significant decreased / increased...

Among groups, we did not find any changes in the levels of...

... was significantly elevated in... in comparison to...

The number of... in... was significantly smaller in... group than in... group

Something did not differ between (among) groups.

There was (were) (no) (significant) difference (s) in… between (among) groups at time 1, as compared with time 2.

Something was greater or less in group A than in group B.

Something in group A was greater or less than that in group B.

Something (esp. a change) was found in group A, as compared with group B…

6.5.5　结果示例

例28

RESULTS

NCCs, but Not Macrophages, Colonize the Trunk during Early Development

Although primitive macrophages are generated in the first wave of yolk sac hemato-poiesis as early as 15 hpf in zebrafish (Lieschke et al., 2001), previous studies demonstrate that these early macrophages do not populate the trunk until 35 hpf or later (Herbomel et al., 1999, 2001). To understand the temporal dynamics of macrophage colonization of the trunk, we crossed Tg (mpeg1:GFP) transgenic fish, where mpeg1 regulatory sequences drive GFP expression in macrophages and microglia, with Tg (olig2:DsRed) transgenic fish, where olig2 regulatory sequences label spinal cord neurons and glia, and counted the number of mpeg1 + macrophages in the trunk of these embryos at 24, 36, and 48 hpf (Figure 1A).

译文：

结果

神经嵴细胞（NCCs），而非巨噬细胞，在早期发育中定植躯干

原始巨噬细胞最早会出现在斑马鱼受精后 15 小时（15 hpf）第一次卵黄囊造血中（Lieschke et al., 2001），然而先前研究表明直到受精后至少 35 小时（35 hpf），这些早期巨噬细胞才会在躯干定植。为了解躯干巨噬细胞定植的时间动态，我们将 Tg（mpeg1:绿色荧光蛋白[GFP]）转基因鱼与 Tg（olig2:红色荧光蛋白[DsRed]）转基因鱼杂交，前者的 mpeg1 调控序列驱动 GFP 在巨噬细胞和小胶质细胞中表达，后者的 olig2 调控序列标记脊髓神经元和神经胶质细胞；并统计 24、36 和 48 hpf 各胚胎躯干中 mpeg1 + 巨噬细胞的数量（图 1A）。

In these studies, we observed an increase macrophage number in both the yolk and trunk between 24 and 36 hpf, and then again from 36 to 48 hpf (Figures 1A and 1B). To better characterize macrophage distribution, we plotted their individual locations into 2D histograms and found that at 24 hpf, macrophages resided in the yolk extension (Figure1C, n = 9fish). By 36 hpf, most macrophages remained in and around the yolk extension, while a few of started to appear near the notochord and the ventral spinal cord, which is referred to as the dorsal trunk below (Figure 1C, n = 9 fish). Ultimately, by 48 hpf, macrophages fully colonized the trunk with an equal distribution in both the yolk extension and dorsal trunk (Figure 1C, n = 9 fish).

在这些研究中,我们观察到在 24~36 hpf 和 36~48 hpf 期间,卵黄和躯干中的巨噬细胞数量增多(图 1A 和 1B)。为更好表征巨噬细胞的分布,我们将它们的单个位置绘制到二维直方图中,发现 24 hpf 巨噬细胞存在于卵黄区(图 1C,鱼 n = 9)。到 36 hpf,大多数巨噬细胞仍停留在卵黄区及周围区域,而有一小部分开始出现在脊索和腹侧脊髓附近,这一区域在下文被称为背侧干(图 1C,鱼 n = 9)。最终 48 hpf 时,巨噬细胞完全定植躯干,且在卵黄区和背侧干中均匀分布(图 1C,鱼 n = 9)。

Because we did not observe any macrophages in the dorsal trunk in 24 hpf embryos, we sought to determine whether dead cells were present at this stage. To visualize apoptotic cells in live animals, we created a transgenic line, Tg (bactin2:Gal4), which has Gal4 under the control of β-actin regulatory sequences and crossed it with Tg (UAS:secA5-YFP) zebrafish, to drive expression of secreted human annexin V protein fused to YFP (secA5-YFP), which binds to the membrane of apoptotic cells (van Ham et al., 2010).

由于在 24 hpf 胚胎背侧干中未观察到巨噬细胞,所以我们需明确在此阶段是否存在死亡细胞。为了可视化活体动物中的凋亡细胞,我们建立了一个斑马鱼转基因品系 Tg (bactin2:Gal4),其 Gal4 表达由 β-肌动蛋白基因调节序列驱动,然后将该斑马鱼品系与转基因斑马鱼 Tg (UAS:secA5-YFP) 杂交,从而使 Gal4 驱动分泌型 AnnexinV-YFP 荧光融合蛋白(secA5-YFP)表达。secA5-YFP 荧光融合蛋白可与凋亡细胞膜结合,从而使斑马鱼体内的凋亡细胞可视化。

In Tg (bactin2:Gal4);Tg (UAS:secA5YFP) embryos at 20 hpf, we observed secA5+ cells in the yolk extension and intermediate cell mass (Figure 1D) (Sarvothaman et al., 2015; Stachura and Traver, 2016). Additionally, we also found secA5+ cells in the dorsal trunk (Figure 1D) at both 20 and 36 hpf (Figure 1D). Quantification of the percentage of somites with secA5+ cells in the dorsal trunk at 20 and 36 hpf (n = 65/56 so-mites in 6/9 embryos for 20/36 hpf) showed that the presence of dead cells was robust and consistent among embryos at these stages (Figure 1E). Using a newly created line, Tg (sox10:TagRFP), where TagRFP is expressed in NCCs under sox10 regulatory sequences, we found that sox10+ NCCs were spatially correlated with apoptotic cells near the spinal cord (Figure 1D), which is consistent with a previous study demonstrating the presence of apoptotic cells around the neural tube during NCC migration in mice (Massa et al., 2009). These data demonstrate that migratory NCCs colonize the dorsal trunk in zebrafish when macrophages are absent but apoptotic debris is present.

20 hpf,在 Tg (bactin2:Gal4);Tg (UAS:secA5YFP) 胚胎的卵黄区和中间细胞群中观

察到 secA5+细胞（图 1D）。此外，20 hpf 和 36 hpf 在背侧干中也发现了 secA5+细胞（图 1D）。定量 20 hpf、36 hpf 背侧躯干中含 secA5+细胞体节的百分比（20/36 hpf，n＝6/9 胚胎中 65/56 体节），结果显示这两个阶段的胚胎中一直存在大量死亡细胞（图 1E）。使用新建株系 Tg（sox10：TagRFP），其中 TagRFP 受 sox10 序列调控在 NCCs 中表达，我们发现 sox10+ NCCs 与脊髓附近的凋亡细胞具有空间相关性（图 1D）。这与先前一篇文献的报道一致，该文献证实了小鼠 NCC 在迁移过程中，神经管周围存在凋亡细胞。这些数据表明，巨噬细胞还没形成而胚胎中存在凋亡碎片时，迁移性 NCC 在斑马鱼的背侧干中定植。

The association of migratory NCCs with dead cells at early developmental stages (Figure 1D) prompted us to investigate whether NCCs expressed genes implicated in phagocytosis. To do this, we performed RNA-sequencing of foxd3＋/sox10＋ NCCs collected from the trunk of Gt（foxd3：mCherry）；Tg（sox10：mEGFP）embryos at 36 and 72 hpf, which represent developmental stages before and after the full colonization of macrophages into the trunk（Figure 1C）（Simo~es-Costa and Bronner, 2015）. Using Gene Ontology（GO）enrichment analysis and KEGG pathway analysis, we found that 36 hpf NCCs were highly enriched in cellular components related to debris clearance such as the endoplasmic reticulum, lysosomes, endosomes, and V-ATPase（Figures S1A and S1B）. Lysosome and endosome pathways were also upregulated（Figures S1C and S1D）. Moreover, many genes required for phagocytosis were highly expressed in 36 hpf NCCs （Figures S1E and S2F；Table S2）（Ashburner et al., 2000；Villani et al., 2019）. Taken together, we hypothesize that NCCs have the capacity to clear debris at developmental stages before the appearance of professional phagocytes.

在发育早期，迁移性 NCC 与死亡细胞之间的这种关系（图 1D）促使我们探究 NCC 是否表达有吞噬作用的基因。为此，我们分别收集了 36 hpf（巨噬细胞定植躯干之前的发育期）和 72 hpf（巨噬细胞定植躯干之后的发育期）Gt（foxd3：mCherry）；Tg（sox10：mEGFP）胚胎躯干中的 foxd3+/sox10+ NCCs，并对其进行 RNA 测序（图 1C）。使用 GO 富集分析和 KEGG 通路分析，我们发现 36hpf 的 NCC 高度集中于与清除碎片有关的细胞成分中，如内质网、溶酶体、核内体和 V-ATP 酶等（图 S1A 和 S1B）。溶酶体和核内体的通路均上调（图 S1C 和 S1D）。此外，许多吞噬相关的基因在 36 hpf 的 NCC 中都有高表达（图 S1E 和 S2F；表 S2）。综上所述，我们假设在"专职"吞噬细胞出现之前，NCC 有能力清除发育阶段的凋亡碎片。

NCCs Migrate away from Their Segmental Stream of Origin to Engulf Cellular Debris
神经嵴细胞（NCCs）迁移出原有节段以吞噬细胞碎片

To monitor the migration and behavior of NCCs and investigate whether they contribute to debris clearance during development, we performed in vivo, time-lapse imaging. To do this, we used Tg (sox10: nls-Eos) embryos that express nuclear-localized Eos to track the movement of individual NCCs and a Tg (nkx2.2a: nls-mCherry) transgene to label lateral floorplate cells as a reference for the location of the ventral spinal cord (Figures 2A and 2B) (Kucenas et al., 2008). In time-lapse movies of Tg (sox10: nls-Eos); Tg (nkx2.2a: nls-mCherry) embryos from 19 to 40 hpf, we observed that the majority of newly delaminated trunk NCCs migrated ventrally around the neural tube, reaching MEP (motor exit points) TZs (transition zones) in the middle of each hemi-segment, and then migrated along motor axons (Figures 2A and 2B), as previously described (Banerjee et al., 2011; Vega-Lopez et al., 2017). (Banerjee et al., 2011; Vega-Lopez et al., 2017). We also observed ~ 1 to 2 NCCs per hemi-segment undergo apoptosis during their migration (Figure 2B; Video S1). When cell death occurred, individual NCCs migrated away from their innate streams and moved toward these dying cells, and NCCs that associated with dying cells were observed both dorsal and ventral to MEP TZs (Figures 2B and S2A; Videos S1 and S2).

为了监测 NCC 的迁移和表现,并探究它们在发育过程中是否发挥清除凋亡碎片的作用,我们进行了体内延时成像。我们用表达核定位 Eos 蛋白的 Tg(sox10:nls-Eos) 胚胎来追踪单个 NCC 的运动,并用 Tg(nkx2.2a:nls-mCherry) 转基因标记侧底板细胞以定位脊髓腹侧(图 2A 和 2B)。从 Tg(sox10:nls-Eos);Tg(nkx2.2a:nls-mCherry) 胚胎从 19 hpf 到 40 hpf 的延迟视频中,我们观察到大多数新分层的躯干 NCC 沿神经管腹侧迁移,到达每半个横断面中间的运动神经出口点过渡区(MEP TZs),然后再沿运动轴突迁移(图 2A 和 2B),这与之前相关文献描述一致。我们还观察到每半个横断面约有 1 至 2 个 NCC 在迁移过程中发生凋亡(图 2B;视频 S1)。当细胞死亡发生时,个别 NCC 偏离原先迁移路径,移向这些垂死细胞;在 MEP TZs 的背侧和腹侧,我们也观察到与垂死细胞有关的 NCC(图 2B 和 S2A;视频 S1 和 S2)。

We next examined whether NCCs that migrated toward dying cells engulfed them. In order to better visualize NCC behavior, we used a Tg (sox10: Eos) line to label NCC cytoplasm with Eos, a photoconvertible protein that when exposed to ultraviolet (UV) light, shifts its emission wavelength from a neutral state emitting green fluorescence (516 nm), to an anionic state emitting red fluorescence (581 nm) (Prendergast et al., 2012). Recent studies demonstrate that the Eos protein settles in a pH-dependent equilibrium between these two states: the neutral form (green) favors lower pH (6-8), and the anionic state (red) favors physiological pH (8-10) (Berardozzi et al., 2016; Turkowyd et al., 2017). Considering the acidification that occurs during apoptosis and inside engulfment vesicles (Gottlieb, 1996; Levin et al., 2016), we hypothesized that healthy and apoptotic NCCs could be differentially labeled by the two forms of Eos protein. To verify this, we exposed Tg (sox10: Eos) embryos to UV light at 20 hpf, photoconverting existing Eos protein in NCCs to the anionic state (red), and performed time-lapse imaging. As expected, NCCs labeled with high levels of photoconverted (red) Eos switched to yellow upon apoptosis (Figures S2B and S2C). Yellow NCC corpses were then quickly engulfed by neighboring red NCCs that formed large engulfment vesicles with green debris inside (Figures 2C, S2B, and S2C). Moreover, these engulfment vesicles were positive for LysoTracker Deep Red (Figures 2C and 2D), a dye that labels acidic organelles (Fogel et al., 2012), and measured-2 to 8 μg in diameter (Figure 2E, n = 95vesicles), similar to the size of phagosomes in professional phagocytes (Champion et al., 2008). From these data, we conclude that migratory NCCs engulf apoptotic neighbors and form acidic engulfment vesicles.

接下来,我们检测迁移至垂死细胞的 NCC 是否吞噬它们。为了更好地观察 NCC 的表现,我们利用 Tg(sox10:Eos)株系,用 Eos 标记 NCC 细胞质;Eos 是一种见光可转换的蛋白质,紫外线(UV)照射时,其发射波长会从发绿色荧光的中性状态(516 nm)转变为发红色荧光的阴离子态(581 nm)。最近的研究表明,Eos 蛋白随着环境 pH 值不同,在两种状态之间动态平衡。当 pH 值较低时(6~8)呈中性状态(绿色),而生理 pH 值(8~10)时呈阴离子状态(红色)。考虑到细胞凋亡时和吞噬囊泡内部的酸化现象,我们假设正常和凋亡的 NCC 分别可通过两种 Eos 蛋白进行差异标记。为了验证这一结论,我们将 Tg(sox10:Eos)胚胎(20 hpf)暴露于紫外线下,把 NCC 中现有的 Eos 蛋白光转化为阴离子状态(红色),并延时摄像。与预期的一致,光转化(红色)Eos 高水平标记的 NCC 在凋亡时变为黄色(图 S2B 和 S2C)。随后,黄色 NCC 残骸很快被周围红色的 NCC 吞噬,形成含有绿色碎片的吞噬囊泡(图 2C,S2B 和 S2C)。此外,这些吞噬囊泡用 LysoTracker Deep Red 染色呈阳性(图 2C 和 2D),该染料用于标记酸性细胞器,直径约为 2 至 8 μg(图 2E,囊泡 n = 95),大小与"专职"吞噬细胞中的吞噬体相似。通过这些数据,我们判定迁移的 NCC 可吞噬周围的凋亡细胞,并形成酸性吞噬囊泡。

We next asked whether these NCCs could engulf non-NCC debris. To do this, we treated Tg(sox10:Eos);Tg(nkx2.2a:nlsmCherry) embryos with 20 μM LysoTracker Red DND-99, which stains both dying cells and acidic organelles (Fogel et al., 2012), and time-lapse imaged from 19 to 40 hpf. In these movies, we observed NCCs migrate away from motor axons toward LysoTracker + debris located between two spinal motor nerves in neighboring so-mites (Figure 2F; Video S3). In one instance, we observed a NCC first send dynamic protrusions toward LysoTracker+ debris and then quickly engulf it (Figure 2F; Video S3). When NCCs tried to engulf large debris, like dead muscle fibers, they exhibited a behavior similar to frustrated phagocytosis, where one or many NCCs circled the dead cell for hours without successful engulfment (Figure S2D)(Cannon and Swanson, 1992). In spite of being highly active in response to cellular debris, NCCs do not engulf frequently in healthy embryos. Quantification of NCCs with engulfment vesicles showed that 1 to 2 cells per hemi-segment between 24 to 36 hpf had engulfment vesicles（Figure 2G，n = 17 fish），which is ~5%-10% of all NCCs in a hemi-segment. Taken together，these data demonstrate that NCCs can migrate away from motor axons and engulf debris.（Migratory Neural Crest Cells Phagocytose Dead Cells in the Developing Nervous System，*Cell*.，2019 Sep 19，179）

接下来，我们探究这些 NCC 是否会吞噬非 NCC 残骸。为此，我们使用对死亡细胞和酸性细胞器均可染色的 20 μM LysoTracker Red DND-99 染料处理 Tg（sox10∶Eos）；Tg（nkx2.2a∶nlsmCherry）胚胎，并从 19 hpf 到 40 hpf 延时成像。在这些视频中，我们观察到 NCC 从运动轴突移向 LysoTracker+的碎片，这些碎片位于相邻体节的两个脊髓运动神经之间（图 2F；视频 S3）。在一个视频中，我们观察到 NCC 首先向 LysoTracker+ 的碎片动态投射，然后迅速将其吞没（图 2F；视频 S3）。当 NCC 吞噬较大碎片（如死亡肌纤维）时，它们的表现类似于无效吞噬，一个或多个 NCC 围绕死亡细胞数小时却无法成功吞噬（图 S2D）（Cannon and Swanson，1992）。尽管对细胞残骸反应异常活跃，但在健康的胚胎中 NCC 并不会经常发挥吞噬作用。对含吞噬囊泡的 NCC 进行定量分析，结果显示 24 至 36 hpf，每半个横断面中有 1 至 2 个细胞有吞噬囊泡（图 2G，鱼 n = 17），占该半段所有 NCC 的 ~5%~10%。综上，这些数据表明 NCC 可以迁移至运动轴突外吞噬碎片。（迁移性神经嵴细胞吞噬神经系统发育期的死亡细胞）

例29

Results

Of the 370 children treated for Kawasaki disease at both sites during the study period，133（36%）did not qualify because they failed to meet strict eligibility criteria（n = 86）or had one or more exclusion criteria（n = 47；figure）. Of the 237 study-eligible patients，the parents of 196（83%）gave written consent，and these patients were randomly assigned to either the infliximab or placebo group（n = 98 in each group）. Of the 196 patients enrolled，183（93%）had at least four clinical criteria for Kawasaki disease，whereas 12（6%）and one（0.5%）qualified with two or more clinical criteria plus supporting laboratory values or an abnormal echocardiogram，respectively.

译文：

结果

研究期间共有 370 例川崎病儿童在两所医院接受了治疗，其中不合格患者 133 例（36%），包括 86 例不符合严格的纳入标准，47 例符合 1 条及以上的排除标准。在 237 例符合标准的患者中，196 例（83%）患者的父母签署了书面知情同意书，随后这些患者被随机分入英夫利昔单抗组或安慰剂组（每组 98 例）。纳入的 196 例患者中，183 例（93%）至少符合川崎病临床诊断标准中的 4 项；12 例（6%）和 1 例（0.5%）除符合临床标准中的两项及以上，还分别具有实验室诊断指标或心电图异常。

One patient in the placebo group was withdrawn from the study because of hypotension before receiving the study drug and was considered too ill by the study investigators to participate. All 196 patients were successfully contacted by telephone and reported no adverse events since the last study visit.132 of the 196 patients have returned for a 1-year follow-up assessment by one of the investigators and none have reported a serious illness since completion of the study.

安慰剂组中 1 例患者在接受研究药物前出现低血压被研究人员判定病情严重不能参与随后的试验,因此退出了研究。所有的 196 例患者均成功接受电话随访,并且在最后一次随访后再未出现不良事件。132 例患者已经接受了研究员为期 1 年的随访评估,研究结束后未出现严重疾病。

Baseline characteristics were similar between the two groups (table 1). The primary endpoint, treatment resistance, was similar in both groups, irrespective of site, with 11 (11.3%) of 97 patients in the placebo group and 11 (11.2%) of 98 in the infliximab group resistant to treatment (table 2). Four of the re-treated patients (two in the placebo and two in the infliximab group) were given a second intravenous immunoglobulin infusion before the 36 h timepoint specified in the protocol because of the clinical severity of their illness. A logistic regression model, with adjustment for illness day at enrolment and baseline alanine transaminase, γ-glutamyl transferase, percent bands, and age-adjusted haemoglobin, showed no difference in the treatment resistance rates between study groups ($p = 0.81$). The median days of fever in the infliximab group was 1 (range 0-4) compared with 2 days (range 0-6) in the placebo group ($p < 0.0001$; table 2). No patients receiving infliximab had intravenous immunoglobulin infusion reactions, compared with 13 (13.4%) of those receiving placebo ($p < 0.0001$).

两组的基线临床特征相似 (表 1)。主要终点,即治疗抵抗,在两所医院的两组中均相似,其中安慰剂组 97 例患者中出现 11 例 (11.3%),英夫利昔单抗组 98 例患者中出现 11 例 (11.2%) (表 2)。4 例接受再次治疗的患者 (每组各 2 例) 因出现严重的临床症状,按方案规定在 36 h 内予第二次 IVIG 输注治疗。调整入组时的患病天数、基线时的丙氨酸氨基转移酶、γ 谷氨酰转移酶、和中性粒细胞带状百分比及按龄期调整血红蛋白后,logistic 回归分析显示研究组的治疗抵抗率无显著差异 ($P = 0.81$)。英夫利昔单抗组发热天数的中位数为 1 天 (范围 0~4),安慰剂组为 2 天 (范围 0~6) ($P < 0.0001$;表 2)。英夫利昔单抗组无 1 例患者发生 IVIG 输注反应,而安慰剂组有 13 例 (13.4%) 患者 ($P < 0.0001$)。

Table 3 shows the coronary artery Z scores and classification for the study population by treatment group. Compared with baseline, there was a two-fold greater decrease in the mean Z score of the proximal left anterior descending coronary artery in the infliximab group compared with placebo at week 2 ($p = 0.045$; table 4, appendix), but no significant difference at week 5. There were no differences in the left main coronary artery or proximal right coronary artery Z scores compared with baseline at week 2 and week 5, or in the Z_{max}

between treatment groups (table 4). A post-hoc analysis of the mean change from baseline of the left main coronary artery and proximal right coronary artery Z scores of the 45 patients (25 in infliximab group, 20 in placebo group) with a baseline Z score of 2.5 or higher showed no difference between treatment groups.

表3显示治疗组研究人群的冠状动脉 Z 值和分类。与基线期相比,在第 2 周,英夫利昔单抗组患者的左冠状动脉前降支近端平均 Z 值的降低幅度是安慰剂组患者的两倍(P = 0.045;表4),但在第5周两组间无显著差异。在第 2 周和第 5 周,两治疗组的左冠状动脉主干或右冠状动脉近端 Z 值或 Z 最大值均无差异(表4)。基线期,45 例患者(英夫利昔单抗组 25 例,安慰剂组 20 例)的左冠状动脉主干和右冠状动脉近端 Z 值≥2.5。对 Z 值的平均变化进行析因分析,结果显示两治疗组间无差异。

The reduction in the concentration of C-reactive protein and absolute neutrophil count from baseline to 24 h after completion of intravenous immunoglobulin was greater in patients in the infliximab group than in the placebo group (p = 0.0003 for C-reactive protein and p = 0.024 for absolute neutrophil count) but similar at week 2 (table 5). There was also a greater reduction in erythrocyte sedimentation rate at week 2 compared with baseline in the infliximab group than in the placebo group (p = 0.009). There were no statistically significant differences at week 5 compared with baseline for any of the laboratory values.

从基线期到 IVIG 治疗后 24 h,英夫利昔单抗组比安慰剂组的 C 反应蛋白浓度和中性粒细胞绝对值降低更显著(C 反应蛋白浓度 P = 0.0003,中性粒细胞绝对值 P = 0.024),但在第 2 周时相似(表5)。与基线相比,在第 2 周,英夫利昔单抗组比安慰剂组的红细胞沉降率减少也更为显著(P = 0.009)。与基线相比,在第 5 周,实验室检查数据方面无统计学意义上的显著差异。

The adverse events are summarised by group in table 6. The number of patients who had one or more adverse events did not differ significantly between the groups (56 [57.1%] infliximab vs. 66 [67.4%] placebo, p = 0.18). No serious adverse event was related to the study drug. (Infliximab for intensification of primary therapy for Kawasaki disease: a phase 3 randomised, double-blind, placebo-controlled trial, *Lancet.*, 2014 Feb 24, 383)

表6总结了各组患者的不良事件。发生不良事件≥1 种的患者数量两组间未见显著性差异[英夫利昔单抗组 56 例(57.1%)vs. 安慰剂组 66 例(67.4%),P = 0.18]。没有与研究药物相关的严重不良事件。(注:图表省略)(英夫利昔单抗用于川崎病的初始强化治疗:一项 3 期、随机、双盲、安慰剂对照试验)

Exercise

1. Read the samples of "Results" and analyze their contents and structures. Recognize the signal markers and sentence patterns to realize these contents. Note the use of tenses for different contents in the writing.

2. Translate the following sentences in the "Results" into English.

1) 为证实经 GLP 和洋甘菊油（chamomile oil）处理后的细胞向胰岛素生成细胞（insulin-producing cells）分化，我们采用 RT-PCR 分析法测定了 NKX-2.2，PAX4，INS 和 PDX1 的 mRNA 水平。结果表明，尽管经 GLP 或洋甘菊油处理后的细胞均显著表达 NKX-2.2，PAX4，INS 和 PDX1，但在 GLP + 洋甘菊油处理的细胞中，这些标记物的表达最高。

2) 接受尿囊素（allantoin）治疗的大鼠中过氧化氢酶（catalase）活性、超氧化物歧化酶（superoxide dismutase）活性和谷胱甘肽（glutathione）水平明显高于接受顺铂（cisplatin）治疗的大鼠。接受顺铂治疗的大鼠中丙二醛（malonaldehyde）水平和一氧化氮（nitric oxide）浓度高于正常大鼠。

3) 用顺铂治疗的大鼠（第 2 组）的缩尾潜伏期（tail withdrawal latency）明显低于正常大鼠（第 1 组），表明出现痛觉过敏（hyperalgesia）。与顺铂组相比，尿囊素治疗显著延长了缩尾潜伏期。

4) 与对照组相比，完全弗氏佐剂（CFA）显著增加了大鼠脊髓组织中 NLRP3 的表达。但是，定量逆转录聚合酶链反应（qRT-PCR）分析法表明，丙泊酚治疗后，以 CFA 诱导的大鼠脊髓组织中 NLRP3 的表达显著降低。

5) 为了评估细胞的功能，我们检测了细胞对不同浓度的葡萄糖反应时所分泌 C 肽的水平。如图所示，在无葡萄糖的情况下，各组间未发现显著差异。而细胞对 15 和 30 mM 浓度的葡萄糖反应有显著差异。

6) 低温组（hypothermia group）90 天之内死亡的患者人数为 231 例，正常体温组为 247 例。在两组的存活患者或死亡患者中，机械通气（mechanical ventilation）的持续时间或 ICU 住院时间都没有显著差异。

6.6　讨论

6.6.1　讨论的功能

讨论（Discussion）是研究论文中最重要也是最难写的部分，包括作者对研究或实验结果的综合分析、理论说明及逻辑推理。论文的讨论与结果部分联系紧密，但又完全不同。结果部分叙述研究获得的依据（evidence），即结果和数据，并表明数据的统计学意义。而讨论部分是对结果和数据的阐释（interpretation），表明数据和结果与研究命题的相关性。讨论部分主要有三方面功能：解答"引言"中提出的命题，解释支持或不支持答案的依据和利用现有知识背景解释答案的合理性。

6.6.2　讨论的内容

在验证假设型论文中,讨论部分的内容可归纳为四部分:应答、论证、补充、结论。应答即"引言"中提出的命题的答案或展示整体结局。论证是对命题答案或结局提供的支持、解释和论证。补充内容视具体研究,有则写之,无则省之,包括研究的不支持依据,本研究的意外发现,本研究的不足之处或本研究的可靠性;并说明有待解决的问题,提出今后的研究方向。结论则揭示本研究的价值和重要性。

尽管在写作内容上相似,各期刊对讨论部分呈现形式的要求存在差异。比如,*JAMA* 要求"结论"从"讨论"部分独立出来,并用小标题标示;*Lancet* 和 *The New England Journal of Medicine* 则将结论置于讨论的最后,用信息标记语体现,如"in conclusion"。除对结论的呈现存在差异外,各期刊在讨论的体例上也存在差异,部分期刊允许使用小标题对讨论内容进行标示,具体如下例:

Cell

Discussion

A Cascade of Signals Directing the Patterning of Sequential Smooth Muscle Layers

Multiple Roles of Signals in Gut Morphogenesis

Common Pathways Control Muscle Differentiation in Tubular Organs

A New paradigm for Understanding the Development of Muscle Alignment through Mechanical Control

British Medical Journal

Discussion

Interpretation and implications

Strengths and weakness of this study

Conclusion

从以上示例也不难发现,讨论部分小标题的设定既可以是针对具体的内容,如 *Cell* 一例,也可以是针对讨论的层次,如 *BMJ* 一例。

6.6.3　讨论的结构

6.6.3.1　讨论的开启

命题答案或整体结局是讨论部分最重要的内容,是作者在提出研究问题、完成研究步骤、获得研究结果之后得出,是整篇论文的高潮(culmination)。因此,应该放在讨论最重要的位置——开始部分,并且用信息语标记。表达命题答案的信息语有 This study shows that…; Our results indicate that …; In this study, we provided evidence that …; In this study, we have shown that…; 和 In this study, we have found that…等。具体写作时,有三种方式。

1. 直接叙述命题答案或展示整体结局

例1

In this 15-year follow-up study, we found that 5.6 years of intensive glucose lowering that led to a median separation of 1.5 percentage points in the glycated hemoglobin curves did not result in a significantly lower risk of major cardiovascular events than standard therapy.

译文:在这项为期 15 年的随访研究中,我们发现,5.6 年期强化降糖导致糖化血红蛋白曲线中位数差异 1.5 个百分点,但并没有使主要心血管事件的风险显著低于标准治疗。

例2

In two parallel trials, one involving patients who underwent knee arthroscopy (POT-KAST) and one involving patients who were treated with casting of the lower leg (POT-CAST), we found that treatment with anticoagulants, either for the 8 days after arthroscopy or during the complete period of immobilization due to casting, was not effective for the prevention of symptomatic venous thromboembolism.

译文:在两项平行试验中,一项研究纳入行膝关节镜检查的患者(POT-KAST),另一项研究纳入接受小腿石膏固定治疗的患者(POT-CAST),我们发现抗凝剂治疗,无论在关节镜检查后持续 8 日还是石膏固定制动的全程,均不能有效地预防症状性的静脉血栓栓塞。

例3

Our data indicate that the interaction of B and T cells leads to activation and growth, i.e., AP, which appears to play an important role in the autoimmune response in MS. The study extends our previous findings that myelin-specific T cells can be activated, show TCR signaling, and proliferate upon contact with fully activated dendritic cells and in the absence of exogenously added antigen.

译文:我们的数据表明,B 细胞和 T 细胞的相互作用可致活化和生长,如自身增殖,该现象在多发性硬化病人的自身免疫反应中似乎起着重要作用。本研究拓展了我们之前的研究发现。之前的研究发现髓鞘特异性 T 细胞可被激活,传递 TCR 信号,并在与完全激活的树突状细胞接触和无外源添加抗原的情况下发生细胞增殖。

2. 重述研究问题后给出命题答案或展示整体结局

例4

In this study, we examined the role of transmission in the ongoing epidemic of XDR tuberculosis by combining multiple genotyping methods with social-network and epidemiologic analysis. We found that XDR tuberculosis remains widespread throughout KwaZulu-Natal and that transmission is the primary driver of the epidemic.

译文:在这项研究中,我们将多种基因分型方法与社交网络和流行病学分析相结合,评价了传播在 XDR 结核病的持续流行中发挥的作用。我们发现 XDR 结核病仍然在

KwaZulu-Natal 广泛传播,并且传播是其流行的主要驱动因素。

例5

We previously reported that the peptide based on Cx43, TAT-Cx43$_{266-283}$, inhibits c-Src activity and exerts important effects in different types of glioma cells in vitro, including freshly removed surgical specimens of glioblastoma. In this study, we explored the possibility of using this peptide for the therapy against malignant gliomas by studying its effect on healthy brain cells and by evaluating its anti-tumor effects in vivo.

译文:我们以前报道过基于 Cx43 的肽,即 TAT-Cx43$_{266-283}$,抑制 c-Src 活性,并对体外不同类型胶质瘤细胞产生重要作用,包括刚切除的胶质母细胞瘤手术标本。在本研究中,我们通过分析这种肽对健康脑细胞的作用以及评估它在体内的抗肿瘤作用,探讨使用这种肽治疗恶性胶质瘤的可能性。

The present study showed that the effect of TAT-Cx43$_{266-283}$ is cell-selective. Thus, while GSC viability was strongly decreased, neuron and astrocyte viability was not greatly affected by TAT-Cx43$_{266-283}$. Moreover, the morphology, expression of differentiation markers and motility of these normal brain cells were unaffected by TAT-Cx43$_{266-283}$. Conversely, TAT-Cx43$_{266-283}$ reduced stemness, proliferation, survival, invasion, and migration in GSCs.

本研究表明 TAT-Cx43$_{266-283}$ 的作用具有细胞选择性。因此,尽管 GSC 活性大幅度下降,TAT-Cx43$_{266-283}$ 对神经元和星形胶质细胞的影响不大。并且,TAT-Cx43$_{266-283}$ 也不影响这些正常脑细胞的形态学、分化标志物的表达以及活性。相反,TAT-Cx43$_{266-283}$ 降低 GSCs 的干性、增殖、存活、浸润和迁移。

在写作时,重述研究问题必须注意与引言部分一致,关键词、动词、语态要保持一致。有些作者在重述研究命题之后,可能还会重述研究设计,但一定要注意详略得当,否则会喧宾夺主,读者无法在最醒目的地方找到最重要的信息。

3. 简述研究背景后给出命题答案或展示整体结局

例6

Scar formation by astrocytes (Anderson et al., 2016; Faulkner et al., 2004; Herrmann et al., 2008; Sabelström et al., 2013; Sil-ver, 2016) and type A pericytes (Göritz et al., 2011) is crucial for sealing off the injured tissue and regaining tissue integrity after CNS lesions. At the same time, scar tissue is considered a major block for axonal regeneration. Most attention has been focused on astrocytes forming the glial component of the scar, and reactive astrocytes have long been thought to inhibit axonal regeneration (Cafferty et al., 2007; Xu et al., 2015; Yiu and He, 2006), although this notion has recently been questioned (Ander-son et al., 2016; Silver, 2016). Pericytes give rise to fibroblast-like cells that constitute the fibrotic compartment of the scar and are required for the generation of fibrosis and extracellular matrix deposition. We demonstrate that pericyte-derived scarring represents a major barrier for axonal regrowth and that moderate inhibition of this process preserves intact wound healing and dampens inflammation and reactive astrogliosis while enabling axonal regrowth and improved functional recovery.

译文：星形细胞和 A 型周细胞的疤痕形成对于在中枢神经系统损伤后封闭损伤组织和恢复组织完整性至关重要。同时，瘢痕组织被认为是轴突再生的主要障碍。相关研究主要关注形成疤痕胶质成分的星形细胞，反应性星形细胞也长期被认为能抑制轴突再生，然而这一观念最近却受到质疑。周细胞产生成纤维样细胞，这些细胞构成疤痕的纤维间室，也参与纤维化的形成和细胞外基质的沉积。我们证明，周细胞源性的疤痕形成是轴突再生的主要障碍；这一过程能维持伤口愈合、抑制炎症和反应性星形胶质细胞形成，同时促进轴突再生和功能恢复。

例7

Previously treated squamous-cell NSCLC represents an area of unmet need, with little progress made since the approval of docetaxel in 1999. A retrospective review of recent U. S. Medicare data indicates that survival remains poor among patients receiving second-line treatment for squamous-cell NSCLC, with a median overall survival of 6.4 months and survival rates of 22% at 1 year and 5% at 2 years. 17 Here we report results of an international, prospective, randomized, phase 3 trial that showed superior survival and an improved safety profile with nivolumab versus standard-of-care docetaxel in patients with advanced, previously treated squamous-cell NSCLC.

译文：此前对鳞状细胞 NSCLC 的治疗效果并不令人满意。自 1999 年多西他赛获批以来，该疾病治疗上的进展乏善可陈。对美国 Medicare 最近发布的数据进行回顾性研究，结果表明，接受二线药物治疗鳞状细胞 NSCLC 患者生存率较低，中位总生存期为 6.5 个月，1年生存率为 22%，2 年生存率为 5%。我们在此报告一项国际性、前瞻性、随机化的三期临床试验的结果，显示在此前治疗过的晚期鳞状细胞 NSCLC 患者中，与标准治疗方案多西他赛相比，接受纳武单抗治疗的患者生存期更长，用药安全性更好。

值得注意的是，虽然讨论开始可适当回顾研究背景，但切忌在讨论开始部分再现引言，或扩展引言，甚至重写一个不同的引言，而是对引言中的背景信息或相关研究进行重点回顾。

6.6.3.2　讨论的主体

应答研究命题之后，就开始展开讨论。讨论的顺序从最重要到次重要，即根据讨论内容与命题答案的相关程度依次展开，例如，对命题答案的支持、解释和论证通常置于最重要的位置。另外，涉及不同讨论内容时，应多使用主题句及信息标记语以提高文字的可读性和逻辑性，如：The results of… in the present study are in accordance with…；The present study extends these observations…；While we confirm these reports, we also show that…；The discrepancies between the results of our study and those of other studies may be due to…等。具体参见以下各例。

1. 用本研究结果或数据支持命题答案

给出命题答案之后，用本研究结果加以支持，增强答案的说服力。根据需要，选择性重述结果部分的重要结果或数据。

例8

Inadequate treatment of MDR tuberculosis accounted for, at most, 31% of cases of XDR tuberculosis. Genotyping methods also showed the clonal nature of this epidemic and provide further support for the predominant role of transmission. Social-network analysis showed connections among participants with XDR tuberculosis; these connections created numerous opportunities for transmission not only in hospitals, but also in community settings. Our finding of the role of transmission in the epidemic of XDR tuberculosis provides insight as to why the epidemic continues, at least in this community, as efforts to control tuberculosis to date have not sufficiently addressed the interruption of transmission.

译文：MDR 结核病治疗不足在 XDR 结核病病例中最多占 31%。基因分型方法也表明了这种流行病的克隆属性，并进一步证明了传播的主导作用。社交网络分析显示 XDR 结核病患者之间存在联系，这些联系不仅在医院，而且在社区环境制造了大量的传播机会。我们发现了传播在 XDR 结核病流行中发挥的作用，这一发现有助于解释为什么这一疾病至少在这一地区持续流行，原因是迄今为止控制结核病的努力尚未充分阻断传播。

2. 用同类研究解释和支持命题答案

除了用本研究结果支持外，以公认知识或同类研究结果对命题答案给予解释（explanation）、支持（support），说明其可靠性（reliability）。

例9

Our finding that dairy intake was not associated with lower risk of mortality is also consistent with mendelian randomization studies using lactase persistence genotype rs4988235 as the instrumental variable. Two studies conducted in a Danish population of 97811 participants found that the T allele of rs4988235 was not associated with lower risks of type 2 diabetes, total mortality, and mortality due to cardiovascular disease and cancer. (56,57) Two studies conducted within the CHARGE consortium involving more than 171000 participants showed that the T allele of rs4988235 was associated with slightly higher body mass index and systolic blood pressure, two important risk factors of mortality. (58 59)

译文：我们的研究发现，乳品摄入与较低的死亡率无关联。这一发现与使用乳糖酶持续性基因型 rs4988235 为工具变量的孟德尔随机化研究结果一致。在丹麦 97811 名受试者中进行的两项研究发现，rs4988235 的 T 等位基因与 2 型糖尿病患病风险、总死亡率以及心血管疾病和癌症致死率的降低无相关性。两项 CHARGE 联合体开展的研究纳入超过 171000 名受试者，研究表明 rs4988235 的 T 等位基因与稍高的体重指数和收缩压有关，二者均是死亡的重要危险因素。

3. 与同类研究相比，论证本研究的创新之处

如果本研究的答案或结果与国内外同类研究的答案或结果不同，则需要辩证（defense）。辩证时需从正反两方面进行。首先找出不一致的原因，如研究人群不同，研究方法不同，或是数据质量的等级不同等。然后再阐述本研究和他人研究相比存在的优势，或他人研究存在的不足。论证时应注意公正客观，切忌夸大或隐瞒。

例10

Despite similar dietary assessment methods and calculation of gluten intake, discrepancies in results among the studies are likely attributable to study design and population size. In the randomized clinical trial, the time of gluten introduction was not accounted for and gluten amounts were fixed, [11] which differed from the present observational study consisting of a larger population that reflected the natural variations of gluten intake in real life. Other contributing factors may be differences in exposures to various triggering environmental factors, such as gastrointestinal infections or rotavirus vaccination status, [4,5] which could partly explain why Swedish children are more prone to develop celiac disease compared with children from other countries.

译文：尽管饮食评估方法和谷蛋白摄入量计算相似，研究结果却表现出差异。这可能归因于研究设计和人群规模。在一项随机临床试验中，谷蛋白的引入时间未予考虑，谷蛋白的量也是固定的。这些与本文的观察研究不同，本研究人群较大，能反映现实生活中谷蛋白摄入量的自然差异。其他影响因素可能是暴露于不同的环境诱因，如胃肠道感染或轮状病毒疫苗接种的情况。因此，某种程度上，瑞典儿童比其他国家的儿童更容易患小肠吸收不良症。

6.6.3.3　讨论的补充内容

1. 不支持命题答案的结果

除了对本研究的答案进行陈述、支持、解释和（或）与相关研究进行比较之外，讨论部分还可能叙述不支持研究答案的结果（un-supporting finding）并尽可能给予合理解释，通常使用标记语 contrary to，unexpectedly，interestingly 等。

例11

The main finding of the present study is that β-adrenergic blockade does not impair performance of maximal or submaximal exercise at high altitude. As expected, treatment with the β-blocker propranolol substantially decreased heart rate at high altitude. However, contrary to our hypothesis, propranolol-treated subjects were able to maintain levels of oxygen uptake during maximal and submaximal exercises as great as those in placebo-treated subjects. This finding cannot be attributed to increased arterial oxygen saturation or hemoglobin concentration, since values for propranolol-treated subjects were not different from those for placebo-treated subjects. Rather, it appears that oxygen uptake was maintained by increasing stroke volume.

译文：本研究的主要发现是 β-肾上腺素能阻滞不减损在高海拔的极量或亚极量运动能力。不出所料，β-阻断剂心得安大幅降低高海拔心率。然而，与我们假设不同的是，在极量或亚极量运动时，经心得安治疗的受试者跟安慰剂组的受试者一样能维持摄氧水平。这一结果的原因不可能是动脉血氧饱和度或血红蛋白浓度增加,因为两组受试者的这些指标值没有差异。相反,很有可能是心搏出量增加维持了氧的摄入。

2. 研究的意外发现

意外发现(unexpected findings)可大可小。重大的意外发现能发人深思,激发新的研究思路。描述时应尽量给出合理解释。

例12①

Unexpectedly, we also found great variability in the response of fetal pulmonary blood flow to the effects of lung distention. In one-half of the fetuses, the mean increase in pulmonary blood flow during lung distension was maximal, whereas in the other half it was only about 20% of the cumulative response. Interestingly, Cook et al. found similar variability in their study of nitrogen and air ventilation: of the six fetuses studied, two showed no effect of nitrogen ventilation but a large effect upon changing to air, two showed a small effect of nitrogen and a larger response to air, and two showed a large increase in pulmonary blood flow during nitrogen ventilation with no further change upon exposure to air. To explain these findings, Cook et al. noted that nitrogen had the greatest effect on the smallest fetuses. However, we were unable to identify the reasons for the variability we found. It was not on a purely arithmetic basis. That is, the major responders did not begin with lower control flows or have lower maximal flows. In fact, the two groups had remarkably similar pulmonary blood flows both during baseline measurements and during ventilation with 100% oxygen. The groups were also not different in their overall maturity, with respect to either gestational age or weight. In addition, differences in p_{O_2} were not responsible for the differences between major and minor responders, since both during baseline measurements and during lung distension, the minor responders were neither more hypoxic nor more hypercapnic than the major responders. Lastly, adequacy of alveolar ventilation was probably not responsible for the difference between the groups. Although we were not able to determine the adequacy of alveolar ventilation during lung distension, during oxygenation, PO_2 and PCO_2 values were similar in the two groups, without the method of ventilation having been changed in either group.

译文:作者还意外地发现胎羊(注:原文中的胎儿意指胎羊,以下胎儿都译为胎羊)肺血流对肺膨胀反应有很大的差异性。在肺膨胀时,一半胎羊的肺血流平均量达最高值,而另一半胎羊的肺血流的平均增加值只占累积反应的20%。有趣的是,Cook 等人在一项应用氮气和空气通气的研究中也发现了类似的差异性。在 6 只胎羊中,2 只显示对氮气通气无反应而转换空气通气后反应增大,另 2 只对氮气通气反应较小而对空气通气反应较大;还有 2 只在氮气通气时肺血流明显增加而接触空气时无进一步变化。为了解释这些结果,Cook 等人注意到氮气对胎龄最小的胎羊影响最大。然而,我们未能确定本研究发现的这一差异性的

---

① 杨明山,《医学英语新教程》,上海:世界图书出版公司,2005 年,第 205-206 页。译文基于原译文有调整。

原因。这并非是一个单纯的数字计算。因为主要反应组起始控制流量不低,最大流量也不低。事实上,两组间基线测量与纯氧通气时的肺血流量非常相似。两组间胎龄和体重相关的成熟度无差异。此外,氧分压差异并非导致了主要及次要反应组间的差异,因为在基线测定与肺膨胀时,次要反应组出现低氧血症或高碳酸血症不比主要反应组多。最后,肺泡通气的充足程度可能不会造成两组间的差异。虽然在肺膨胀、氧合中我们无法测定肺泡通气的充足程度,但两组间氧分压与二氧化碳分压值相似,且任何一组都没有改变通气方式。

3. 研究的可靠性

如果研究方法、研究设计存在任何不足,或研究是建立在某种假设之上,讨论中应该指出并阐明其对研究的影响以表明研究的可靠性(validity),也可以特别强调本研究设计上的优点,以增强研究的可靠性。常用句型有:The study has several weaknesses still; There are still some unanswered questions…; Such an assumption still needs further investigation using…等。

例13

Our study has several strengths. Firstly, dairy intake was measured repeatedly in all three cohorts, and we calculated cumulative averages for dairy intake to minimize the random measurement error caused by within-person variation. Furthermore, we stopped updating dairy intake on the diagnosis of potential intermediate conditions, which minimized the potential for reverse causation due to change of lifestyle factors because of chronic diseases. Secondly, our study included 217755 participants with 51438 deaths. The large sample size and number of deaths provided sufficient power for the analyses.

译文:我们的研究有如下优点。首先,在所有三个队列中重复测量乳制品摄入量,并计算乳制品摄入量的累积平均值,以最小化由个体差异引起的随机测量误差。并且,一旦诊断出受试者处于潜在的慢性病前期,我们则停止更新乳品摄入量的数据,以此将由于慢性病引起的生活方式因素改变而导致的逆转的可能性降至最低。其次,我们的研究纳入了217755名受试者,其中51438例死亡。大样本量和死亡例数都为分析提供了足够的统计学效能。

例14

Some limitations of our trial should be considered. First, although the reduction in the dose of tranexamic acid during the course of the trial provided an opportunity to test for a dose effect, this analysis was underpowered. Second, our trial included few patients who were at the highest risk for bleeding or thrombosis; however, we did not identify a subgroup effect that would suggest different findings among patients with overall higher risk. Third, in this trial, the attending anesthesiologists were sometimes aware of the treatment-group assignment; however, sensitivity analysis and the analysis of truly blinded data on postoperative blood loss and transfusion were consistent with the analysis of postoperative trial outcomes data. Finally, our trial included only a small proportion of patients undergoing off-pump surgery, and although the point estimates of effects among those patients were generally consistent with the point estimates of effects among patients undergoing on-pump surgery and although there were no significant interactions between subgroups, clinically important differences cannot be ruled out.

译文:应该考虑到我们的试验有一些局限性。第一,尽管在试验过程中降低氨甲环酸剂量提供了测试剂量效应的机会,但该分析效能不足。第二,我们的试验纳入了少数出血或血栓形成最高危的患者,然而我们没有发现能够提示总体风险较高的患者中有不同结果的亚组效应。第三,在本试验中,主管麻醉医师有时知晓治疗组的分配情况,然而敏感性分析和对手术后失血和输血进行的全盲数据分析均与术后试验结局数据的分析结果一致。最后,我们的试验只包括了一小部分接受非体外循环手术的患者,并且尽管这些患者治疗效果的点估计值通常与接受体外循环手术患者治疗效果的点估计值一致,且亚组间没有显著的交互作用,但仍不能排除临床上有重要的差异。

6.6.3.4 研究的意义

通过表明研究的应用价值(applications),揭示研究的含义(implications),提出建议(recommendations)或作出推测(speculations)、展望(expectation)等方式来揭示研究意义。写作时,可使用不同的信息语表达不同的意义,如下所示:

结尾	信息语	情态动词
应用价值	apply, use	can, will
建议	recommend, suggest	should
含义	suggest, imply	may, might
推测	speculate	may, might

例15

研究的应用价值

This is the first large randomized controlled trial on the value of ACT for advanced rectal cancer patients, receiving CRT and surgery based on postoperative pathological stage. This is of great significance that ACRNaCT will provide novel and individualized adjuvant treatment strategies for rectal cancer patients following neoadjuvant CRT and surgery.

译文:这是探讨 ACT 治疗晚期直肠癌患者效果的第一项大样本随机对照试验,选取的患者均基于术后病理分期进行了 CRT 和手术。研究表明 ACRNaCT 有望成为结肠癌患者在行新辅助 CRT 和手术之后的一种新的个体化辅助治疗策略,研究发现具有重大意义。

例16

建议

This study provides strong evidence to support influenza vaccination of care home staff even when vaccine uptake by residents is high. Results are likely to be generalisable to other care homes in the United Kingdom and abroad and may also be applicable to acute hospital settings, in particular elderly care and rehabilitation wards. It has proved difficult to achieve high uptake rates in healthcare workers owing to perceptions that influenza is a relatively trivial illness, concern about side effects, beliefs that the vaccine is ineffective, and lack of time and motivation.[29] Campaigns to promote influenza vaccination among healthcare workers or staff of long term care facilities should emphasize the protection of vulnerable patients and residents as well as the benefits to the individual.

译文：本研究用有力的证据证明，即使疗养人员的疫苗接种率高，也应对养老院的工作人员接种疫苗。这一发现有可能适用于英国和国外的其他养老院，也有可能适用于急诊医院，特别是医院里的老年和康复病房。由于认为流感无关大碍，顾虑其副作用，怀疑疫苗的效果，以及缺少时间和动机等因素，在医疗工作人员中不易达到高疫苗接种率。在医疗或长期护理机构的工作人员中倡导疫苗接种时，应该同时强调对个人的益处及对易感患者和疗养人员的保护作用。

例17

研究的含义

Our findings in dogs, together with findings from studies of human coronary arteries, suggest that H_1 blockers may antagonize histamine-mediated vasoconstriction and vasospasm in patients with atherosclerotic coronary artery disease and thus may have therapeutic value. Conversely, H_2 blockers may permit unopposed H_1-mediated vasoconstriction of epicardial arteries and may also limit vasodilation and thus may not have therapeutic value.

译文：犬类实验以及人冠状动脉的其他研究结果提示，在冠状动脉粥样硬化患者中 H_1 受体阻断剂可以对抗组织胺介导的血管收缩和血管痉挛，因此可能具有治疗价值。相反，H_2 受体阻断剂不会对抗 H_1 介导的心外膜动脉血管收缩，还可限制血管扩张，因此可能不具有治疗价值。

例18

展望研究的价值

Our studies show that MYCi induces ICD in tumor cells and allows increased T cell infiltration and subsequent upregulation of PD-L1 in the tumor microenvironment. Accordingly, MYCi treatment sensitized otherwise refractory tumors to immune checkpoint blockade. One may envision a future treatment regimen in which an MYC inhibitor is given to patients for a limited period of time followed by immune checkpoint blockade, thus avoiding potential toxicities to normal tissues that may arise from prolonged MYC inhibition.

译文：我们的研究表明 MYCi 诱导肿瘤细胞内的 ICD，导致肿瘤微环境中 T 细胞浸润增加随后上调 PD-L1 表达。因此，对难治性肿瘤，MYCi 增加了其对免疫检查点阻断的敏感性。人们可以设想一种未来的治疗方案：患者出现免疫检查点阻断后，短期服用 MYC 抑制剂，从而避免可能因 MYC 抑制延长对正常细胞造成的潜在毒性。

6.6.3.5　讨论的结尾

讨论部分的结尾也是论文的结尾，应该起到画龙点睛的作用，常常被标注为结论。通常包含三方面内容：重述命题答案，表明本研究的重要性和新颖性，展望进一步研究的方向。写作时，可视研究的具体情况选择性地加以描述。

重述命题答案时，常用 In summary, we have shown that…; In conclusion, this study shows that…; In conclusion, our results indicate that…等结论语作为信息标记。提示尚待解决的问题及下一步的研究方向时，常用 Further work may be needed to…; Further study is needed to…; In the future, we will extend the present studies to…和 Further studies are needed to answer these questions.等作为信息标记语。

例19

In conclusion, we have proved that the tested drug, HC, has protective effects against MI and stroke in such severe conditions. The current study could be a reference for stroke post-MI experimentation on animals. It reproduces the same cascade of events that leads to the stroke and its complications in human. This study is pioneer research: it will open new horizons for the management of stroke and myocardial infarction and it will improve dramatically the life of human patients. Thus, human trials on this new coumarin are strongly recommended to confirm this study findings.

译文：综上所述，我们已经证明测试药物 HC 对危重情况下的心肌梗死和卒中有保护作用。本研究可为心梗后卒中的动物实验提供参考。再现了导致人群卒中及其并发症同样的系列事件。这项研究具有开创性：它将为卒中和心肌梗死的治疗开辟新的视野，并将显著改善人类患者的生活质量。因此，强烈建议对这种新香豆素进行人体试验，以证实这一研究结果。

例20

In conclusion, osimertinib was more effective than combination platinum-based chemotherapy in patients with T790M-positive non-small-cell lung cancer (including those with CNS metastases) after disease progression with first-line EGFR-TKI therapy.

译文：总之，对 T790M 阳性的非小细胞肺癌患者（包括出现 CNS 转移的患者），一线 EGFR-TKI 治疗后出现疾病进展，奥希替尼的疗效显著优于铂类为基础的联合化疗。

例21

In summary, our data link B and T cells with MS pathogenesis and show that the interactions of these two cell types probably occur in conjunction with the MS-associated DR15 molecules and that B cells may express antigens, which are also upregulated in the brain and recognized by AP CD4+ T cells. We expect that our data will be instrumental for further studies about MS pathomechanisms, as *in vitro* drug finding platform and to guide the search for the specificity of B and T cells. Furthermore, they provide a plausible explanation for the high efficacy of anti-CD20 therapy in a T cell-mediated disease such as MS. Future studies should address whether AP is influenced by antigen-specific tolerization (Lutterotti et al., 2013).

译文：总之，我们的数据显示了 B 细胞和 T 细胞与 MS 发病的关联性，并表明这两种细胞类型的相互作用可能与 MS 相关的 DR15 分子一起发生；B 细胞可能表达抗原，这些抗原在大脑中也被上调，并被 AP CD4+T 细胞识别。作为体外药物研发平台，我们的数据有望推动 MS 的病理机制的进一步研究，并对 B 细胞和 T 细胞特异性研究具有指导意义。此外，这些数据合理解释了抗 CD20 治疗 T 细胞介导性疾病（如 MS）的高效性。未来的研究应探讨 AP 是否受到抗原特异性耐受性的影响。

6.6.4　讨论的写作要点

6.6.4.1　讨论部分的时态

讨论部分的时态比较复杂。陈述具有普遍意义的答案或结论时，用现在时。展示整体结局或局限于本研究的结论时，用过去时。讨论中的分析、比较和推理则有过去时和现在时的交替使用，涉及本研究的问题、方法和结果方面的描述、与以往研究的比较用过去时；而分析、推理后得出的论点则用现在时。

6.6.4.2　讨论部分的模糊限制语

论文的讨论部分存在较多基于研究发现的主观论断。这种具有主观测度的表达要求准确精密，避免绝对武断。为了达到这一目的，作者可能会使用模糊限制语。模糊限制语指一些把事物弄得模模糊糊的词语，可以表达话语的真实程度，也可以表明作者对话语内容的主观态度，或者提出客观根据，对话语作出间接的评估。即使看法不全，观点有错误，也能得到读者的理解，从而起到保护自己的作用。下面就生物医学期刊论文中模糊限制语的使用作简要介绍。

1. 表达"准确"的模糊限制语

作者在阐述某种见解或提出某种论断时，用模糊限制语把一些接近准确、但又不敢肯定完全正确的话语，说得跟实际情况更接近一些，避免了论断中语言的绝对化和武断性。另外，对一些不必准确或不能准确的内容进行表述时，通过模糊限制语来修饰和限制以达到确切表达思想内容的目的。表达"准确"的模糊限制语主要有以下两种。

（1）情态动词

用情态动词 will, can, would, could, should, may, might 表示作者的推测。多用于分析、推理等论述中，使肯定的语气得到适当的缓和，以表示一种不完全肯定的估计或推测。上述情态动词所表达的肯定程度按所排列顺序递减。

例22

While MMP-9, specifically, does not appear to be involved in facilitating early dissemination of the M. tuberculosis bacilli, the data presented here suggest that this degradative enzyme plays a causative role in granuloma development. As shown in Fig. 7A to C, in the absence of MMP-9 cells appeared trapped in visibly condensed alveolar septa at day 60 of infection, a phenomenon observed by other investigators using MMP-2KO（7） and MMP-9KO (23) mice in allergen challenge models. In addition, lymphocytes accumulated around the perivascular region, suggesting that they were unable to migrate into and around the granuloma. In contrast, visible septa were absent in the FVB wild-type lung, and granulomas were well formed as in Fig. 7D and 7E. Interestingly, similar to lung sections from the MMP-9KO mice, the susceptible CBA/J mouse strain also exhibited visibly thickened alveolar septa within loosely associated cellular accumulations at day 28 of infection, whereas granuloma formation in resistant C57BL/6 mice was marked by a decrease in alveolar septal wall integrity (Fig. 6A and 6B). As granuloma formation progressed to day 40, it was evident that the susceptible strain of mouse was unable to form well-organized granulomas compared to the resistant strain, which formed tight granulomas (Fig. 6C and 6D). The failure by the susceptible mouse strain to form tight, well-organized granulomas may be the result of an inability to remodel tissue sufficiently, due to reduced MMP-9 activity. In fact, when MMP-9 was absent, macrophage recruitment into the lungs was significantly reduced compared to that observed in the FVB wild-type lungs (Fig. 8A), and there were fewer F4/80-positive cells within the lung lesions of the knockout strain (data not shown). With fewer host cells present in which to multiply, the reduced number of macrophages in the lungs of the MMP-9KO mice may have accounted for the decreased bacterial load in the mice lacking MMP-9 compared to the FVB wild-type strain (Fig. 5). Interestingly, although there were fewer macrophages in the lungs of the MMP-9KO mice, there were similar levels of TNF-and IFN-in the lungs between the FVB wild-type and the knockout mice (data not shown), indicating that the reduced CFU numbers in the knockout strain were not the result of reduced production of these two cytokines. The knockout mice, however, produced significantly less MCP-1 (Fig. 8C), and they recruited fewer macrophages to the lungs (Fig. 8A), suggesting that MMP-9 may play a role with MCP-1 in recruiting macrophages to the lungs during granuloma development. In addition, it seems likely that macrophage-derived MCP-1, previously shown to strongly recruit monocytes and Th1-type lymphocytes in response to products of M. tuberculosis (8), played a role in facilitating cellular organization within the granuloma since this chemokine was up regulated in the resistant C57BL/6 mice compared to the susceptible CBA mice (Fig.3C). Based on these data together with the histologic findings, it is probable that the inability of the susceptible strain to form tight granulomas was based on a lack of MMP-9 activity in the lungs and therefore a lack of tissue remodeling and cellular recruitment that must occur in order for protective granulomas to form.

　　译文:MMP-9似乎不特定参与促进 M.肺结核杆菌的早期播散,但本文所显示的数据提示该降解酶促使肉芽肿的形成。如图 7A-C 所示,MMP-9 酶缺乏的细胞在感染第 60 天聚集于明显压缩的肺泡隔,其他研究者用变应原激发模型 MMP-2 敲除 (7) 与 MMP-9 敲除 (23) 小鼠实验观察到同样现象。另外,淋巴细胞聚集到血管周围,提示它们无法迁移至肉芽肿内或其附近区域。相反,FVB 野生型肺中未出现明显肺泡隔,但肉芽肿却成型良好,如图 7D 和 7E 所示。有趣的是,与 MMP-9 敲除鼠肺切片相似,感染第 28 天,敏感 CBA／J 鼠株在结构松散的细胞聚集中也呈现明显增厚的肺泡隔,而肉芽肿形成在抗性 C57BL／6 小鼠却表现为肺泡隔的壁完整性下降 (图 6A 和 6B)。当肉芽肿发育至第 40 天,易感鼠株明显不能形成结构良好的肉芽肿,与之相比较,抵抗株却有结构致密的肉芽肿形成 (图 6C 和 6D)。易感鼠株不能形成结构良好且致密的肉芽肿可能系 MMP-9 活性减低从而不能充分重塑组织所致。事实上,与 FVB 野生型肺相比,当 MMP-9 缺失时,募集至肺部的巨噬细胞明显减少 (图 8A),且敲除株的肺损伤部位的 F4／80-阳性细胞较少 (数据未显)。与 FVB 野生型株相比,随着可供繁殖的宿主细胞减少,MMP-9 敲除鼠肺中巨噬细胞的数量减少则有可能导致 MMP-9 缺乏小鼠中细菌荷载量减少 (图 5)。有趣的是,尽管 MMP-9 敲除鼠肺中巨噬细胞的数量减少,但 FVB 野生型与敲除型肺中的 TNF-与 IFN-水平却相似 (数据未显),表明敲除株中 CFU 数量减少并非因为这两种细胞活素分泌减少所致。然而敲除鼠中 MCP-1 分泌量显著减少 (图 8C),募集至肺中的巨噬细胞减少 (图 8A),提示在肉芽肿形成时,MMP-9 与 MCP-1 共同募集巨噬细胞至肺部。另外,有研究证实在 M.肺结核产物的作用下,巨噬细胞源性 MCP-1 具有较强的募集单核细胞与 Th1-型淋巴细胞的能力 (8),其很可能参与促进肉芽肿内细胞构成,因为与易感 CBA 鼠相比,该趋化因子水平在抵抗 C57BL／6 鼠中上调 (图 3C)。基于以上数据及组织学发现,易感株不能形成致密的肉芽肿很可能是因为肺中 MMP-9 活性不足,从而缺乏形成保护性肉芽肿所需的组织重塑及细胞募集。

(2) 副词及形容词

用起到限制作用的副词,如 certainly, undoubtedly, clearly, apparently, remarkably, notably, markedly, pronouncedly, probably, possibly, likely 等,及其相应的形容词构成模糊语,或强调结论的肯定性,或使结论的肯定语气得以缓和,不再绝对,而是相对和留有余地,从而使论断更臻严密而科学。

例23

During seasons with higher levels of activity, such as years when there are severe epidemics, the benefits of vaccination would undoubtedly be greater.

译文:在流感活动水平更高的季节,比如流感严重流行的年份,接种的益处无疑会更大。

例24

The relatively low proportion of patients in the device group who had an ischemic stroke during follow-up is probably related to the unique textured surfaces of the device we used.

译文:随访中装置组的病人发生缺血性休克的比例相对较低,可能与我们使用的装置表面的特殊材质有关。

例25

Vaccination against influenza markedly decreases the numbers of hospitalization and deaths due to complications of influenza among the elderly. It is probable that vaccination is of similar benefit in younger persons.

译文:流感疫苗接种显著降低老年人入院次数和因流感并发症导致的死亡率。有可能在年轻人中,接种也有类似的益处。

2. 表达"客观"的模糊限制语

讨论部分关于研究答案或整体结局属于基于本研究的证据性事实,表达这一事实时作者会同时传递其主观态度。用 study,results,data,findings 等作主语,以显示论点的客观性,而非作者杜撰,大多以 confirm, prove, demonstrate, show, indicate, find, suggest, imply, seem, appear 等动词作谓语,按所排列顺序递减,表达作者对研究答案的不同肯定程度。

例26

This pilot study demonstrates that air is a suitable substitute for barium in the diagnosis and reduction of intussusception.

译文:这项试验性研究证实空气可以替代钡用于肠套叠的诊断与复位。

例27

The results of this placebo-controlled trial show the benefits that vaccination against influenza offers for healthy, working adults.

译文:这项安慰剂对照试验表明流感疫苗接种对健康从业成年人有益处。

例28

The present study finds that the prevalence of H pylori in children is higher if the social conditions are lower.

译文:本研究发现社会条件越差,儿童幽门螺旋杆菌的感染率越高。

例29

The fact that an effect was shown in a year with below average influenza activity suggests that a protective effect would be observed in most years.

译文:流感活动低于平均水平年份有效果,这一事实揭示多数年份中也会观察到疫苗的保护效果。

例30

Of the 40 to 50 percent mortality found in acute myocardial infarction, over half occurs prior to hospitalization and seems to be sudden in onset and related to ventricular fibrillation.

译文:在40%~50%急性心肌梗死的死亡病例中,一半以上发生在住院前,似乎发病突然,并且与心室纤维性颤动有关。

3. 表达"谦虚"的模糊限制语

论文的读者大多为同行,作者应注意使用适当的模糊限制语来突出作者的作用,敬重读者的反馈,同时也表现出作者的谦逊态度。这种模糊限制语的典型标志是用第一人称或含有第一人称的短语作主语,如 we believe, to our knowledge, as far as we know, we conclude 等。一方面表明作者勇于承担责任,同时在一定程度上缓和语气,给读者留有探讨的余地,避免把自己的观点强加于人;另一方面,即使看法不全,观点有错误,也能得到读者的理解,从而起到保护自己的作用。

例31

We suggest that acute exertion should be added as a potential risk factor for plaque rupture, along with elevated serum cholesterol level.

译文：我们建议把急性劳累与血清胆固醇水平增高均视为斑块破裂的潜在因素。

例32

We believe our findings are a good basis for further molecular genetic research on drug-resistance in treatment of intractable epilepsy.

译文：我们相信本研究发现为难治性癫痫治疗中的药物耐受现象进行进一步分子遗传学研究奠定了良好的基础。

例33

We can conclude from these results that the bisulfate anion has a protective effect and prevents photo dissociation of the complex in two manners.

译文：我们可以从这些结果得出结论，硫酸氢钠阴离子具有保护作用，并以两种方式防止复合物的光离解。

例34

This is the first study to our knowledge to use a convolution neural network to identify the electrocardiographic signature of atrial fibrillation present during sinus rhythm.

译文：据我们所知，这是第一项利用卷积神经网络识别窦性心律期间心房纤颤的心电图特征的研究。

例35

As far as we know, TARDIS is the first trial designed to use ordered categorical primary and safety outcomes according to fatal event, severe non-fatal event, mild non-fatal event, or no event.

译文：据我们所知，TARDIS 是第一个根据致命事件、严重非致命事件、轻度非致命事件或无事件使用有序分类的主要和安全转归的试验。

6.6.4.3　讨论部分的常用表达

1. 表达整体结局或命题答案

Our present results indicated that...

The findings strongly suggest that...

The present data confirm that...

Our results suggest that...

The experimental evidence suggests that...

In the present study, we show for the first time that...

One of the major insights to emerge from the study is...

Based on these results we propose that...

These results support the hypothesis that...

We showed a strong association between / among…

Strong evidence from animal studies and clinical trials shows that…

We did identify a significant relationship between… and…

There is substantial evidence that…

There is substantial pre-clinical evidence to support…

Our assessment identified clinical important differences in…

These results suggest a possibility that…

Based on the present data and on those available in the literature, we hypothesize that…

These findings lend support to the hypotheses…

Our study revealed the existence of…

Using… analysis, we found that…

Our evidence indicates that…

Our study led to the discovery of…

Here, we report… as…

These findings provide an explanation for…

The trial showed no evidence that… was associated with…

The results of this study seem to indicate that…

2. 表达与同类研究的比较

The strengths of our investigation include…

The results of… in the present study were in accordance with…

The present study extends these observations…

While we confirm these reports, we also show that…

These findings are in agreement / line / accordance / with…

Previous findings indicate that…

Numerous studies have indicated…, others report that…

A number of differences between these previous studies and present design may help explain the conflicting results.

This result is in agreement with previous data, showing that…

A recent study confirms our previous findings and findings in this study.

The overall rate of… in this study was compared to the result of other studies.

These figures are all higher / lower than those of some other studies.

To our knowledge, this is the first time that…

To our knowledge, this is the first study to assess and demonstrate a relation between…

In contrast to the findings described above, …

Currently, no firm conclusion can be drawn, but the following statements represent the consensus view that...

Our findings extend the conclusion of observational studies.

Although much progress has been made in recent years, all previous attempts at... have met limited success.

Previous... studies have focused on... suggesting that... is associated with...

Many researchers have described an association between... and...

However, the majority of studies in developed countries have been conducted in...

Previous analysis of... has found that... plays a greater role than... in...

In contrast to the current studies, the study showed...

3. 表达研究的局限性及对未来研究的展望

Further work may be needed to definitely determine...

Further study is needed to establish...

Further studies are required to clarify this issue.

The present data leave open the possibility that...

Our study has several limitations.

Further work will also be necessary to demonstrate that...

Several limitations of our study should be addressed.

Future studies may be hoped to standardize the...

The study has several weaknesses still.

There are still some unanswered questions on...

Our goal for the future is to determine if...

We have not yet been able to identify that...

In the future, we will extend the present studies to...

We anticipate / expect that...

Further studies are needed to answer these questions.

Some obvious reservations about our results must be addressed.

The crucial point of future studies has to be...

Further study should help to optimize the use of... in clinical practice

Such an assumption still needs further investigation using...

Further development of accurate and rapid methods to identify... is still needed.

Although the results of this trial are encouraging, further research remains essential to find a short, simple regimen for...

Currently, our understanding of the... is very limited.

Further surveillance is necessary to monitor the development and spread of...

We have not been able to identify... that meets these three requirements but continue to study this possibility.

Nevertheless, further studies should be performed to evaluate these above limitations if our methods were to be used for patients.

4. 表达结论及研究意义

This study is, therefore, a stepping-stone to future efforts seeking to...

... provided new insights into...

Although many factors undoubtedly play a role, our results imply that..., which is crucial for this decision.

The significance... has been established definitively.

We have, thus, concluded that...

From this analysis, we conclude that...

Overall, we feel our data are generalizable regarding...

This finding is biologically plausible and may have significant implications for...

Our observations may have potential implications for...

Collectively these and other findings strongly implicate...

It could be speculated that...

Our study adds more information to understand the relationship of...

In conclusion, we found a significant association between...

Thus, our studies may help elucidate the mechanism for... in...

These findings support the hypothesis that...

In conclusion, the findings of this study suggest that...

We also demonstrate that the combination of... with... may provide a promising alternative therapy for...

6.6.5 讨论示例

例36

Disscussion

Scar formation by astrocytes (Anderson et al., 2016; Faulkner et al., 2004; Herrmann et al., 2008; Sabelstrōm et al., 2013; Sil-ver, 2016) and type A pericytes (Gōritz et al., 2011) is crucial for sealing off the injured tissue and regaining tissue integrity after CNS lesions. At the same time, scar tissue is considered a major block for axonal regeneration. Most attention has been focused on astrocytes forming the glial component of the scar, and reactive astrocytes have long been thought to inhibit axonal regeneration (Cafferty et al., 2007; Xu et al., 2015; Yiu and He, 2006), although this notion has recently been questioned (Ander-son et al., 2016; Silver, 2016). Pericytes give rise to fibroblast-like cells that constitute the fibrotic compartment of the scar and are required for the generation of fibrosis and extracellular matrix deposition. We demonstrate that pericyte-derived scarring represents a major barrier for axonal regrowth and that moderate inhibition of this process preserves intact wound healing and dampens inflammation and reactive astrogliosis while enabling axonal regrowth and improved functional recovery.

译文：

讨论

源于星形细胞和 A 型周细胞的瘢痕形成对于在中枢神经系统损伤后封闭损伤组织和恢复组织完整性至关重要。同时，瘢痕组织被认为是轴突再生的主要障碍。相关研究主要关注形成疤痕胶质成分的星形细胞，反应性星形细胞也长期被认为能抑制轴突再生，然而这一观念最近却受到质疑。周细胞产生成纤维样细胞，这些细胞构成疤痕的纤维间室，也参与纤维化形成和细胞外基质的沉积。我们证明，周细胞源性的疤痕形成是轴突再生的主要障碍；这一过程能维持伤口愈合、抑制炎症和反应性星形胶质细胞形成，同时促进轴突再生和功能恢复。

Using lineage tracing, we previously identified a small pericyte subset as the origin of scar-forming fibroblast-like cells following spinal cord injury (Gõritz et al., 2011). Similarly, pericytes have also been implicated in dermal scarring and kidney fibrosis as the source of ECM-producing (myo) fibroblasts (Lin et al., 2008; Sundberg et al., 1996). However, a recent fate mapping study (Guimaraes-Camboa et al., 2017) targeting Tbx18-expressing pericytes and smooth muscle cells showed little proliferation and no contribution of this lineage to scar-forming cells in response to cortical stab wounds. There are two important points that may explain the discrepancy between the aforementioned studies. First, type A pericytes and Tbx18-expressing mural cells might represent non-overlapping populations. Our previous study established functional heterogeneity among pericytes, with scar formation being restricted to a small subset accounting for 10% of all pericytes (Gõritz et al., 2011). Second, in contrast to spinal cord injuries, cortical stab lesions do not give rise to extensive fibrotic tissue, indicated by the absence of a substantial increase in Col1a1-GFP expressing cells post-injury (Guimaraes-Camboa et al., 2017).

利用谱系追踪，我们之前确认了一个小的周细胞亚群，该亚群是脊髓损伤后形成瘢痕的成纤维样细胞的来源。类似地，周细胞作为产生 ECM 的成（肌）纤维细胞的来源，也参与真皮瘢痕形成和肾纤维化。然而，最近一项细胞谱系追踪研究显示，表达 Tbx18 的周细胞和平滑肌细胞，在皮层刺伤后，几乎没有增殖，对形成疤痕细胞的增殖也没有贡献。以下两点可以解释上述研究之间的差异。首先，A 型周细胞和表达 Tbx18 的壁细胞可能代表不同的群体。我们之前的研究确认了周细胞之间的功能异质性，仅有占周细胞总量 10% 的一个亚群形成疤痕。其次，与脊髓损伤不同，皮质刺伤不会产生广泛的纤维组织，表现为损伤后表达 Col1a1-GFP 的细胞不会显著增加。

Scar tissue is composed of different cell types with distinct cellular origin (Barnabé-Heider et al., 2010; Gõritz et al., 2011; Meletis et al., 2008; Zhu et al., 2015a) and reduction of a specific cellular scar component will influence the contribution of other scar-forming cells. Prevention, deletion or attenuation of astrocyte scarring leads to increased neurotoxic inflammation and expansion of fibrotic scarring, compromising axon regeneration and worsening functional recovery (Anderson et al., 2016; Faulkner et al., 2004; Herrmann et al., 2008; Sabel-ström et al., 2013; Silver, 2016). Conversely, the decreased reactive astrogliosis and inflammation associated with reduced pericyte-derived scarring we describe here may contribute to the beneficial effect on axonal regeneration and functional recovery.

瘢痕组织由具有不同细胞起源的细胞类型构成,特定细胞瘢痕成分的减少将影响其他瘢痕形成细胞的作用。预防、消除或减轻星形胶质细胞瘢痕形成,会导致神经毒性炎症增加和纤维化瘢痕扩大,损害轴突再生并恶化功能恢复。相反,本文描述反应性星形胶质细胞增生减少和炎症缓解与周细胞源性瘢痕减少相关,从而可能促进轴突再生和功能恢复。

That fibrosis inhibits axonal regeneration is consistent with indirect observations in previous studies. For example, when promoting inherent neuronal regenerative capacity by experimentally reducing PTEN, CST axon regrowth is observed along glial bridges and in fibrotic tissue-free regions (Zukor et al., 2013). Moreover, microtubule stabilization was shown to reduce scarring and impact axon regeneration of serotonergic and growth-competent sensory neurons after spinal cord injury (Hel-lal et al., 2011; Ruschel et al., 2015). However, these studies did not distinguish between the effects of reduced scarring and axonal stabilization and targeted various cell types and cellular mechanisms. Using a cell-type-specific targeting strategy, we show that a moderate reduction of pericyte-derived scar tissue facilitates CST and RST axon regeneration and functional recovery.

纤维化抑制轴突再生,这与之前研究的间接观察结果一致。例如,通过实验性减少 PTEN 来提升固有的神经元再生能力时,可观察到 CST 轴突沿着神经胶质桥和在无纤维组织区域再生。并且,脊髓损伤后微管稳定可减少瘢痕形成,并影响 5-羟色胺和具有生长能力的感觉神经元的轴突再生。但是,这些研究没有区分轴突再生和功能恢复是瘢痕减少和轴突稳定,还是靶向细胞类型与细胞机制作用的结果。采用细胞类型特异性靶向策略,我们发现适度减少周细胞源性瘢痕组织有助于 CST 和 RST 轴突再生和功能恢复。

CST axons, which show the greatest resistance to regeneration, mediate voluntary fine motor movement, a function that is much desired in spinal cord injury patients (Liu et al., 2011; Wel-niarz et al., 2017). As in most studies focusing on CST regeneration, we have used a dorsal hemisection model to ensure transection of CST projections. This lesion model spares main descending brainstem motor systems such as the vestibulospinal and reticulospinal tracts. Although not being directly responsible for most aspects of gross locomotor hind limb recovery, the CST/ 5-HT regenerated fibers could ultimately contribute via (inter) segmental, propriospinal, and other indirect relay-circuits to the observed improvement in functional recovery in Tam animals (Filli and Schwab, 2015; Flynn et al., 2017; Hou, 2014; Ueno et al., 2012).

除了表现出对再生具有最强的抵抗性外,CST 轴突还介导自主精细运动,这一功能是脊髓损伤患者缺失的。和大多数聚焦 CST 再生的研究一样,我们使用了背侧半切模型确保 CST 投射的横切。这一损伤模型保留了主要的下行脑干运动系统,比如前庭脊髓和网织脊髓束。尽管 CST/5-HT 再生纤维与大运动后肢恢复大多没有直接关联,但最终可以通过(跨)节断、本体脊髓和其他间接中继回路明显改善 Tam 动物的功能恢复。

While being more clinically relevant, severe injury models such as contusion lesions (commonly combined with BMS scoring to follow functional recovery), are not the preferred injury models to study CST regeneration, as not all the CST axons are destroyed by the lesion, making it difficult to distinguish between bona fide regeneration and sprouting of spared axons. Dense fibrotic scarring is seen following both dorsal hemisection and contusion injury (Zhu et al., 2015b) in rodents. Humans also form a fibrous extracellular matrix rich non-neural lesion core following traumatic spinal cord injury (Buss et al., 2007; Norenberg et al., 2004), suggesting that attenuation of pericyte-derived scarring may be explored as a therapeutic target to facilitate regeneration following CNS injury. (Reducing Pericyte-Derived Scarring Promotes Recovery after Spinal Cord Injury *Cell*, 2018 March 22, 173)

尽管更具临床意义,像挫伤这样的严重损伤模型(通常结合 BMS 评分来跟踪功能恢复)并不是研究 CST 再生的首选损伤模型,因为并不是所有的 CST 轴突都被病灶破坏,因此很难区分到底是真正的再生还是残存的轴突发芽。啮齿动物在背侧半切和挫伤后均可见致密的纤维瘢痕形成。人类在外伤性脊髓损伤后也形成纤维细胞外基质丰富的非神经损伤核心,提示周细胞源性瘢痕形成的衰减可能是促进中枢神经损伤后再生的治疗靶点,应进一步研究。(减少周细胞源性瘢痕形成促进脊髓损伤后康复)

例37

Discussion

In this trial, we found no evidence that the use of tranexamic acid resulted in a higher risk of death or thrombotic complications than that with placebo among patients undergoing coronary artery surgery. We also found that the tranexamic acid group had a lower risk of blood loss, blood transfusion, and reoperation but a higher risk of postoperative seizures than did the placebo group. Subgroup analyses of the primary outcome showed no significant interactions. The results were consistent among patients who were being treated with aspirin and those who were not.

译文:

讨论

在这项试验中,对于行冠状动脉手术的患者,我们未发现证据表明使用氨甲环酸导致死亡或血栓性并发症的风险高于使用安慰剂。我们还发现，与安慰剂组相比，氨甲环酸组的失血、输血和再次手术的风险更低，但是术后惊厥的风险较高。主要转归的亚组分析表明没有显著的交互作用。无论患者是否接受阿司匹林治疗，结果一致。

Patients in the tranexamic acid group received 46% fewer units of blood products than did those in the placebo group. In a cardiac surgical practice similar to the practices in which our trial population was treated, the use of tranexamic acid would save approximately 57 units of blood products for every 100 patients treated. The observed blood-sparing effects are consistent with those reported in meta-analyses.[4,5,12] The results of our trial have extended the reported findings by showing a significantly lower rate of reoperation with tranexamic acid than with placebo and robust estimates of the blood-sparing effects (including a lower risk of blood loss, decrement in hemoglobin levels, transfusions, and reoperations) associated with the use of tranexamic acid.

氨甲环酸组患者使用的血液制品单位数比安慰剂组少 46%。在与我们试验群体治疗实践相似的心脏外科实践中，每 100 例接受氨甲环酸治疗的患者节省约 57 单位的血液制品。该研究中观察到的节血效应与荟萃分析中报道的一致。我们的试验结果拓展了现有报道，表明氨甲环酸组的再手术率显著低于安慰剂组，并用高质量证据证明使用氨甲环酸的节血效应（包括失血、血红蛋白水平降低、输血和再手术的较低风险）。

Although many observational studies have linked blood transfusion with poor outcomes after cardiac surgery, we did not identify a beneficial reduction in the risk of myocardial infarction, stroke, or death despite the blood-sparing effects of tranexamic acid. In addition, the lower risk of bleeding with tranexamic acid than with placebo did not translate into shorter surgery times, and the slightly shorter duration of mechanical ventilation did not translate into earlier discharge from the hospital.

虽然已经有许多观察性研究将输血和心脏手术后的不良结局联系起来，但是除了节血效应我们并没有发现（氨甲环酸治疗后）心肌梗死、卒中或死亡危险的有益降低。另外，氨甲环酸比安慰剂的出血风险更低并没有缩短手术时间，略短的机械通气持续时间也没有缩短住院时间。

Tranexamic acid is commonly administered at a dose of 30 to 100 mg per kilogram for a 4-hour procedure.[4,26,27] We used a dose of 100 mg per kilogram at the beginning of the trial but later reduced this dose because of the growing number of reports of seizures associated with tranexamic acid that were believed to be dose-related.[13,20,21] The smaller dose (50 mg per kilo-gram) did not reduce the risk of seizure.[28] There is a strong association between seizures and stroke after cardiac surgery, even without the use of tranexamic acid.[20,29] The relationship of postoperative seizures with stroke and death observed in this trial suggests a possible underlying thromboembolic cause of the seizures.

4 小时的手术通常使用 30 ~ 100 mg / kg 剂量的氨甲环酸。我们在试验开始时使用了 100 mg / kg 的剂量，但随后减少了剂量，因为越来越多的报道指出使用氨甲环酸所致的惊厥与剂量相关。较小的剂量（50 mg / kg）并未降低惊厥的风险。即使不使用氨甲环酸，心脏手术后的惊厥和卒中之间也存在强相关性。本试验中观察到的术后惊厥与卒中和死亡的关系提示，血栓栓塞是惊厥的可能潜在原因。

Some limitations of our trial should be considered. First, although the reduction in the dose of tranexamic acid during the course of the trial provided an opportunity to test for a dose effect, this analysis was underpowered. Second, our trial included few patients who were at the highest risk for bleeding or thrombosis; however, we did not identify a subgroup effect that would suggest different findings among patients with overall higher risk. Third, in this trial, the attending anesthesiologists were sometimes aware of the treatment-group assignment; however, sensitivity analysis and the analysis of truly blinded data on postoperative blood loss and transfusion were consistent with the analysis of postoperative trial outcomes data. Finally, our trial included only a small proportion of patients undergoing off-pump surgery, and although the point estimates of effects among those patients were generally consistent with the point estimates of effects among patients undergoing on-pump surgery and although there were no significant interactions between subgroups, clinically important differences cannot be ruled out.

值得一提的是，我们的试验有一些局限性。第一，尽管在试验过程中降低氨甲环酸剂量提供了测试剂量效应的机会，但该分析效能不足。第二，我们的试验纳入了少数出血或血栓形成最高危的患者，然而我们并未发现有亚组效应能够提示总体风险较高的患者具有不同的结果。第三，在本试验中，主管麻醉医师有时知晓治疗组的分配情况，然而敏感性分析和对手术后失血和输血进行的全盲数据分析均与术后试验结局数据的分析结果一致。最后，我们的试验只包括了一小部分接受非体外循环手术的患者，尽管这些患者治疗效果的点估计值通常与接受体外循环手术患者治疗效果的点估计值一致，且亚组间没有显著的交互作用，仍不能排除临床上有重要的差异。

In summary, we found no evidence that tranexamic acid increases the risk of death and thrombotic complications after coronary-artery surgery. Tranexamic acid was associated with a lower risk of bleeding complications than placebo but also with a higher risk of postoperative seizures. (Tranexamic Acid in Patients Undergoing Coronary-Artery Surgery *The New England Journal of Medicine*, 2017 Jan.12, 376 (2))

总之，我们未发现氨甲环酸会增加冠状动脉手术后死亡和血栓性并发症的危险。与安慰剂组相比，氨甲环酸组出血并发症的风险更低，但是术后惊厥的风险更高。（氨甲环酸在行冠状动脉手术患者中的应用）

Exercise

1. Read the samples of "Discussion" and analyze their contents and structures. Recognize the signal markers and sentence patterns to realize these contents. Note the use of tenses for different contents in the writing.

2. Translate the following sentences in the "Discussion" into English.

1）这项试验证明，用左心室辅助装置（assist device）长期支持显著改善患有严重心力衰竭但不适合接受心脏移植术病人的生存率。药物治疗组病人接受了心力衰竭专科医师给予的地高辛（digoxin）、利尿剂（diuretics）、血管扩张素转换酶抑制剂（angiotensin-converting-enzyme inhibitors）和 β 受体阻滞剂（β-blockers）的最佳药物治疗。这组病人的 1 年死亡率为 75%，超过了获得性免疫缺陷综合征和乳腺癌、肺癌和结肠癌的死亡率，是 β 受体阻滞剂试验中死亡率的 4 倍多。

2）我们进行了一项随机试验，用金标准高胰岛素正血糖钳夹（gold-standard hyperinsulinemic euglycemic clamp）检查咖啡对超重亚洲个体胰岛素敏感性的影响。试验表明在 24 周内每天喝 4 杯咖啡对胰岛素敏感性、空腹血糖（fasting glycemia）指标或其他心脏代谢生物标志物均没有显著影响，但会使 FM 轻微下降。

3）我们的研究表明，两种方法都是有效的治疗方案，尽管内镜方法的一个重要临床优势是减少胰腺外瘘（external pancreatic fistulas）和缩短住院时间。在我们看来，有感染性坏死的患者应该由多学科小组在三级转诊中心（tertiary referral centers）进行治疗，因为其中一些病人可能需要联合治疗，而中心可同时提供内镜和手术阶梯式治疗（step-up approach）。

4）我们的结果与其他纳入危重（critically ill）儿童的多中心试验的结果一致。儿童心脏手术中安全血糖（Safe Pediatric Euglycemia in Cardiac Surgery，SPECS）试验和儿科重症监护治疗中的高血糖控制（Control of Hyperglycaemia in Paediatric Intensive Care，CHiP）试验均表明，不论是否接受心脏手术的儿童在 ICU 住院天数或死亡率方面没有显著差异。CHiP 试验表明，在未接受心脏手术的患儿中，分配至较低血糖控制目标组的患儿与分配至常规血糖控制组的患儿相比，其 12 个月的平均医疗花费较低，该结果出现的原因很可能是在那些分配至较低控制目标组的患儿中，有入院指征（index addmission）而住院的时间较短。值得注意的是，我们试验中的住院天数在两治疗组中没有显著差异。

5）以前的研究曾比较了脐带血供体（cord-blood donors）和其他来源供体移植的结局。由于曾经报道的移植前微小残留病（minimal disease）对非脐带血移植结局的严重影响，我们仔细检查了该变量。与所有回顾性分析的数据一样，我们的数据可能容易出现偏倚，因为哪些患者接受了哪种治疗是非随机选择的结果（例如临床优先）。

6）这项研究的一个主要优势是它的前瞻性设计，从具有不同婴儿喂养习惯的 4 个国家纳入具有相同一般风险（same generic risk）的大规模儿童队列（a large cohort），并遵循相同的研究方案。另一个优势是研究采用的饮食评估方法。该方法允许重复测量,以捕捉在发病前一段时间内正处于发育阶段的婴幼儿饮食习惯的变化。前瞻性设计还降低了饮食习惯改变带来的影响,因为在收集饮食信息时,父母并不知道孩子的自身抗体状况(autoantibody status)。

7)我们的研究存在一些局限性。第一,知情同意(informed consent)是在高血糖得到确认之后才签署,因此在高血糖发病和治疗之间产生了延迟。第二,床旁医师团队(bedside team)不可能不知晓研究组别分配方案(study-group assignment)。明确定义的干预和主要结局减少了对这种偏倚的顾虑。第三,为在常规医疗的范围内比较两种严格的血糖控制目标,我们没有纳入第三个分组,即不接受高血糖治疗组。因此两个研究组进行了明确的血糖管理和胰岛素调整(insulin adjustment)。

8)总之,在根治性前列腺切除术(radical prostatectomy)后因前列腺癌生化(PSA)复发(biochemical [PSA] recurrence)接受治疗的患者中,与放疗联合安慰剂相比,挽救性放疗(salvage radiation therapy)联合抗雄激素制剂(antiandrogen agent)可以提高总生存率、疾病特异性生存率(disease-specific rate)以及无转移生存率(metastasis-free survival rate)。与安慰剂相比,抗雄激素疗法的较高总生存率在治疗后第二个十年中才显现出来。

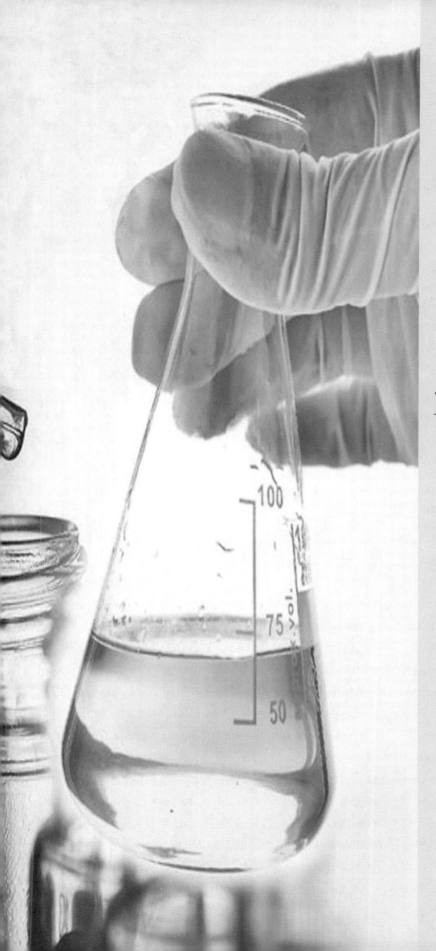

第

7

章

文献综述

7.1 何谓文献综述

文献综述（review article）是对某一方面进行专题搜集,经综合分析写成的一种学术论文,旨在报道某一领域中某分支学科或重要专题的历史、现状、最新进展、学术见解和建议等。

7.2 文献综述写作指要

文献综述的格式与一般研究性论文的格式有所不同。这是因为研究性论文注重研究的方法和结果,而文献综述则是向读者介绍与主题有关的详细资料、动态、进展、展望以及对以上方面的评述。因此文献综述的格式相对多样,但总的来说,主体部分一般都包含三部分,即引言（Introduction）、主体（Body）和总结（Summary）。

7.2.1 引言

7.2.1.1 引言的内容和结构

文献综述的引言主要包括研究的理由、目的、背景,前人的工作和知识空白,理论依据和实验基础,预期的结果及其在相关领域里的地位、作用和意义。

例1

Introduction

Drug resistance **remains** the greatest challenge to improving outcomes for cancer patients. （主题句,引出主题,指出目前存在的问题和挑战。） **Although** significant strides towards more effective cancer treatments have been made over the past few decades, most current treatments simply delay the inevitable. （研究背景和理由：已知信息、未知信息、研究空白,标记语：although。） There is no doubt that genetic mutations are responsible for many cases of therapeutic resistance.[1,2,3] **However,** our focus on cataloguing these mutations and their functional consequences has caused us to largely overlook the fact that non-genetic / epigenetic changes—that is, changes to gene activity states that occur independently of changes to the underlying DNA sequence[4]—can also play an important role in drug resistance.[5,6] （研究背景、或研究空白、或研究理由,标记语：**However** 。）

The power of epigenetics to modulate changes in cell fate should come as no surprise to any biologist. （主题句,引出主题。） During the process of development, epigenetic changes enable our entire range of cell types to originate from essentially the same genetic sequence.7,8 By comparison with these developmental changes, the epigenetic differences required for a cancer cell to acquire drug resistance appear relatively subtle. Although cancer does not arise through a physiological developmental pathway, epigenetic differences are still present within cancer cell populations and can be stably maintained through cell division. In fact, these differences form the basis of the cancer stem cell (CSC) hypothesis, which refers to normal development to explain the existence of heterogeneous subpopulations within a tumour.9,10 Even what might initially appear to be phenotypically homogenous populations of cancer cells are actually heterogeneous, with fluctuations between metastable gene expression programmes reported across a range of cancer types.11,12,13,14 **Taken together**, the prevalence of non-genetic heterogeneity in cancer and the ability for epigenetic changes to mediate major differences in cell fate **implicate** non-genetic evolution as a potential driving force for therapeutic resistance. A number of studies **support** this hypothesis, clearly demonstrating that non-genetic resistance occurs across a range of cancer and treatment contexts. (通过引用文献支持主题观点,最后,对文献进行总结评价。表示总结的标记语:**Taken together**;表示观点的标记语:**implicate, support**。)

In this review, we **begin by** outlining the evidence for pervasive non-genetic resistance in cancer and highlight the different forms of resistance that have been observed. We **then** define the two key variables epigenetic heterogeneity and epigenetic plasticity, **before** exploring exactly how they influence the capacity for non-genetic resistance through Darwinian selection and/ or Lamarckian induction. **Finally,** we discuss the potential interaction between genetic and non-genetic adaptation and define the important factors that dictate which pathway cancer cells follow to acquire resistance. Many of these ideas and concepts will also apply to other aspects of cancer biology, such as metastasis and immune evasion, but for simplicity here we focus on the acquisition of drug resistance. (表示综述内容的标记语:**In this review, we** …;表示综述结构的标记语:**begin by, then, before, finally**。) Altogether, **this review aims to** synthesise our current knowledge into a conceptual framework that assists future investigations of non-genetic resistance in cancer. (表示综述目的的标记语:**this review aims to**…。)

(Principles and mechanisms of non-genetic resistance in cancer, *British Journal of Cancer*, 2019 December 13, 122 (6))

译文:

引言

耐药性仍然是改善癌症患者结局的最大挑战。尽管在过去的几十年,癌症治疗方法取得了长足的进步,但当前大多数的方法只是推迟了不可避免的最终结局。毫无疑问,基因突变是造成治疗耐药性的主要原因。然而,我们关注编目这些突变及其功能后果使得我们很大程度上忽略了一个事实:非遗传性/表观遗传的改变,即独立于潜在 DNA 序列变化的基因活性状态的改变也可能在耐药性中发挥重要作用。

生物学家普遍认为,表观遗传学具有调节细胞命运变化的能力。在发育过程中,表观遗传的变化使我们的整个细胞类型本质上起源于相同的基因序列。与这些发育变化相比,癌细胞产生耐药性所需的表观遗传差异似乎相对微妙。虽然癌症不是通过生理发育途径产生的,但表观遗传差异仍然存在于癌细胞群中,并且可以通过细胞分裂得以稳定维持。事实上,这些差异构成了癌症干细胞假说的基础,该假说用正常发育来解释肿瘤内异质亚群的存在。即使最初看起来是表型一致的癌细胞群实际上也是异质的,据报道,在一系列癌症类型中,亚稳态基因表达程序之间存在波动。总之,癌症具有普遍的非遗传异质性,表观遗传变化能介导细胞命运的主要差异,这些发现暗示非遗传进化是耐药性发生的潜在驱动力。许多研究支持这一假设,清楚地表明一系列癌症类型和治疗手段都可产生非遗传耐药性。

在这篇综述中,我们首先概述了癌症中普遍存在的非遗传耐药性的证据,并强调了已观察到的不同形式的耐药性。然后,我们定义了表观遗传异质性和表观遗传可塑性这两个关键变量,然后通过达尔文选择和/或拉马克诱导来探索它们如何影响非遗传性耐药能力的。最后,我们讨论了遗传和非遗传适应之间的潜在相互作用,并确立了决定癌细胞获得耐药性途径的重要因素。许多这些想法和概念也将适用于癌症生物学的其他方面,如转移和免疫逃避,但为了简单起见,本综述重点讨论耐药性的发生。总之,这篇综述的目的是将我们目前的知识综合成一个概念框架,以帮助未来对癌症中非遗传耐药性的研究。(癌症非遗传耐药性的原则和机制)

7.2.1.2 引言的写作要点

在引言部分,作者提出问题、进行定义性解释或介绍研究背景等,常用一般现在时或现在完成时。引言部分最后一段的最后一句需指明研究目的,用一般现在时。

1. 介绍研究背景

例2

Developments in 3D bioprinting **have been** mostly motivated by the limited availability of organs globally,[1] which are needed for the rehabilitation of lost or failed organs and tissues. The most challenging and demanding applications for engineered tissues **include** the skin,[2,3] cartilage,[4] hard tissues such as bones,[5] cardiac tissue,[6] and vascular grafts.[7]

说明:在引言部分,提出问题和介绍研究背景常用一般现在时或现在完成时。

译文:全球器官供应有限推动了3D生物打印的发展,这些器官和组织是器官缺失或衰竭者康复所必需的。工程化组织最具挑战性的应用范围包括皮肤、软骨、诸如骨头的硬组织、心脏组织和血管移植物。

2. 指明研究目的

例3

Our aim is to review the literature and **provide** surgeons with evidence based data to improve decision making regarding antidepressant drugs that directly impact the clinical outcomes of patients undergoing spine surgery.

说明:引言部分最后一段的最后一句指明研究目的。描写研究目的用一般现在时。

译文：本综述旨在回顾相关文献，为外科医生提供循证数据，以改善抗抑郁药的使用决策，从而直接影响行脊柱手术患者的临床结局。

3. 引言部分的常用表达

The purpose / aim / objective of this review is to…

The pertinent literature is reviewed.

This article reviews…

This review will concentrate on…

In the following, a brief review is given of…

In this review, we aim to highlight…

7.2.2　主体

7.2.2.1　主体的内容和结构

综述的正文部分（Body），主要包括论据和论证。通过提出问题、分析问题和解决问题，比较各种观点的异同点及其理论根据，提出作者自己的观点和见解。为把问题说得明白、透彻，可分为多个部分，以小标题标注。可按年代顺序综述，也可按不同的问题进行综述，还可按不同的观点进行比较综述。

例4

例 1 来源的综述主体部分包含以下六方面的内容。

2.1　Evidence for pervasive non-genetic resistance

2.2　Epigenetic heterogeneity and epigenetic plasticity

2.2.1　Epigenetic heterogeneity

2.2.2　Epigenetic plasticity

2.2.3　The interplay between heterogeneity and plasticity

2.3　Potential mechanisms of non-genetic resistance

2.4　Sources of epigenetic heterogeneity

2.4.1　Deterministic and stochastic heterogeneity

2.4.2　Active maintenance of epigenetic heterogeneity?

2.5　Interaction between genetic and non-genetic resistance

2.6　The path of most resistance

以下对其中有代表性的 2.2 部分内容进行阐述。

2.2　Epigenetic heterogeneity and epigenetic plasticity

Before we can explore the potential mechanisms that mediate non-genetic resistance, a clear picture of the factors that contribute to adaptive potential is required. The two key variables that dictate the capacity for a given cancer cell population to undergo non-genetic evolution are epigenetic heterogeneity and epigenetic plasticity. （对本节内容的概述，指出该

主题中的两个关键变量。)

2.2.1　Epigenetic heterogeneity（第一个变量）

Epigenetic heterogeneity **refers to** the variability in epigenetic state across a cell population.（对关键词 Epigenetic heterogeneity 进行定义，标记语：… **refers to** …）It is influenced by both cell-intrinsic and cell-extrinsic factors and **therefore** the degree of heterogeneity will vary according to cancer type, mutational profile and tissue microenvironment. 6**Analogous to** genetic heterogeneity, epigenetic heterogeneity can act as a substrate for Darwinian selection, with a greater degree of diversity increasing the chance that certain cells will display a state capable of surviving and/or adapting to the therapeutic pressure. 36, 41, 42, 43, 44 **For example**, in patients with acute myeloid leukaemia（AML）or breast cancer, individuals with higher epigenetic heterogeneity（independent of genetic heterogeneity）display a poorer prognosis and/or shorter time to relapse. 40, 41（通过推断［标记语：therefore…］、比较［标记语：**analogous to**］、举例［标记语：**For example**］等方式对主题进行综述。）

2.2.2　Epigenetic plasticity（第二个变量）

Epigenetic plasticity **refers to** the capacity of a cell to alter its epigenetic state with a degree of heritability in response to internal or external stimuli.（给定义，标记语：… **refers to**…）Plasticity is **therefore** critical for the drug-induced cellular reprogramming that can cause non-genetic resistance. Drug-induced cellular reprogramming can be considered a form of Lamarckian adaptation, as the adaptive changes occur as a direct response to an environmental stimulus. **Therefore**, plasticity is the driving force for Lamarckian adaptation. For the most part, the nature of epigenetic plasticity is largely unknown, but given that chromatin plays a key role in cell type stability, it appears that the chromatin landscape is likely to be important. 45, 46 Different cell types appear to display different degrees of plasticity, which is likely to influence the capacity of different cancer types to acquire non-genetic resistance.（对主题进行评述，发表作者自己的观点和见解。）

2.2.3　xThe interplay between heterogeneity and plasticity（第一个变量和第二个变量之间的关系）

In instances where plasticity contributes to resistance, heterogeneity must also be involved, as not all cells are capable of surviving and adapting to treatment（see the section on mechanisms of epigenetic resistance, below）.（主题句，引出观点。）**For example**, in melanoma, heterogeneous, stochastic expression of BRAF inhibitor resistance markers enables the initial survival of a subpopulation of cells, which also has the necessary epigenetic plasticity required to undergo transcriptional adaptation and form a stably resistant population. 31 **We also observed similar results** in our model of BET inhibitor resistance in AML: 29, 30 although not intrinsically resistant, the drug-naïve leukaemic granulocyte macrophage progenitor population enriched for leukaemia stem cells showed a greater capacity to adapt than the bulk population.（结果与其他研究结果进行比较，标记语：… similar results …）Interestingly , in both of these scenarios, and others, less-differentiated subpopulations acquire drug resistance.（指出先前研究有趣的发现，标记语：Interestingly。）17,18,22,23 These populations **might** have increased plasticity due to the less-restrictive chromatin landscape associated with a stem cell-like state（reduced heterochromatin and DNA methylation）, which **could** facilitate activation of a broader range of gene expression programmes in response to therapy. **As a result** , epigenetic heterogeneity in the form of more plastic, less-differentiated subpopulations might be a common source of non-genetic drug resistance.（通过举例、比较、文献引用、推理等方式对主题进行论证，发表作者自己的观点和见解。）

It is important to note that heterogeneity and plasticity are not completely independent variables.（主题句，引出观点。）**For example,** cells that display greater heterogeneity might do so because the epigenetic state of the population is more plastic. **In fact,** as mentioned above, plasticity itself can also be a form of epigenetic heterogeneity, whereby different subpopulations have different degrees of plasticity. **However,** it is conceivable that a population could be highly heterogeneous, but not possess a high degree of plasticity. **Likewise,** the entire population could be highly plastic, without a high degree of baseline epigenetic heterogeneity. **Therefore,** epigenetic heterogeneity and plasticity must be viewed as interrelated, yet distinct, variables.（通过举例、摆事实、比较、推理等方式对主题进行评述，发表作者自己的观点和见解；使用句首标记语 For example，In fact，However，Likewise，Therefore 进行评述。句子结构清晰，逻辑清楚。）

译文：

2.2 表观遗传异质性和表观遗传可塑性

在探索介导非遗传耐药的潜在机制之前，需要对影响适应性潜力的因素有一个清楚的认识。决定癌细胞群进行非遗传进化的能力有两个关键变量：表观遗传的异质性和表观遗传的可塑性。

2.2.1 表观遗传的异质性

表观遗传异质性是指整个细胞群中表观遗传状态的变异性。它受细胞内和细胞外因素的影响，因此异质性的程度将取决于癌症类型、突变特性和组织微环境。与遗传异质性相似，表观遗传异质性可作为达尔文选择学说的基础，多样性程度越高，某些细胞表现出存活和／或适应治疗压力能力的几率也就越高。例如，急性髓细胞白血病（AML）或乳腺癌患者中，表观遗传异质性越高（独立于遗传异质性）的个体预后更差和／或复发时间更短。

2.2.2 表观遗传可塑性

表观遗传可塑性是指细胞在受到内部或外部刺激时，以一定程度的遗传力改变其表观遗传状态的能力。因此，可塑性对于药物诱导的细胞重编程至关重要，这种重编程会导致非遗传耐药。药物诱导的细胞重编程可以被认为是拉马克适应学说的一种形式,因为适应性变化是对环境刺激的直接反应。因此,可塑性是拉马克适应学说的驱动力。在很大程度上,对表观遗传可塑性知之甚少,但是鉴于染色质在细胞类型稳定性中起着关键作用,染色质图谱似乎很可能具有重要性。不同的细胞类型表现出不同程度的可塑性,这可能会影响不同癌症类型获得非遗传耐药性的能力。

2.2.3 异质性与可塑性的相互作用

可塑性促进耐药性的情况一定与异质性有关,因为并非所有细胞都能存活并适应治疗(请参见下文有关表观遗传耐药性机制章节)。例如,在黑色素瘤中,BRAF 抑制剂耐药标记物的异质随机表达能使细胞亚群初始存活,该亚群还具有进行转录适应和形成稳定耐药群体所必需的表观遗传可塑性。我们在 AML 患者 BET 抑制剂耐药的模型中也观察到了相似的结果,尽管不是固有耐药,但未经药物治疗的富集白血病干细胞的白血病粒细胞巨噬细胞祖细胞群,其表现出比其他多数种群更强的适应能力。有趣的是,在这两种情况以及其他情况下,分化程度较低的亚群都具有耐药性。由于与干细胞样状态(异染色质减少和 DNA 甲基化)相关的染色质图谱限制性较少,这些种群可能具有更高的可塑性,由此可能促进治疗后更广泛的基因表达程序的激活。因此,以可塑性更强而分化程度更低的亚群为表现形式的表观遗传异质性可能是非遗传药物耐药性的常见来源。

值得注意的是异质性和可塑性并不是完全独立的变量。例如,细胞之所以表现出更大异质性可能是因为群体的表观遗传状态更具可塑性。实际上,如上所述,可塑性本身也可以是表观遗传异质性的一种形式,因而不同的亚群具有不同程度的可塑性。然而可以理解的是,一个种群可能具有高度异质性,但不具备高度可塑性。同样,整个种群可能具有很高的可塑性,而不具有高度的基线表观遗传异质性。因此,表观遗传异质性和可塑性必须被视为相互关联但又截然不同的变量。

7.2.2.2 主体的写作要点

文献述评部分需要有作者的见解。段落组织要有序,可以通过使用转换语和主题句对文献进行比较和对比。正文部分通常采用一般现在时态。

1. 在段落开始提供总括句

例5

Along with their impact on sodium handling, AT1 receptors also **seem to play** a critical role in controlling urinary concentrating mechanisms.

说明:在段落的开头提供强有力的总括句子,引出新的主题。

译文:AT1 受体不仅对钠处理有影响,似乎在控制尿液浓缩机制中也起着关键作用。

2. 在段落中使用连接语表明句子间逻辑关系

例6

Moreover, cell-specific deletion of AT1 receptors from the collecting duct is sufficient to cause a urinary concentrating defect (345). In this case, epithelial levels of aquaporin-2 protein were significantly diminished in the inner and outer medulla, **whereas** localization to the apical membrane was unaffected.

说明：段落中通过使用连接词如 Moreover 和 whereas，使句子之间逻辑关系一目了然。

译文：此外，集合管中 AT1 受体的细胞特异性清除足以引起尿液浓缩不足。在这种情况下，在内髓和外髓中水通道蛋白-2 的上皮水平显著下降，而顶膜的定位则不受影响。

3. 比较、对比文献并提出见解

例7

Similarly, AT1A receptor deficient mice with preservation of inner medullary architecture also have a urinary concentrating defect due to a relative resistance to vasopressin, and this defect can be reproduced in wild-type mice by administration of an AT1 receptor blocker.

译文：同样，保留了髓内结构的 AT1A 受体缺陷型小鼠也由于对血管加压素的相对耐药而存在尿浓缩不足，这种缺陷可通过野生型小鼠使用 AT1 受体阻滞剂重现。

4. 在评论中使用总结性标记语

例8

Thus, direct effects of AT1 receptors in epithelial cells of the collecting duct modulate aquaporin-2 levels and these actions are required to achieve maximal urinary concentration.

说明：在评论中使用含 Thus 标记语的总结句。

译文：因此，集合管上皮细胞中 AT1 受体的直接作用调节了水通道蛋白-2 的水平，而这些作用是最大化浓缩尿液所必需的。

5. 述评部分的常用表达

It is (has been) found that…

It has been reported that…

It has been showed / proved that…

It is generally recognized / agreed / accepted that…

It is thought / regarded / considered that…

It may be safely said that…

It has been observed that…

It must be pointed out that…

It can be asserted that…

It should be added that…

It must be admitted that…

It need not be said that… / it goes without saying that… / It is understood that…

It will be seen from this that…

It is (not) possible / probable / likely that…

It must be emphasized / stressed that…

It should be made clear that…

It stands to reason that…

Nothing is more important than the fact that…

It is apparent / clear / evident that…

There is no doubt that…

A more important fact is that…

But there is no conclusive evidence so far about…

There is as yet no clinical proof of…

There is ample evidence that…

By… we mean…

… is (has been) defined as…

7.2.3 总结

7.2.3.1 总结的内容和结构

总结部分（Summary），是对全文主题进行扼要总结，作者最好能提出自己的见解。本部分内容通过总结现有文献的重要方面，指出前人工作的不足、并突出进一步研究的必要性和理论价值。总结的写作应该明确、完整和精练，其内容一般应包括以下几个方面：

1. 本文研究结果说明了什么问题；

2. 对先前研究的观点作了哪些修正、补充、发展、证实或否定；

3. 本文研究的不足之处或遗留未解决的问题，以及解决这些问题的可能关键点和方向。

例9

Conclusions

Antidepressants are used for various purposes in the field of spine surgery：（1）Antidepressants, including ami-triptyline and duloxetine, are among the first line drugs to treat neuropathic pain, which is common in patients with degenerative diseases of the spine. Venlafaxine **can** be used for cases with SCI-related disabilities presenting with depression or nociceptive pain. （2）Preoperative treatment of depression **should be** considered in patients with intractable spine disease as it may improve patients satisfaction postoperatively by ameliorating postoperative pain and reducing risk of postsurgical delirium and, thus, improving overall QOL. （总结抗抑郁药在脊柱手术外科中的各种用途；按顺序（1）、（2）列成条文，写作明确完整。）

By contrast, antidepressants may have disadvantages：（1）They **may** result in prolonged hospital stay and increased cost. （2）SSRIs **may** increase the risk of intraoperative bleeding up to 2.5-fold and allogenic blood transfusion by 2-fold. Bupropion may also be involved. （3）PFA is warranted preoperatively for major procedures to avoid unexpected significant intraoperative bleeding in patients taking serotonergic antidepressants. （4）The impact of antidepressants on BMD remains controversial；**therefore**，strict monitoring of BMD in elderly and high-risk group patients **is recommended.**（按顺序（1）、（2）、（3）、（4）总结抗抑郁药的副作用，最后提出建议；标记语：…**therefore，… is recommended.**）

（Antidepressants in Spine Surgery：A Systematic Review to Determine Benefits and Risks，*Asian Spine J.*，2019 Dec，13（6））

译文：

结论

抗抑郁药在脊柱外科领域具有多种用途：（1）抗抑郁药，包括阿米替林和度洛西汀，是治疗神经性疼痛的一线药物，而神经性疼痛常见于脊柱退行性疾病的患者。文拉法辛可用于伴有抑郁症或伤害性疼痛的脊髓损伤的残疾患者。（2）对顽固性脊柱疾病患者应考虑术前抗抑郁治疗，因为这样可以减轻术后疼痛和降低术后谵妄的风险，改善患者的总体生活质量，从而提高患者的术后满意度。

然而另一方面，抗抑郁药也有以下缺点：（1）可导致住院时间延长和费用增加。（2）SSRIs可使术中出血的风险增加2.5倍，同种异体输血的风险增加2倍。可能会使用安非他酮。（3）对于服用5-羟色胺能抗抑郁药的患者，应术前使用PFA，避免术中意外大出血。（4）抗抑郁药对骨密度的影响尚存争议；因此，建议对老年人和高危人群进行严格的骨密度监测。（抗抑郁药在脊柱外科的使用：一项确定获益和风险的系统性回顾）

7.2.3.2 总结的写作要点

结论部分的写作要求措词严谨、逻辑严密、表达具体。用语肯定但又不应夸大，对尚不能完全肯定的内容应注意留有余地。在总结部分，表述作者建设性意见或展望，常用一般现在时或一般将来时。

1. 指出不足之处

例10

There are some limitations to the present systematic review that warrant discussion. First，all included studies were case series，and none were randomized controlled trials ［46］. Therefore，the current evidence is still of relative low quality. **Second**，the sample size was still small，although our study represents the largest number of patients with a minimum of 2-year follow-up in the literature. **Third**，some identical cases may have inadvertently been included in different studies，even though authors attempted to exclude known identical cases from the same clinical site.

说明：指出不足之处，按顺序1、2、3列成条文，采用一般现在时。

译文：本系统综述存在一些局限性，值得探讨。首先，所有纳入的研究均为病例系列研究，无随机对照试验。因此，目前的证据质量仍然相对较低。其次，尽管我们的研究代表了文献中随访至少2年的最大数量的患者，样本量仍然很小。最后，即使作者试图从同一临床地点排除已知的相同病例，也可能无意中将相同病例纳入不同的研究。

2. 对不足之处的处理

例11

To address this, we performed a sensitivity analysis to diminish this effect. Due to the apparent and now obvious advantages of magnetically controlled growing rods, it would be scientifically and medically unethical to conduct a randomized controlled study.

说明:本段描写为了减少不足之处造成的影响,采取的具体措施。使用标记语 To address this…; 与本研究方法相关的内容,采用一般过去时。

译文:为了解决这个问题,我们进行了敏感性分析以减少这种影响。由于磁控生长棒具有明显的优势,因此,进行随机对照研究是不符合科学和医学伦理的。

3. 结论性评价

例12

Therefore, our present study provides the best evidence regarding clinical outcomes and reduced complications of magnetically controlled growing rods for the treatment of pediatric scoliosis at this time.

说明:结论部分的最后一句往往是结论性评价,标记语常为 Therefore, … 。时态多为一般现在时。

译文:因此,本研究为磁控生长棒在治疗小儿脊柱侧弯的临床结局和减少并发症方面提供了最佳证据。

4. 指出未来的研究方向

例13

Further studies should be conducted across multiple centers and include a full long-term follow-up of patients from implantation of magnetically controlled growing rods to final fusion.

说明:指出今后研究的方向,使用标记语:Further studies should be…用情态动词表达研究建议。

译文:下一步应进行多中心研究,包括对患者进行从植入磁控生长棒到最终融合的长期随访。

7.3 文献综述示例

例14

Treatment of Hypertension in Patients with Asthma

Asthma and hypertension are common chronic diseases, each with attendant morbidity, mortality, and economic effects. It is estimated that 300 million people worldwide have asthma, and an increase in prevalence to 400 million is anticipated by 2025. Approximately 250,000 asthma-related deaths occur yearly, many of which are believed to be avoidable. 1 In the United States, more than 8% of adults have asthma, with disproportionate representation among women, ethnic minorities, and people who are economically disadvantaged. Asthma-related health expenditures in 2013 were estimated at $80 billion. 2 The presence of hypertension with asthma creates an additional health burden; hypertension is the world's most common modifiable risk factor for cardiovascular disease and death. Worldwide estimates suggest that 874 million adults have a systolic blood pressure higher than 140 mm Hg, 3, 4 and the prevalence of hypertension, like that of asthma, is increasing, along with costs, morbidity, and mortality. 5 Elevated systolic blood pressure was the leading global contributor to preventable death in 2015. 6 In the United States, approximately one in three adults has high blood pressure. 7 Since current hypertension guidelines incorporate new evidence that has led to lower thresholds for treatment, the number of persons considered to have hypertension will expand, and the attendant costs will escalate. 3

Patients with asthma are more likely to have hypertension than those who do not, independent of traditional risk factors. 8 A diagnosis of hypertension is associated with augmented asthma severity, 9 and reduced lung function has been correlated with heightened cardiovascular mortality. 10 Given the bidirectional relationship between compromised lung function and compromised cardiovascular function, the rationale for treating and controlling hypertension in persons with asthma is compelling. Although the effect of blood-pressure control on asthma is largely unexplored, the risk of death from cardiovascular disease is decreased when systolic blood pressure is reduced to levels below 130 mm Hg. 11-14 In this review, we discuss the potential mechanistic links between hypertension and asthma, the influence each condition has on the other, and approaches to the treatment of hypertension in adult patients with asthma.

Mechanistic Relationship between Hypertension and Asthma

Predisposing factors (genetic profile, stress, and age), dietary and lifestyle choices, and inflammatory mechanisms all contribute to the hypertensive asthmatic phenotype. These factors may be important in understanding the development of the condition (Fig.1).

Systemic inflammation serves as an underpinning for the burden of disease that accrues from hypertension and asthma. 15 Inflammation is widely accepted as being both fundamental to the pathogenesis of asthma 16 and central to the development of hypertension and its deleterious consequences. 17, 18 A large cross-sectional study of middle-aged persons with asthma showed that the prevalence of hypertension was higher among those with lower values for forced expiratory volume in 1 second (FEV1), with the risk of hypertension increasing as the FEV1 decreased. 19 Furthermore, C-reactive protein levels, a marker of systemic inflammation related to interleukin-6 and hypertension, were correlated with the rate of loss of FEV1. 20 Such findings may imply a reciprocal relationship, wherein systemic inflammation influences the disease course for both hypertension and asthma.

Asthma is currently understood as a disorder that is characterized by two main endotypes: type 2 high inflammation and type 2 low inflammation. These subtypes are broadly defined by their predominant underlying mechanism, which is largely determined by the T cells or innate lymphocytes and cytokines that are involved.21 Each endotype can be further subdivided into multiple phenotypes that are distinguished by clinical features, pathological findings, and biomarkers (chemokines) (Table 1). Owing to the lack of uniform criteria for classifying types of asthma, estimates of the prevalence of type 2 high- and type 2 low-inflammation endotypes vary; however, each endotype appears to represent approximately half the population with asthma.16

The Severe Asthma Research Program conducted multiple studies in which patients with asthma were grouped into discreet clusters on the basis of a hierarchical analysis of variables that included clinical characteristics, biomarkers, cellular profiles, lung function, atopic status, responses to treatment, gene expression, and coexisting conditions.22-24 It is notable that two studies that included hypertension as a variable showed cosegregation of hypertension with asthmatic profiles that are typical for the type 2 low-inflammation endotype.22,23 Patients with features of the type 2 low-inflammation endotype (older age, later onset of asthma, higher body-mass index [BMI], greater severity of disease, and low atopy) were also more likely to have hypertension (48 of 175 patients [27%]) than patients with the type 2 high-inflammation endotype (50 of 551 patients [9%]).22 The results of a separate study based on clinical characteristics and assessments of inflammatory cells in blood and sputum showed a significantly higher incidence of hypertension in clusters distinguished by severity of disease, older age, later onset of disease, higher BMI, and greater resistance to treatment with glucocorticoids: 31% (51 of 164 patients) as compared with 11% (28 of 259 patients).23 These observations suggest that type 2 low inflammatory pathways may provide a pathogenic mechanism that links these two diseases.

The degree of inflammation in patients with hypertension and asthma reflects the conjoint effect of both conditions. Hypertension skews T cells toward a proinflammatory (type 1 helper T-cell [Th1 cell]) phenotype, characterized by increased interferon-γ responses and decreased type 2 helper T-cell (Th2 cell) responses.25 In asthma, enhanced airway hyperresponsiveness and severe disease are associated with elevated levels of interferon-γ.26 Correspondingly, in hypertension, interferon-γ and Th1-cell polarization contribute to blood-pressure elevation and its sequelae.17 Interleukin-17 has also been shown to play a major role in the development of hypertension and its related end-organ damage in both studies in animals and in vitro models.

Interleukin-17 induces a proinflammatory phenotype in vascular smooth-muscle cells by enhancing the release of mediators, including interleukin-6, CXCL8 and CXCL10, and C-reactive protein.27 Both anti-interleukin-17 treatment and genetic deletion have been shown to reduce hypertension in studies in animals.17,27 A role for interleukin-17 is also evident in some patients with severe asthma in whom an elevated level of interleukin-17 is correlated with neutrophil infiltration, airway hyperresponsiveness, and a lack of sensitivity to glucocorticoids. In these patients, interleukin-17 is capable of inducing secretion of proinflammatory cytokines from lung structural cells and airway smooth muscle, including tumor necrosis factor α, interleukin-1β, granulocyte colonystimulating factor, and interleukin-6 as well as the chemokines CCL11 (eotaxin) and CXCL8 (interleukin-8), which are important in airway inflammation and remodeling.28,29 Surprisingly, in one trial, the targeting of interleukin-17 failed to ameliorate symptoms in patients with severe asthma30; however, a subgroup analysis identified patients with highly reversible depression in FEV1 who had some improvement, as reflected by the Asthma Control Questionnaire. The functional role of interleukin-17 in the contraction of smooth-muscle cells may offer a partial explanation for the more favorable response in this subgroup.31

Experimental evidence supports the concept that elevated interleukin-6 levels can drive the differentiation of CD4+ T cells through interaction with transforming growth factor β to promote skewing toward type 17 helper cells (Th17 cells), leading to a reduction of regulatory T cells (Tregs). Tregs play a protective role in the development of hypertension that is related in part to production of interleukin-10 27 and play a critical role in the regulation of asthma development.32

Interactions among interferon-γ, interleukin-17, and interleukin-6 have the potential to affect disease expression for both hypertension and asthma (Fig. 2). Together, these cytokines stimulate the inflammation, smooth-muscle activation, and fibrinogenesis that are fundamental to airway and cardiovascular disease. Thus, persons who have both hypertension and asthma appear to compose a patient subgroup with difficult-to-treat disease who are at increased risk for end-organ damage.

Obesity and Metabolic Dysfunction

Elevated interleukin-6 levels and systemic inflammation result in metabolic dysfunction that increases the morbidity associated with both hypertension and asthma. Secretion of proinflammatory cytokines, notably interleukin-6, by adipocytes and inflammatory macrophages in white adipose tissue is of pathogenic importance in asthma,33 a condition in which interleukin-6 appears to be a biomarker for metabolic dysfunction and severe disease. 34 Elevation of interleukin-6 levels has been identified in association with hypertension in studies in humans and animals, in which it has been shown to be related to disease development.35,36

Smooth-Muscle Remodeling and Vascular Biology

Smooth-muscle remodeling, driven in substantial part by inflammatory cytokines, is a critical component of both asthma and hypertension. 37-39 Hyperplasia and abnormal contracture of the smooth-muscle cells surrounding the airway play an important role in airway obstruction in asthma. Similarly, the abnormal contraction and proliferation of smooth-muscle cells are well recognized as features of the vascular remodeling and endothelial abnormalities associated with hypertension.

Genetic factors clearly affect the expression of asthma and hypertension; however, the relevant interrelations are complex and difficult to dissect. Polymorphisms in β-adrenergic receptors on smooth-muscle cells have been reported in patients with both hypertension and asthma, but their importance in disease manifestation may lie in their modulation of the response to antagonists and agonists, which could have more influence on treatment outcomes than on disease causation.40 In contrast, modification of the vascular smooth-muscle cell phenotype in response to local environmental influences is thought to play a critical role in the pathogenesis of hypertension and asthma as well as atherosclerosis.41

Dietary Salt

Dietary salt intake has long been considered to be relevant to the development of cardiovascular conditions. Early observations associating higher salt intake with blood-pressure elevation have been refined to identify subpopulations of saltsensitive and salt-insensitive persons.42 The responsiveness of the kidneys, sympathetic nervous system, and vasculature to salt has been observed. 43 The immune system may be important in responsiveness to salt. For example, Th17 cells appear to play a role in mediating the relationship between salt exposure and hypertension.17,18,27 In a mouse model, high-salt diets promoted the generation of Th17 cells through alterations in the gut microbiome, with depletion of *Lactobacillus murinus*. Saltsensitive hypertension is prevented by treatment with *L. murinus*, which has a modulating effect on Th17 cells. Evidence suggests that the effect is related to the tryptophan metabolites produced by this organism.44 Healthy persons on a highsalt diet are also reported to have reduced levels of lactobacillus, elevated levels of Th17 cells, and elevated blood pressure, all of which support the proposition that higher salt intake plays a role in inflammation in humans.44-46 At present, similar information related to dietary salt content in patients with asthma is lacking.

Management of Disease in Patients with Asthma and Hypertension

The mechanisms linking asthma and hypertension not only are of theoretical interest but also have implications for therapy and disease management. The treatment of hypertension in a patient with asthma should involve a multifactorial approach that involves control of both conditions, treatment of coexisting conditions, and the institution of lifestyle modifications (Fig.3).

Pharmacologic Treatment of Hypertension in Patients with Asthma

In the 2017 report of the American College of Cardiology-American Heart Association Task Force on clinical practice guidelines for the prevention, detection, evaluation, and management of high blood pressure in adults, hypertension was categorized as either stage 1 (130-139 / 80-89 mm Hg) or stage 2 (>140 / >90 mm Hg).3 Pharmacotherapy was recommended for patients who have or who are at high risk for cardiovascular disease at stage 1 and for all patients at stage 2. It is noteworthy that the threshold for a diagnosis of hypertension was lowered in the 2017 guidelines, a development that has led to substantial controversy, since it has expanded the percentage of adults in the United States with a diagnosis of hypertension from 32% to 46%.

What does the treatment of hypertension generally accomplish, and how might that treatment affect patients with asthma? To date, allcause mortality has not differed significantly among patients with hypertension treated with any of the four major classes of first-line antihypertensive agents (Table 2). The degree of bloodpressure reduction rather than the choice of antihypertensive medication appears to be the major determinant of outcome. 47 In patients with asthma, however, additional issues related to various pharmacologic agents should be considered.

Beta-Blockers

Some caution should be used when introducing beta-blockers to patients with asthma owing to concerns regarding both unopposed bronchoconstrictive signals and therapeutic response to $\beta2$-agonists. Furthermore, beta-blockers are not generally recommended as monotherapy for the treatment of hypertension in patients with most conditions, although there may be specific indications for patients with congestive heart failure who have arrhythmias or who have had myocardial infarction. 3, 4 Beta-blockers may be either nonselective, targeting both the $\beta1$ and $\beta2$ adrenergic receptors, or relatively cardioselective, predominantly targeting the $\beta1$ receptor. Selective beta-blockers differ in their relative potency against $\beta1$ and $\beta2$ receptors, and their selectivity may be decreased at higher doses. Asthma exacerbations and even fatal outcomes have been reported after treatment of glaucoma with eyedrops that contain nonselective beta-adrenergic blockers.48, 49 A metaanalysis of randomized, blinded, placebo-controlled trials reported relatively small but significant declines in FEV1 in patients who had received short-term treatment with a selective or nonselective beta-blocker, but a significant increase in symptoms was reported only in patients who received nonselective blockers.50 A subgroup of patients did have a decline in FEV1 of 20% or more after short-term exposure to selective betablockers. A decrease in the response to shortacting $\beta2$ agonists (SABAs) was noted, with selective beta-blockers blunting the response and nonselective blockers abrogating the response.50 Long-term exposure to beta-blockers is associated with a lower risk of bronchospasm than short-term exposure. In clinical practice, betablockers have been used in patients who had disease that was stable, who did not have evidence of reduced FEV1, did not increase use of SABAs, and did not have an increase in symptoms with continued treatment. 9, 51

Nevertheless, the use of beta-blockers in patients with unstable disease or those with severe airway obstruction requires vigilance.

Angiotensin-Converting-Enzyme Inhibitors

As is the case in the general population of patients with hypertension, angiotensin-converting-enzyme (ACE) inhibitors are useful in patients with asthma and hypertension—they are not contraindicated. However, clinical confusion regarding asthma control can arise during treatment, because an ACE inhibitor-related cough may develop in exposed patients. 52 The incidence of this side effect is unclear, ranging from 2.8 to 40% depending on ethnicity, genotype, presence of underlying cardiovascular disease, methodology of assessment, and the specific ACE inhibitor used. 52-56 ACE inhibitors have also been associated with escalating severity of asthma in some patients with hypertension. 57 In a case-control trial involving patients with hypertension and asthma, ACE inhibitors were associated with increased asthma morbidity, including increased use of SABAs, increased emergency-department visits or hospitalizations, and increased use of systemic glucocorticoids. 9 Given that ACE inhibitors are considered to be a major drug class for the treatment of hypertension, clinicians should be alert to the fact that the use of these drugs can be deleterious in a minority of patients with asthma.

Angiotensin-Receptor Blockers

Angiotensin-receptor blockers (ARBs) may be the preferred drugs that act on the renin-angiotensin system for use in patients with asthma who have hypertension. Levels of circulating angiotensin II and renin were found to be increased in patients with severe asthma during exacerbations as compared with those without exacerbation. 58 Experimental infusion of angiotensin II also led to a decrease in FEV1 and an increase in symptoms of chest tightness or cough in patients with mild asthma. 58 Inhibition of angiotensin II type 1 receptors has resulted in slight abatement in bronchial hyperresponsiveness. 59 ARBs appear to target pathways that would address both hypertension and asthma. ARBs do not appear to result in either cough or increased airway responsiveness, even in patients who are unable to take an ACE inhibitor. 60,61

Calcium-Channel Blockers

There are theoretical benefits associated with the use of calcium-channel blockers in patients with asthma who have hypertension. This class of medication decreases smooth-muscle contraction; alleviates the bronchoconstriction that may occur in response to a variety of stimuli, including certain antigens, exercise, histamine, and cold air; and induces mild bronchodilation. 62 In clinical practice, however, calcium-channel blockers have not been shown to have a salutary effect on asthma outcomes. 63,64 Nonetheless, given their physiological profile and efficacy, calcium-channel blockers are a favored treatment for persons with asthma who have hypertension. 3,4,65,66

Thiazides

Low-dose thiazides, used alone or in combination with other agents, such as calcium-channel blockers, are often prescribed for the treatment of hypertension.67 In asthma, high doses of a β2 agonist can be associated with hypokalemia, which appears to be more severe in patients who take diuretics and are thus subject to the resultant arrhythmogenic potential.68 For a patient with asthma and hypertension who is receiving diuretics as well as a β2 agonist, the addition of a glucocorticoid or theophylline may further enhance the risk of hypokalemia.

Pharmacologic Treatment of Asthma in Patients with Hypertension

Hypertension is a leading cardiovascular complication of the use of systemic glucocorticoids.69 Since persons with asthma who have hypertension often have a severe asthma phenotype and receive long-term or high-dose treatment with systemic glucocorticoids, blood-pressure control may become an issue. Similarly, frequent use of SABAs as a rescue medication is also of concern with respect to cardiovascular risk.70 Adjusting pharmacologic management in this patient population to minimize the required dosages of systemic glucocorticoids and SABAs is therefore of particular importance. Approaches to the treatment of severe, difficult-to-treat asthma have recently been reviewed.21 Current biologic therapies predominantly target the type 2 high-inflammation endotype, but agents for the treatment of the type 2 low-inflammation endotype are also under investigation.21,71

Obstructive Sleep Apnea

Obstructive sleep apnea is associated with hypertension and is thought to promote the inflammatory cascades involved in both cardiovascular disease and asthma.72 The intermittent hypoxia that typifies obstructive sleep apnea activates pathways mediated by nuclear factor kappa lightchain enhancer of activated B cells (NF-κB), releasing mediators integral to systemic inflammation and vascular pathology.19,72 Although the effect of treatment for obstructive sleep apnea on blood-pressure control has yet to be clearly delineated,3,4 treatment appears to effect a reduction in inflammatory markers that may contribute to the development of hypertension.72

Obesity

The global obesity epidemic has coincided with the growing prevalence of hypertension and asthma.6,73 In the United States, two thirds of the population are considered to be overweight or obese.74 For every 5% increase in weight, the risk of hypertension rises by 20 to 30%.75 Obesity has also been directly associated with asthma severity.76,77 Conversely, weight loss improves multiple outcomes in obese persons with asthma.78 Thus, weight loss is important for obese persons who have both asthma and hypertension. However, the treatment of obesity is extremely difficult, requiring a multidisciplinary approach.79

Lifestyle

Trends in the general population, including increases in dietary salt intake, ingestion of calories from sources other than vegetables and fruits, obesity, and reductions in physical activity have likely contributed to the increased prevalence of hypertension and, possibly, of asthma. 6, 73 Patients with both conditions may benefit from lifestyle modifications, including changes in diet, restriction of salt intake, and increased physical activity. 80-82 Weight loss can effect decreases of approximately 1 mm Hg in blood pressure for each kilogram lost as well as reductions in carcologic interventions has the potential to reduce systolic blood pressure by 3 to 8 mm Hg and diastolic blood pressure by 1 to 4 mm Hg. 4,83-85 A healthful diet and exercise can also have a favorable influence on asthma outcomes, even in nonobese patients. 86 Stress has been linked to increased susceptibility to a variety of diseases, including hypertension and asthma. 87-89 Although controlled outcome studies of the effect of stress reduction on patients with hypertension and asthma are lacking, it would be of interest to investigate nonpharmacologic approaches, such as transcendental meditation and mindfulness-based stress reduction.

Conclusions

Persons with both hypertension and asthma represent an important subset of the globally escalating number of persons with cardiovascular and airway disease. Experimental evidence from studies in animals and observations in human disease highlight smooth-muscle activation, vascular dysfunction, and systemic inflammation as unifying characteristics within this cohort. The influence of type 1 and type 17 inflammatory pathways is noteworthy for increasing the severity of disease in patients who have hypertension and severe asthma who are also obese and have metabolic dysfunction. The treatment of patients with both hypertension and asthma should involve an integrated approach that includes pharmacotherapy and changes in lifestyle. A combination of interventions—including diet modification, salt restriction, stress reduction, and weight loss—that target shared pathophysiological mechanisms may be of value for these patients. (Treatment of Hypertension in Patients with Asthma, *N Engl J Med.*, 2019 Dec. 5, 381 (23))

译文：

哮喘患者的高血压治疗

哮喘和高血压是常见慢性病,均可致病、致死并造成经济负担。据估计,全世界有 3 亿人患哮喘,预计到 2025 年将增至 4 亿。每年约有 25 万人死于哮喘,其中许多被认为是可以避免的 1。美国有超过 8% 的成人患哮喘,其中女性、少数族裔和经济状况不佳的人群所占比例较高。2013 年与哮喘相关的医疗支出估计为 800 亿美元 2。高血压合并哮喘造成额外的健康负担。在全球范围内,高血压是心血管疾病和死亡最常见的可缓控危险因素。据估计,全球有 8.74 亿成人的收缩压高于 140 mmHg 3,4,而且和哮喘一样,高血压的患病率、相关费用、发病率和死亡率持续增加 5。2015 年,收缩压升高是全球可预防死亡的首要促发原因 6。美国约 1/3 的成人患高血压 7。由于现行高血压指南纳入了支持较低治疗阈值的新证据,因此我们认为患高血压的人数将增加,随之而来的费用也将增多 3。

哮喘患者比非哮喘患者更易患高血压,这与常规危险因素无关 8。高血压诊断与哮喘加重相关 9,并且肺功能下降与心血管死亡率增加相关 10。鉴于肺功能受损和心血管功能受损之间的双向关系,对哮喘患者进行高血压治疗和控制的理据充分。虽然血压控制对哮喘的影响基本未获研究,但当收缩压降至 130 mmHg 以下时,心血管疾病引起的死亡风险会降低 11-14。在本综述中,我们讨论了高血压与哮喘潜在的机制关联,高血压和哮喘的相互影响,以及成人哮喘患者的高血压治疗方法。

高血压和哮喘之间的机制关联

易感因素(遗传特征、压力和年龄)、饮食和生活方式的选择以及炎症机制都是高血压哮喘表型的促发因素。这些因素可能对理解病情的发展具有重要意义(图 1)。

全身性炎症是高血压和哮喘造成疾病负担的基础 15。目前普遍认为炎症既是哮喘发病机制的基础 16,也是高血压及其不良后果产生的关键因素 17,18。一项在中年哮喘患者中进行的大型横断面研究表明,在第一秒用力呼气量(FEV1)值越低的人群中,高血压患病率越高,并且高血压患病风险随着 FEV1 值的降低而增加 19。此外,C 反应蛋白水平(与白细胞介素-6 和高血压相关的全身炎症标志物)与 FEV1 的减少率相关 20。这些发现可能暗示了高血压和哮喘之间的相互关系,而在这一相互关系中,全身炎症影响两种疾病的病程。

目前认为哮喘表现为两种内型:2 型高炎症和 2 型低炎症。这些亚型主要根据其基础机制进行定义,而基础机制主要由参与应答的 T 细胞或固有淋巴细胞和细胞因子决定 21。每个内型可以进一步细分为多个表型,并根据临床表现、病理检查结果和生物标志物(趋化因子)加以区分(表 1)。由于目前缺乏统一的哮喘分型标准,因此 2 型高炎症和 2 型低炎症内型的患病率估计值不一致,但每种内型在哮喘患者人群中约占一半 16。

重症哮喘研究计划(Severe Asthma Research Program)开展了多项研究,依据临床特征、生物标志物、细胞特性、肺功能、特应性状态、疗效、基因表达和合并症等变量的分层分析结果,哮喘患者分成不同群组 22-24。值得注意的是,两项纳入高血压为变量的研究表明,高血压与典型的 2 型低炎症内型的哮喘特征存在共分离 22,23。与 2 型高炎症内型患者(551 例患者中的 50 例[9%])相比,具有 2 型低炎症内型特征(老龄、哮喘较迟发、体质指数[BMI]较高、较严重和特应性低)的患者也较易患高血压(175 例患者中的 48 例[27%])22。另外一项基于临床特征以及血液和痰液炎性细胞指标的研究表明,按疾病严重程度、老龄、疾病较迟发、BMI 较高和对糖皮质激素耐药性较严重进行区分的群组中,高血压发生率显著较高:31%(164 例患者中的 51 例)vs. 11%(259 例患者中的 28 例)23。这些观察结果提示,2 型低炎症通路可能提供了将这两种疾病的病理关联机制。

高血压合并哮喘患者的炎症程度反映了两者的共同作用。高血压使 T 细胞偏向促炎(1 型辅助 T 细胞[Th1 细胞])表型,表现为干扰素-γ 应答增加和 2 型辅助 T 细胞(Th2 细胞）应答降低 25。哮喘中，气道高反应性增强和重度哮喘与干扰素-γ 水平升高相关 26。相应地，高血压中，干扰素-γ 和 Th1 细胞极化导致血压升高及引起后遗症 17。动物和体外模型研究中，也证明白细胞介素-17 在高血压发生及其相关性终末器官损伤中发挥重要作用。

白细胞介素-17 通过增加介质（包括白细胞介素-6、CXCL8、CXCL10 及 C 反应蛋白）释放在血管平滑肌细胞中诱导促炎表型 27。动物研究表明，抗白细胞介素-17 治疗和基因缺失可以减少高血压发生 17,27。白细胞介素-17 的作用在一些重度哮喘患者中也很明显，其白细胞介素-17 水平升高与中性粒细胞浸润、气道高反应性和对糖皮质激素不敏感相关。在这些患者中，白细胞介素-17 能够诱导肺结构细胞和气管平滑肌分泌促炎性细胞因子，包括肿瘤坏死因子 α、白细胞介素-1β、粒细胞集落刺激因子、白细胞介素-6 及趋化因子 CCL11（嗜酸性粒细胞趋化因子）和 CXCL8（白细胞介素-8），这些细胞因子在气道炎症和重塑中起重要作用 28,29。令人惊讶的是，在一项试验中，靶向白细胞介素-17 未能改善重度哮喘患者的症状 30；然而，一项亚组分析发现某些患者 FEV1 下降的情况高度可逆，病情因此得以改善［哮喘控制问卷（Asthma Control Questionnaire）反映出病情改善］的患者。白细胞介素-17 在平滑肌细胞收缩中发挥功能部分程度上提高了亚组的应答 31。

实验证据支持以下观点，白细胞介素-6 水平升高可以通过与转化生长因子 β 的相互作用来驱动 CD4+ T 细胞分化，从而促进向 17 型辅助细胞（Th17 细胞）偏移，导致调节性 T 细胞（Treg 细胞）减少。Treg 细胞在高血压发生过程中起保护作用，而高血压的发生与白细胞介素-10 27 的生成部分相关，此外 Treg 细胞在调节哮喘发生过程中也起着至关重要的作用 32。

干扰素-γ、白细胞介素-17 和白细胞介素-6 之间的相互作用有可能影响高血压和哮喘的疾病表现（图 2）。这些细胞因子共同刺激炎症，导致平滑肌激活和纤维蛋白生成，而这些是气道和心血管疾病的基础。因此，同时患高血压和哮喘的人群似乎构成了一个难治性亚组，患者的终末器官损伤风险增加。

肥胖和代谢功能障碍

白细胞介素-6 水平升高和全身炎症可导致代谢功能障碍，从而增加高血压和哮喘相关性发病率。白色脂肪组织中的脂肪细胞和炎性巨噬细胞分泌促炎细胞因子（尤其是白细胞介素-6），在哮喘发病机制中具有重要作用 33；哮喘中，白细胞介素-6 似乎是代谢功能障碍和重度疾病的生物标志物 34。人类和动物研究已经确定白细胞介素-6 水平升高与高血压相关，这些研究表明白细胞介素-6 水平升高与疾病发生相关 35,36。

平滑肌重塑和血管生物学

平滑肌重塑很大程度由炎性细胞因子驱动，是哮喘和高血压的重要因素 37-39。气道周围平滑肌细胞增生和异常挛缩在哮喘患者气道阻塞中起重要作用。同样，平滑肌细胞的异常收缩和增殖也被认为是与高血压相关的血管重塑和内皮细胞异常的表现。

遗传因素明显影响哮喘和高血压的表现，然而其相互关系复杂且难以解析。据报告，在高血压合并哮喘患者中，平滑肌细胞上的 β 肾上腺素受体存在多态性，但这种多态性在疾病表现中发挥重要作用的原因是调节对拮抗剂和激动剂的应答，因此多态性对治疗结局的影响可能大于对疾病原因的影响 40。相比之下，目前认为血管平滑肌细胞表型受局部环境影响而发生的改变在高血压、哮喘及动脉粥样硬化的发病机制中起关键作用 41。

膳食盐

长期以来，人们一直认为膳食盐摄入量与心血管疾病的发生相关。早期关于高盐摄入量高与高血压之间关系的观察结果已经被细化，确定了盐敏感亚群和盐不敏感亚群 42。我们已经观察到肾脏、交感神经系统和血管系统对盐的反应 43。摄盐后，免疫系统可能发挥作用。例如，Th17 细胞似乎能参与调节盐摄入量与高血压之间的关系 17,18,27。在小鼠模型中，高盐饮食通过减少肠道微生物组中鼠乳杆菌促进 Th17 细胞的生成。盐敏感性高血压可通过对 Th17 细胞具有调节作用的鼠乳杆菌来预防。有证据提示，上述预防作用与鼠乳杆菌产生的色氨酸代谢产物有关 44。据报告，摄入高盐饮食的健康人也出现乳杆菌水平下降，Th17 细胞水平升高，血压升高，所有这些观察结果均支持高盐摄入在人类炎症中起一定作用的观点 44-46。目前缺乏关于哮喘患者膳食盐含量的类似信息。

哮喘合并高血压患者的疾病管理

将哮喘与高血压的关联机制不仅具有理论意义，而且对疾病治疗和管理也具有重要意义。哮喘患者的高血压治疗应该多管齐下，包括控制两种疾病、治疗合并症及改变生活方式（图 3）。

哮喘患者的高血压药物治疗

在美国心脏病学院-美国心脏学会工作组（American College of Cardiology-American Heart Association Task Force）成人高血压预防、检测、评估和治疗临床实践指南的 2017 年报告中，高血压被分类为 1 期（130~139／80~89 mmHg）或 2 期（>140／>90 mmHg）3。对于患心血管疾病或者有心血管疾病高危因素的 1 期患者和所有 2 期患者，建议采用药物治疗。需要注意的是，2017 年的指南降低了高血压的诊断阈值，从而引发了巨大的争议，因为新的阈值将高血压的诊断比例从 32% 提高到了 46%。

高血压治疗一般可达到怎样的效果？这一效果可能对哮喘患者产生怎样的影响？迄今，在接受抗高血压四大类一线药治疗的高血压患者之间，全因死亡率无显著差异（表 2）。结局的主要决定因素似乎是降压程度，而非抗高血压药的选择 47。然而，对于哮喘患者，我们还应考虑与各种药物相关的其他问题。

β 受体阻滞剂

考虑到无对抗的支气管收缩信号和 β2 受体激动剂的疗效，哮喘患者应慎用 β 受体阻滞剂。此外，大多数情况下并不推荐将 β 受体阻滞剂用于高血压的单药治疗，然而对于有心律失常或曾有心肌梗死的充血性心力衰竭患者，可能有特定的适应征 3,4。β 受体阻滞剂可以是非选择性的，即同时靶向 β1 和 β2 肾上腺素能受体，也可以具有相对的心脏选择性，即主要靶向 β1 受体。选择性 β 受体阻滞剂对 β1 和 β2 受体的相对效力不同，并且在较高剂量时它们的选择性可能降低。据报告，患者使用含有非选择性 β 肾上腺素能受体阻滞剂的眼药水治疗青光眼后出现哮喘加重，甚至死亡 48,49。对随机、盲法、安慰剂对照试验进行的一项荟萃分析报告，在接受选择性或非选择性 β 受体阻滞剂短期治疗的患者中，FEV1 有相对小幅但显著的下降，但非选择性 β 受体阻滞剂治疗的患者出现症状显著增多 50。一个患者亚群接受选择性 β 受体阻滞剂短期治疗后，FEV1 下降 ≥20%。我们观察到患者对短效 β2 受体激动剂（SABA）的应答下降，其中选择性 β 受体阻滞剂使应答减弱，而非选择性 β 受体阻滞剂使应答消失 50。长期使用 β 受体阻滞剂的支气管痉挛风险低于短期使用。在临床实践中，β 受体阻滞剂已经被用于病情稳定、无 FEV1 下降证据、SABA 用量未增加并且持续治疗期间症状未增多的患者 9,51。尽管如此，对于病情不稳定的患者或者重度气道阻塞患者，应慎用 β 受体阻滞剂。

血管紧张素转化酶抑制剂

与一般的高血压患者人群情况相同，血管紧张素转化酶抑制剂（ACE）对哮喘合并高血压患者有用，哮喘合并高血压并非禁忌症。然而，因为 ACE 抑制剂用药患者可能出现与 ACE 抑制剂相关的咳嗽，治疗期间的哮喘控制是一大临床难题 52。这一副作用的发生率尚不清楚，取决于族群、基因型、基础心血管疾病、评估方法和具体使用 ACE 抑制剂，发生率在 2.8%~40%之间 52-56。ACE 抑制剂也与一些高血压患者的哮喘逐渐加重相关 57。在高血压合并哮喘患者中进行的一项病例对照试验表明，ACE 抑制剂与哮喘发病率增加（包括 SABA 用量增加、急诊就诊或住院增加以及全身性糖皮质激素用量增加）相关 9。鉴于 ACE 抑制剂被视为治疗高血压的主要药物类别，因此临床医师应注意，使用这些药物可能对少数哮喘患者有害。

血管紧张素受体阻滞剂

对于哮喘合并高血压患者，血管紧张素受体阻滞剂（ARB）可能是作用于肾素-血管紧张素系统的首选药物。与非加重期间相比，我们观察到重度哮喘患者加重期间的循环血管紧张素 II 和肾素水平升高 58。实验性输入血管紧张素 II 还会导致轻度哮喘患者 FEV1 降低，以及胸闷或咳嗽症状增加 58。对血管紧张素 II 1 型受体的抑制作用导致支气管高反应性轻度减弱 59。ARB 所靶向的通路似乎可同时治疗高血压和哮喘。ARB 似乎既不会导致咳嗽，也不会增加气道反应性，而且即使在不能服用 ACE 抑制剂的患者中也是如此 60,61。

钙通道阻滞剂

理论上，钙通道阻滞剂对哮喘合并高血压患者有益。此类药物可减少平滑肌收缩，缓解对各种刺激（包括某些抗原、运动、组胺和冷空气）做出应答时可能出现的支气管收缩，并且诱导支气管轻度扩张 62。然而，我们尚未在临床实践中证明钙通道阻滞剂对哮喘结局有益 63,64。尽管如此，鉴于钙通道阻滞剂的生理特性和疗效，它们是哮喘合并高血压患者的首选治疗 3,4,65,66。

噻嗪类药物

低剂量噻嗪类药物（单独使用或与钙通道阻滞剂等其他药物联合使用）常用于高血压的治疗 67。哮喘的治疗中，高剂量 β2 受体激动剂可能与低钾血症相关，而低钾血症在使用利尿药的患者中似乎更为严重，因此有可能导致心律失常 68。对于接受利尿药和 β2 受体激动剂治疗的哮喘合并高血压患者，加用糖皮质激素或茶碱可能进一步增加低钾血症风险。

高血压患者的哮喘药物治疗

高血压是接受全身性糖皮质激素治疗后的首要心血管并发症 69。由于哮喘合并高血压患者往往具有重度哮喘表型,并接受长期或高剂量的全身性糖皮质激素治疗,因此血压控制可能成为一个问题。同样,频繁使用 SABA(作为挽救药物)也与心血管风险相关 70。因此,调整该患者人群的药物治疗,从而尽可能降低所需的全身性糖皮质激素和 SABA 剂量具有特别重要的意义。最近有文献综述了重度难治性哮喘的治疗方法 21。目前的生物制剂主要针对 2 型高炎症内型,但用于治疗 2 型低炎症内型的药物尚在研究中 21,71。

阻塞性睡眠呼吸暂停

除了与高血压相关,阻塞性睡眠呼吸暂停被认为可促进与心血管疾病和哮喘均相关的炎症级联反应 72。间歇性缺氧作为阻塞性睡眠呼吸暂停的典型特征可激活由活化 B 细胞核因子 κ 轻链增强子(NF-κB)介导的通路,从而释放全身炎症和血管病变过程中的必需介质 19,72。虽然我们尚未明确阻塞性睡眠呼吸暂停治疗对血压控制的影响 3,4,但该治疗似乎可减少可能促发高血压炎症标志物 72。

肥胖

全球范围内肥胖的流行与高血压和哮喘患病率的上升同时发生 6,73。美国有 2 / 3 的人口属于超重或肥胖 74。体重每增加 5%,患高血压的风险就增加 20% ~ 30% 75。肥胖也与哮喘的严重程度直接相关 76,77。减重可以改善肥胖哮喘患者的多种结局 78。因此,对于哮喘合并高血压的肥胖者而言,减重具有重要意义。然而,肥胖的治疗极其困难,需要应用多学科方法 79。

生活方式

大众的生活方式(包括膳食盐摄入量增加,从蔬菜和水果以外的其他来源摄入热量及肥胖、体育活动减少)可能导致了高血压和哮喘患病率的增加 6,73。改变生活方式对上述合并症患者可能有益,包括改变饮食、限制盐摄入量和增加体育活动 80-82。减重产生的效果是,体重每减轻 1 kg,血压可降低约 1 mmHg,此外心血管原因死亡率也会降低。上述每种非药物干预措施都有可能使收缩压降低 3 ~ 8 mmHg,舒张压降低 1 ~ 4 mmHg 4,83-85。健康饮食和锻炼也可能对哮喘结局产生有益影响,即使对非肥胖患者也是如此 86。压力与多种疾病的易感性增加相关,其中包括高血压和哮喘 87-89。虽然目前缺乏探讨减轻压力对于高血压合并哮喘患者的影响的对照研究,但非药物疗法(例如超越冥想和基于正念的减压)值得探讨。

结论

全球的心血管和呼吸道疾病患者不断增多,高血压合并哮喘患者是其中的一个重要亚群。来自动物研究的实验证据和人类疾病观察结果表明,平滑肌激活、血管功能障碍和全身性炎症是这一人群的共同特征。1 型和 17 型炎症通路产生的影响值得关注,对于肥胖且有代谢功能障碍的高血压合并重度哮喘患者,这些炎症通路可加重病情。高血压合并哮喘患者的治疗应采用包括药物治疗和改变生活方式在内的综合方法。针对共同病理生理机制的联合干预措施（包括饮食调整、限盐、减轻压力和减重）对这些患者可能有益①。

参考文献（略）

注：省略图表

Exercise

1. Read the sample of "Review Article" and analyze its contents and structure. Recognize the signal markers and sentence patterns to realize its contents. Note the use of tenses for different contents in the writing.

2. Translate the following sentences in "Review Article" into English.

1）本综述探索了有关癌症基因组（cancer genomes）的系统性测序（systematic sequencing）的经验，讨论了基因组测序的临床应用现状及潜在的前景，并反思了将基因组测序与精准癌症医学（precision cancer medicine）大规模整合（large-scale integration）的前景和挑战。

2）耐药性（resistance）问题仍然是当今癌症治疗面临的最大挑战。有大量的癌症患者，同样也有多种潜在的耐药机制（underlying mechanism），因为每种肿瘤都有自身定义的一系列特征，这些特征决定了肿瘤的进展，并最终导致死亡。

3）虽然有确凿的疫苗接种记录（solid vaccination record），但极少时候也发现青少年中腮腺炎的爆发（outbreak of mump）。这就突出了监测所有年龄组疾病爆发的必要性，并说明爆发可能系原本高效的疫苗产生的保护作用减弱（waning of protection）所导致。

4）尽管关于特定基因与特定疾病的关联性研究取得了长足进步，但是确立这些基因中单个变体（variants）的因果作用仍具困难，许多疑似罕见遗传病（rare genetic diseases）的患者还没有明确的诊断。

5）然而，神经科学家和心理学家已经开始着手研究新技术用以克服这些挑战。这些新方法正被用于这样一个愿景，即对人类记忆进行有目的性的编辑，目标是减少因创伤事件记忆（memories of traumatic events）导致的情感后果，减轻吸毒成瘾者因毒品暗示（drug cues）产生的渴望（cravings）或加强教育。

---

① 本译文基于"NEJM 医学前沿"，http://www.nejmqianyan.cn/article/YXQYra1800345，最后登陆时间：2020 年 6 月 19 日。

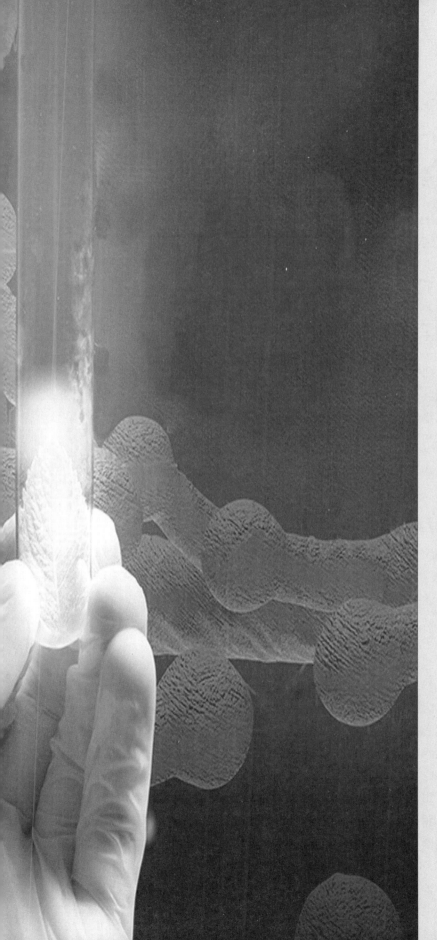

第

8

章

病例报告

8.1 何谓病例报告

病例报告（case report）又称个案报告，是报告临床罕见病例或新发现病例的医学论文。被报告的病例常是临床上罕见的、特殊的，或是认识不清的、新近发现的病例。因此，病例报告对于认识临床上的少见病、发现和掌握疾病诊治过程中的特殊性都有积极意义，并为进一步研究这些疾病提供了临床资料。

8.2 病例报告的写作指要

病例报告一般包括四部分：引言（introduction）或背景（background）、病例介绍（case presentation）或病例报告（case report）、讨论（discussion）和结论（conclusion）。有些期刊还会要求增添一段文献综述。不同期刊对病例报告的格式要求略有不同，因此，投稿前应阅读目标期刊的投稿说明和已发表的病例报告。

8.2.1 引言

8.2.1.1 引言的内容与结构

引言应说明病例报告的背景；介绍病例要处理的问题；在必要处引用相关文献；强调病例报告的目的与意义，以及病例报告的特殊性，如：罕见病例、首例报告、新发病例等。引言通常会在结尾用一句话叙述病患及其遭遇的基本情况。

例1

Background

Trazodone, a triazolopyridine derivative, is a second-generation antidepressant, with a unique chemical structure and a pharmacological profile slightly different from other antidepressants [1]. **It belongs to** the class of serotonin receptor antagonists and reuptake inhibitors (SARIs) [2]. Trazodone can cause reversible AV block [3] and life-threatening arrhythmias that can be fatal. （介绍宏观背景，给出已知信息，指出存在的问题。） **However,** it has been reported to have less severe cardiotoxic effects compared to other antidepressants [4]. To the best of our knowledge, there are no reported cases of omeprazole potentiating the cardiotoxic effect of trazodone. （引用文献，指出研究空白） **We report** a case of 54-year-old man with second degree AV Mobitz type 1 block and syncope after taking a double dose of trazodone while on omeprazole. （最后一句叙述病患及其遭遇的基本情况）

说明：段落首先介绍宏观背景，给出已知信息，然后过渡到存在的药物安全性问题，以及研究空白，最后一句结尾句叙述病患及其遭遇的基本情况。

译文：

背景

三唑并吡啶衍生物曲唑酮是第二代抗抑郁药，有独特的化学结构和与其他抗抑郁药略微不同的药理特性。其类属于 5-羟色胺受体拮抗剂和再摄取抑制剂（SARIs）。曲唑酮可引起可逆性房室传导阻滞和危及生命的心律不齐。然而，据报道，与其他抗抑郁药相比，它对心脏的毒性作用较轻。据我们所知，目前还没有关于奥美拉唑加重曲唑酮心脏毒性作用的报道。在此，我们报告一位 54 岁男性病例，在同时服用奥美拉唑与双倍剂量的曲唑酮后，出现二度莫氏 1 型房室传导阻滞和晕厥。

8.2.1.2 引言的写作要点

1. 突出病例报告的必要性和重要性

例2

Drug-induced thrombocytopenia can result in severe, progressive reductions in platelet counts with resultant sequelae of bleeding [1-3]. In order to associate thrombocytopenia with a medication, recent exposure to the medication should be documented in addition to an investigation excluding all other causes of thrombocytopenia. Identification of drug-induced thrombocytopenia **is important** as the condition is reversible upon discontinuing the medicine [4, 5].

说明：通过引用文献，突出病例报告的重要性和必要性；标记语… is important…，表示重要性。用一般现在时态描述。

译文：药物诱导的血小板减少症可导致血小板计数出现严重的进行性减少，并导致出血后遗症。为了弄清楚血小板减少症与药物使用的关联，除了调查排除血小板减少症的所有其他原因外，还应记录近期该药物的使用情况。药物诱导的血小板减少症的鉴定很重要，因为停药后病情可逆。

2. 介绍病例报告的内容

例3

We report a case of 54-year-old man with second degree AV Mobitz type 1 block and syncope after taking a double dose of trazodone while on omeprazole.

说明：一般在引言的最后一句介绍病例报告的目的，标记语 We report a case of…。

译文：本文报告了一位 54 岁男性病例，在同时服用奥美拉唑与双倍剂量的曲唑酮后，出现二度莫氏 1 型房室传导阻滞和晕厥。

3. 引言的常用表达

… is common, but… is rare.

We report / present one patient with…

We report one (rare) case of…

… is not fully understood / … remains controversial.

No active treatment of… has been advised.

8.2.2 病例报告

8.2.2.1 病例报告的内容与结构

这是病例报告的主体和核心部分。病例报告要清楚地交待病程的必要细节,包括病人的发病、发展、转归及随访的结果等。切忌将原始病历照搬,避免使用各种非客观性、各种怀疑或推测性语句。因病例报告所撰写的是罕见的或是有特殊意义的病例,故应详细描述有特殊意义的症状、体征、检查结果、治疗方法,突出重点。

描述病史时,要交待清楚发病时间 (onset time)、主诉 (chief complaint) 及病情经过 (disease progress)。对反复发作性疾病和先天性疾病要重视既往史和家族史。外伤患者要写明受伤情况。实验室检查及影像学检查通常只列阳性的和必要的阴性结果。无相关意义的其他阴性结果可省略。对有特殊意义的阳性结果要注意前后对比。手术治疗要说明手术名称、术前处理 (preoperative management)、术中发现 (intraoperative finding)、术后处理 (postoperative management) 和术后反应 (postoperative reaction)。治疗结果既要说明疗效,又要说明副作用。

例4

Case Report

A 54-year-old Hispanic man, former smoker, with dyslipidemia, coronary artery disease, and anxiety disorder, **presented to** the emergency room **following an episode of** lightheadedness and syncope as he came out of the bathroom on the morning of admission. (患者基本情况、主诉及入院原因). He **denied** palpitations, dyspnea, chest discomfort, vertigo, nausea, or vomiting. He had an episode of lightheadedness a week **prior to presentation**. He was **taking** trazodone 50 mg **daily**, omeprazole 20 mg daily, and simvastatin 20 mg at bedtime. He **doubled the dose of** trazodone 50 mg the night prior to presentation to calm his anxiety. (用药史) **On admission**, pulse was 65 / minute, irregular and blood pressure was 163 / 116 mm Hg with no orthostatic hypotension. (生命体征) An **electrocardiogram revealed** sinus rhythm at 60 beats per minute, second-degree Mobitz type 1 atrioventricular (AV) block with 5:4 AV conduction, ventricular rate of 52 / minute, narrow QRS, and a normal QTc of 434 milliseconds (Figure 1). **Telemetry revealed** frequent 8:7, 7:6, 5:4, 4:3 AV conductions recurring after every few beats of normal AV conduction (Figure 2). Basic metabolic panel, thyroid-stimulating hormone, and chest radiograph **were normal**. A **transthoracic echocardiogram revealed** aortic valve sclerosis. Lyme disease titer **was negative**, which was tested given his history of hunting in the woods 8 months prior to presentation. (检查结果). **In view of** the probability of omeprazole potentiating trazodone accumulation, both medications **were discontinued**. By the 3rd day of medication discontinuation, **all symptoms had resolved** and the frequency of Mobitz type 1 AV block had decreased to once per hour (Figure 3). (对患者的处理及转归)

说明:病例报告部分首先介绍了病人的基本情况,疾病发生、发展史,用药史;其次介绍了病人的体格检查结果、干预措施与治疗转归。

译文:

病例报告

一位 54 岁的西班牙裔男性,有吸烟史,患血脂异常、冠心病和焦虑症,入院当天早上从浴室出来时头晕和晕厥发作,随后到急诊室就诊。患者否认心悸、呼吸困难、胸部不适、眩晕、恶心或呕吐症状。就诊前一周,患者有过一次头晕发作。每日就寝前服用曲唑酮 50 毫克,奥美拉唑 20 毫克,和辛伐他汀 20 毫克。为了缓解焦虑,就诊前一晚患者服用了双倍剂量的曲唑酮。入院时脉搏不规则,65 次/分钟,血压 163/116 毫米汞柱,无直立性低血压。心电图显示窦性节律为 60 次/分钟,二度莫氏 1 型房室(AV)传导阻滞,AV 传导为 5:4,心室速率为 52 次/分钟,QRS 波变窄,QTc 值正常(434 毫秒)(图 1)。心电遥测显示每几次正常 AV 传导后就会频繁出现 8:7、7:6、5:4、4:3 这样的 AV 传导(图 2)。基础代谢检测组合,促甲状腺激素和胸部放射检查结果均显示正常。经胸超声心动图显示主动脉瓣硬化。莱姆病滴度检测结果为阴性,进行该项检查的原因是就诊前 8 个月患者有过丛林狩猎史。鉴于奥美拉唑会增强曲唑酮积蓄,两种药物均已停用。停药第 3 天,所有症状均得到缓解,莫氏 1 型 AV 传导阻滞的频率已降至每小时一次(图 3)。

8.2.2.2 病例报告的写作要点

这一部分描述病例的病史(history)、体格检查(physical examination)、实验室检查(laboratory tests)和影像学检查(imaging)、治疗(treatment)和随访(follow-up)。

1. 入院原因和主诉摘要

例5

A 25-year-old African American woman **presented** to the emergency department **with** a chief complaint of generalized nonpruritic maculopapular rash.

译文:一名 25 岁的非洲裔美国妇女来急诊科就诊,主诉全身非瘙痒性黄斑丘疹。

2. 病程进展和药物治疗

例6

The rash **was** initially confined to the right antecubital fossa but spread diffusely across the entire body over the course of 2 days. The patient **had** no other complaints and was otherwise in her usual state of health. The patient **had** started taking azithromycin 5 days prior to admission for a tooth extraction. She **was** not taking any other medication.

说明:患者病程进展和药物治疗遵循逻辑顺序和时间顺序。使用表示时间的词语,比如 initially, days, prior to… 时态为一般过去时。

译文:皮疹最初局限于右侧肘前窝,但在 2 天内扩散到全身。该患者没有其他不适,一般身体状况正常。患者入院前 5 天因为拔牙而开始服用阿奇霉素,除此之外无其他药物史。

3. 生命体征及体格检查结果

例7

There was no history of any recent illnesses or sick contacts. **Vitals were within normal limits**. Skin **examination was significant for** generalized petechiae and ecchymoses sparing her head and face. The patient **did not have signs or symptoms of** major bleeding.

说明:生命体征及体格检查结果常用 there be 句型,用一般过去时。

译文:无近期疾病发作或病患接触史。生命体征在正常范围内。皮肤检查发现除头部和脸部外,全身有明显瘀点和瘀斑。该患者无大出血的体征或症状。

4. 辅助检查结果

例8

Blood culture **was negative for** bacterial infection. A blood smear **was performed and ruled out** drug-induced thrombotic microangiopathy. **Bone marrow core biopsy and aspirate smears showed** increased megakaryocytes, myeloid cell hyperplasia, and left-shifted myeloid maturation. **There were no** sideroblasts or increase of blasts, lymphocytes, or plasma cells. **Flow cytometry of bone marrow revealed** no significant immunophenotypic abnormalities.

说明:报告检查结果用一般过去时。标记语有 was negative for…, ruled out, showed / revealed, … were…等。

译文:血液培养显示无细菌感染。进行了血液涂片检查,排除了药物引起的血栓性微血管病。骨髓活检和穿刺涂片检查显示巨核细胞增多、髓样细胞增生和左移性髓样成熟。铁粒母细胞,无母细胞、淋巴细胞或浆细胞未见增多。骨髓流式细胞术未发现明显的免疫表型异常。

5. 治疗用药情况

例9

Azithromycin **was discontinued**. Dexamethasone 40 mg IV daily and intravenous immunoglobulin (IVIG) therapy **were administered.**

说明:描述治疗用药情况用一般过去时和被动语态,药物使用方法标记语如… were administered…。

译文:停用阿奇霉素。每天地塞米松 40 mg 静脉注射和静脉注射免疫球蛋白(IVIG)治疗。

6. 病史、病因、治疗的常用表达

The temperature peaked / dropped to…

A woman / man aged… was admitted with… / for…

… deteriorated…

… complained of…

… were / appeared (ab)normal.

No abnormality was found on…

... was（were）not remarkable / insignificant.

... showed / revealed（ab）normal.

... was（were）（not）detected / noted.

... was diagnosed as having / suffering...

... was given the diagnosis of...

... received...orally

... was subjected to...（a treatment / operation, etc.）

... tolerated the procedure quite well.

... may induce / cause..., induces / causes / leads to / brings about...

... may be due to...

... may be responsible / accountable for...

Once... is diagnosed, the treatment is to... by...

Clinical improvement can be expected within... but full recovery may take...

... indicate a poor / promising outlook.

8.2.3　讨论与结论

8.2.3.1　讨论与结论的内容与结构

　　讨论部分是病例报告最重要的部分,通常也是期刊判定病例是否值得发表的关键章节。叙述内容可从引言已提到的信息开始,着重于为何该病例值得注意及其引发的问题。然后简介同样主题的既有文献,如果期刊要求文献回顾为独立章节,则放在讨论之前。接着讨论病患的主要情况、已有的相关理论和研究发现,整个综述应着重于病例引发疑惑的主要原因以及最主要的挑战。最后将病例与文献联系,阐明本病例与目前对该问题的认知是否一致,以及本病例的证据对未来的临床实践有何价值与贡献。

例10

Discussion

In 2008, trazodone was still **commonly recommended as** an antidepressant [5] and sleep aid [6]. The current clinical use is mainly as a sleep aid [7]. Trazodone is an antidepressant, anxiolytic, hypnotic of the SARIs class [2], predominantly blocking postsynaptic 5-hydroxytrytamine（5-HT2A）receptors with mild presynaptic inhibition of 5-HT reuptake, and an alpha-1 adrenergic blocker causing postural hypotension. In spite of minimal anticholinergic muscarinic receptor blocking action, trazodone-induced 1st degree AV block and complete heart block **have been reported** [1,3,8], the putative mechanism being the blocking of 5-HT4 receptors which facilitate L-type calcium2+ ion-mediated AV nodal conduction [9,10]. **The maximum recommended dose of** trazodone for depression is 400 mg / day and for insomnia it is 50-100 mg / day. The dose of 100 mg / day taken the night before presentation was well within the therapeutic dose limits, yet he developed frequent second-degree Mobitz type 1 AV blocks with syncope. Trazodone is metabolized by liver microsome-based cytochrome P450 enzyme CYP3A4 [7] into m-chlorophenylpiperazine (m-CPP) [11]. Trazodone toxicity in our patient **was attributed to** long-term concomitant use of omeprazole, which is a CYP3A4 inhibitor [12], causing trazodone accumulation. (引用相关文献,介绍已有的理论和研究发现) From among the numerous potential mechanisms of trazodone-induced syncope, **the most probable cause** in this patient was documented frequent second-degree Mobitz type 1 block. Other trazodone-induced mechanisms of syncope were **less likely** because there was no evidence of postural hypotension, atrial fibrillation, ventricular ectopy, or torsades de pointes. (将病例与文献联系,通过分析推理来阐明这个病例与目前认知的异同) To the best of our knowledge, this is **the first report** of reversible second-degree Mobitz type 1 AV block with trazodone, likely potentiated by concomitant use of omeprazole. (突出病例报告的新颖性,标记语:… **this is the first report of** …)

说明: 讨论部分首先简介了相关文献。接着讨论病患的主要情况、已有的理论和研究发现。最后将病例与文献联系,阐明本病例与目前认知的异同。

译文:

讨论

曲唑酮在 2008 年仍然是被普遍推荐使用的抗抑郁药和睡眠辅助药。目前临床主要用于辅助睡眠。曲唑酮是 SARI 类抗抑郁药、抗焦虑药和催眠药,主要通过轻度抑制 5-HT 突触前再摄取来阻滞突触后 5-羟色胺(5-HT2A)受体;曲唑酮还是一种 α1-肾上腺素能阻滞剂,可引起体位性低血压。尽管抗胆碱能毒蕈碱受体的阻滞作用很小,但曲唑酮诱导的一度 AV 传导阻滞和完全性心脏传导阻滞在文献中已有报道,推测可能是因为 5-HT4 受体被阻滞,而该受体可促进 L 型钙离子介导的房室结传导。曲唑酮治疗抑郁的最大推荐剂量为 400 毫克/天;治疗失眠的最大推荐剂量为 50~100 毫克/天。患者就诊前一晚按 100 毫克/天的剂量服用,属于正常治疗剂量范围,但他却频繁出现二度莫氏 1 型 AV 传导阻滞伴晕厥。曲唑酮通过肝微粒体细胞色素 P450 酶 CYP3A4 代谢为间氯苯哌嗪(m-CPP)。我们在此报道的病例中,曲唑酮中毒是由于同时服用 CYP3A4 抑制剂奥美拉唑,导致曲唑酮积蓄。在曲唑酮诱发晕厥的众多潜在机制中,最可能的原因是频发的二度莫氏 1 型 AV 传导阻滞。曲唑酮诱发晕厥的其他机制可能性较小,因为没有体位性低血压、房颤、室性异位或尖端扭转的证据。据我们所知,这是首次报道的由曲唑酮引起的可逆性二度莫氏 1 型 AV 传导阻滞,可能系同时服用奥美拉唑引起。

结论部分是对病例报告的总结,应涵盖病例报告的核心要点。此外,结论部分还可以论述给临床医生、科研人员的建议或推荐方案。目前多数报告将此部分纳入讨论部分,不单设结论部分。

例11

Conclusions

Due diligence and meticulous attention to detail needs to be exercised to uncover drug interactions as potential causes of lethal and nonlethal patient symptomatology, as in this case of syncope caused by concomitant use of trazodone and a widely prescribed medication, omeprazole.

说明:该结论对病例报告进行总结,并分析本病例报告的证据对未来临床实践的启示。

译文:

结论

本文报告了曲唑酮与一种广泛使用的处方药奥美拉唑同时服用引起晕厥的病例。报告提示药物相互作用可能是患者致死和非致死症状的潜在原因,因此,临床实践中需全面问诊并关注细节。

8.2.3.2　讨论与结论的写作要点

讨论部分应突出该病例报告系首例报告;其次将文献与本病例联系起来分析比较;然后分析原因,得出结论性意见。

1. 突出病例报告的新颖性

例12

To the best of our knowledge, these are the first published reports of SMECE associated with the activating mutation in the BRAF gene.

说明:突出病例报告的新颖性,标记语为…the first published reports。时态为一般现在时。

译文:据我们所知,这是 SMECE 与 BRAF 基因激活突变关联性的首次报道。

2. 本病例与文献报道的相关性

例13

BRAF V600E mutation is a **novel** independent molecular prognostic marker in the risk evaluation of thyroid cancer [8, 9]. It **is associated with** a poor clinical outcome with more aggressive, invasive tumors that are less 131I avid. This **is consistent with** the clinical presentation of both our patients.

说明:将本病例与相关文献比较,使用标记语为…be consistent with…。时态为一般现在时。

译文:BRAF V600E 突变是甲状腺癌风险评估中的一种新型独立分子预后标志物。它与对 131 碘摄取较差而更具攻击性和侵袭性肿瘤的不良临床结局有关。这与我们报道的两例患者的临床表现一致。

例14

Our findings **are contrary to** a recent paper that reported five patients with SMECE who did not have BRAF mutation by next-generation sequencing [2]. **However**, none of these cases had distant metastasis. **Thus**, although *BRAF* activating mutation may not be present in all SMECE thyroid cancers, it may be a marker for a subset of SMECE tumors that demonstrate more aggressive behavior, as seen in PTC.

说明:将文献与本病例联系起来分析比较,标记语为… are contrary to…,表示"二者不一致",然后分析原因,得出结论性意见,使用标记语 however, thus。表达结论用一般现在时。

译文:我们的发现与最近的一篇论文报道相反,该论文报道了 5 名 SMECE 患者下一代测序中无 BRAF 突变发现。但是,这些病例均无远处转移。因此,尽管 BRAF 激活突变可能并不存在于所有的 SMECE 甲状腺癌,但它可能是 SMECE 肿瘤亚型的标志物,如 PTC 所示,该亚型的表现更具攻击性。

3. 总结归纳特殊经验或新观点

例15

This observation **opens potential treatment options for** this poorly responsive thyroid cancer.

说明:总结归纳在诊治特殊病例过程中的新经验或新观点,使用标记语… opens potential treatment options for…。用一般现在时描述。

译文:该观察结果为治疗效果较差的甲状腺癌提供了潜在的治疗选择。

4. 讨论的常用表达

In conclusion / To sum up / Therefore…

When…, … is warranted

One lesson of this case is…

… should be remembered when…

It is important to emphasize that…

Any… should be carefully observed for…

8.3 病例报告示例

例16

Sclerosing peritonitis presenting as complete mechanical bowel obstruction: a case report

Introduction

Abdominal cocoon syndrome or sclerosing peritonitis is a rare condition that refers to total or partial encapsulation of the small bowel by a fibrocollagenous membrane resulting in partial or complete mechanical bowel obstruction [1]. The condition is mostly seen in patients with end-stage renal failure requiring peritoneal dialysis (PD) but it can occur without any pre-existing risk factor [2]. We report a case of an adult patient who presented with features of acute intestinal obstruction on a background of intermittent attacks of partial bowel obstruction for the past 6 to 8 months. He was treated surgically followed by a short course of steroids for his relapsing attack of partial bowel obstruction.

Case presentation

A 46-year-old Asian man presented with 5-day history of absolute constipation, vomiting, and central abdominal pain. Besides that he had no known comorbidities and an unremarkable family history. In the past he had similar complaints for which he was managed conservatively. At 4 months prior to his presentation he had a computed tomography (CT) scan of his abdomen for similar symptoms; the CT scan showed ileal thickening for which he was given empirically a 3-month course of anti-tuberculosis therapy (ATT) but his symptoms did not resolve.

On this occasion, an examination revealed a dehydrated patient with pulse of 104 beats/minute and blood pressure (BP) of 130/70 mm. He had abdominal distention and central abdomen tenderness and hyperactive gut sounds. A digital rectal examination was unremarkable and so was a systemic examination. His baseline workup showed blood urea nitrogen of 32 mg/dl and creatinine of 1.2 mg/dl.

Contrast-enhanced CT (CECT) of his abdomen showed mildly dilated thickened jejunal and ileal loops which were encased in a thick fibrocollagenous membrane pushed in the center of his abdominal cavity with collapsed loops of large bowel; the findings were suggestive of sclerosing encapsulating peritonitis/abdominal cocoon (Fig. 1 a, b).

He was initially managed conservatively with intravenously administered fluids and nasogastric tube which resulted in some relief of his symptoms and his pulse of 74 beats/minute. Because of the fact that he came from an area where tuberculosis (TB) is a highly prevalent disease and previously he was empirically treated for abdominal TB, he underwent colonoscopy which showed normal terminal ileum, colon and rectum (Fig. 2 a, b).

His case was discussed in a multidisciplinary team, which included a radiologist, gastroenterologist, and gastroenterology surgeon, and he was planned for diagnostic laparoscopy, followed by laparotomy in case it was not abdominal TB or a malignancy requiring medical management only.

A diagnostic laparoscopy using 10 mm infraumbilical port in a vertical fashion, confirmed that entire small bowel was encapsulated in membrane and it was all plastered in the center of his abdomen. Hence, a decision was made for midline laparotomy, in which thickened sclerosing membrane encapsulating loops of small bowel was removed and whole small bowel was freed and run until ileocecal junction. His stomach appeared thickened while his colon appeared grossly unremarkable (Fig. 3 a, b).

Postoperatively he remained well and was discharged on fourth postoperative day, when he was tolerating an oral soft diet. However, he was again admitted on third day after his discharge with complaints of vomiting and relative constipation. He was kept nil by mouth (NPO) and on parenteral nutrition. Along with conservative management he had a short course of hydrocortisone 50 mg thrice daily for 7 days, which was tapered off later; he responded very well and he was discharged in a stable condition on oral soft diet with normal bowel movements.

He was followed up in clinic after 10 days and he was tolerating a soft diet with normal bowel movements; his stitches were removed in clinic. Later, a histopathology report showed fibrocollagenous tissue with mild chronic inflammation and mild patchy increase in IgG4-positive plasma cells.

He was seen twice as an out-patient at 3-month intervals and appeared asymptomatic; he was advised to have further follow-up only if required.

Discussion

Sclerosing encapsulating peritonitis was first described more than a century ago and was initially termed peritonitis chronica fibrosa incapsulata to describe the membrane encasing the intestine; it has since also been named 'icing sugar', fibroplastic peritonitis, and cocoon abdomen. Sclerosing encapsulating peritonitis has been classified as primary and secondary based on whether it is idiopathic or has a definite cause.

The etiology of the primary form is uncertain with various hypothesis, although it is probably caused by a subclinical peritonitis leading to the formation of a cocoon [3,4,5]. Cytokines and fibroblasts probably influence the development of peritoneal fibrosis and neoangiogenesis in some way [6].

Secondary sclerosing peritonitis, which is more common, has many causes. The predominant cause of sclerosing peritonitis is PD. Patients on PD are predisposed to developing peritoneal deterioration after prolonged exposure to PD fluids and subsequent bacterial peritonitis [7, 8]. Other known causes include: recurrent peritonitis; abdominal TB; autoimmune diseases such as systemic lupus erythematosus, peritoneal shunts, and sarcoidosis; and ovarian disorders such as rupture of dermoid cyst.

The results of baseline investigations are often similar to those found in small bowel obstruction, such as dehydration and decrease in oral intake, and there may be electrolytes imbalance and acute kidney injury with raised creatinine. Abdominal X-ray findings are non-specific. CECT is a useful tool for preoperative diagnosis of abdominal cocoon [9, 10]. The imaging features are, however, not pathognomonic. CT findings of a membrane enveloping loops of small bowel were seen in some paraduodenal hernias, abdominal cocoon, and in peritoneal encapsulation. However, the clinical and pathological features of these entities are different.

Diagnostic laparoscopy is generally confirmatory and rules out other causes [11, 12]; however, laparoscopy is not helpful in management of this condition. Differential diagnosis includes peritoneal encapsulation, which was described as a developmental anomaly where the whole of the small bowel is encased in a thin accessory membrane. The clinical symptoms of this condition differ from those of abdominal cocoon syndrome, in that the patients are mostly asymptomatic and the findings are incidental and late in life.

Treatment, as in this case, is excision of membrane and releasing loops of bowel [7, 13]. Bowel resection is generally not required. However, there is scarce mention in the literature of patients who relapse with symptoms after excision of membrane. As in our case, a short course of steroids may be helpful in relapsing cases because of the inflammatory nature of this condition; however, evidence of use of steroids in cases of sclerosing peritonitis needs to be established.

Conclusion

Sclerosing peritonitis is one of the rare causes of complete mechanical bowel obstruction and it should be in the differential diagnosis when no other obvious cause of bowel obstruction is found. Surgical exploration in which dense sclerosing membrane over the bowel is removed and bowel is straightened is the treatment of choice up until now. A short course of steroids is also helpful in the postoperative period.

References (omitted)

(Sclerosing peritonitis presenting as complete mechanical bowel obstruction: a case report, *Journal of Medical Case Reports*, 2019 October 17, 13)

译文:硬化性腹膜炎表现为完全机械性肠梗阻:一例病例报告

引言

腹茧症或硬化性腹膜炎是一种罕见病,是指纤维胶原膜将小肠完全或部分包裹而导致部分或完全机械性肠梗阻[1]。该病多见于需要腹膜透析(PD)的终末期肾衰竭患者,但也可以在无任何预先危险因素情况下发生[2]。我们报告一例成年患者,该患者在过去 6 至 8 个月内有过几次间歇性部分肠梗阻发作,表现出急性肠梗阻的特征。患者因部分肠梗阻复发而接受了手术治疗,随后使用了短疗程的类固醇治疗。

病例介绍

一位 46 岁的亚裔男子主诉有 5 天的绝对便秘、呕吐和腹部中央痛病史。除此之外,无已知合并症,无明显家族史。患者曾经有过类似的主诉,接受过保守治疗。就诊之前四个月因类似症状行腹部 CT;CT 扫描显示回肠壁增厚,因此接受了 3 个月的经验性抗结核治疗(ATT),但症状未能得到缓解。

这次就诊,检查发现患者有脱水现象,脉搏为 104 次 / 分钟,血压(BP)为 130 / 70 mmHg。患者有腹胀、腹部中央压痛和肠鸣音亢进。直肠指检和全身检查均无异常。基线检查显示血尿素氮为 32 毫克 / 分升,肌酐为 1.2 毫克 / 分升。

腹部增强 CT(CECT)显示,空肠和回肠环有轻度扩张增厚,被一层增厚的纤维胶原膜包裹,腹腔正中受压,大肠环塌陷。该发现提示硬化性包裹性腹膜炎 / 腹部茧(图 1a,b).

静脉内输液和鼻胃插管对患者进行初始保守治疗,症状有所缓解,脉搏 74 次 / 分钟。由于患者来自结核病(TB)高度流行的地区,并且以前曾接受过腹部 TB 的经验性治疗,因此对患者进行了结肠镜检查,结果显示末端回肠、结肠和直肠均正常 (图 2a,b)。

多学科团队对该病例进行了讨论,团队成员包括放射科医生、胃肠病医生和胃肠外科医生。安排了患者进行诊断性腹腔镜检查,如果排除腹部结核或仅需要内科治疗的恶性肿瘤,则行剖腹手术。

诊断性腹腔镜检查以垂直方式使用 10 mm 的脐下端口,检查证实整个小肠都被包裹在膜中,并且全部粘连位于腹部正中。因此,决定行正中线剖腹手术,切除包裹小肠环的增厚硬化膜,游离整个小肠,直至回盲肠交界处。患者的胃壁显示增厚,而肉眼观察结肠无异常 (图 3a,b)。

患者术后情况良好,可以耐受口服软质饮食,于术后第四天出院。但是,出院后的第三天因呕吐和相对便秘再次入院。禁食 (NPO),给予胃肠外营养。给予保守治疗加上 50 mg 氢化可的松,每日 3 次,疗程为 7 天,之后逐渐减量。治疗效果非常明显,出院时情况稳定,能进食软性食物,排便正常。

10 天后门诊随访,患者能耐受软质饮食,排便正常。门诊行手术缝线拆除。随后,组织病理学报告显示纤维胶原蛋白组织有轻度慢性炎症,并伴有 IgG4 阳性浆细胞内轻度斑片状增加。

患者每隔 3 个月两次门诊随访,无症状表现;因此建议患者只在必要时进一步随访。

讨论

硬化包裹性腹膜炎早在一个多世纪前就被首次描述,最初被称为慢性纤维化包膜性腹膜炎,用以描述肠膜包裹;后来一直被称为"糖粉"、纤维增生性腹膜炎和茧腹。硬化包裹性腹膜炎根据其是否具有特发性或明确病因分为原发性和继发性两种。

原发性硬化包裹性腹膜炎病因学尚不确定,有各种假说,可能是由导致茧形成的亚临床腹膜炎引起[3,4,5]。细胞因子和成纤维细胞可能以某种方式影响腹膜纤维化发展和新生血管生成[6]。

继发性硬化腹膜炎更为常见,有多种病因。硬化性腹膜炎的最主要原因是腹膜透析。长时间暴露于 PD 液继而引起细菌性腹膜炎后,腹膜透析患者更易发生腹膜恶化[7,8]。其他已知发病原因包括:复发性腹膜炎、腹部结核、自身免疫性疾病 (如系统性红斑狼疮)、腹膜分流和结节病以及卵巢疾病 (如皮样囊肿破裂)。

基线调查的结果通常与小肠梗阻 (例如脱水和进食减少) 中发现的结果相似,并且可能存在电解质失衡和急性肾脏损伤伴肌酐升高。腹部 X 线检查结果无特异性。CECT 是术前诊断腹茧症的有效手段[9,10]。然而,成像特征不具有病理性。在一些十二指肠旁疝,腹部茧和腹膜包囊中发现了小肠膜包膜环的 CT 表现。但是,这些病种的临床和病理特征并不相同。

诊断性腹腔镜检查通常用于排除其他病因,具有确诊价值[11,12];但是,该检查无助于腹茧症的治疗。鉴别诊断包括腹膜包囊,这是一种发育异常,被描述为整个小肠被包裹于一层薄薄的附膜中。腹膜包裹与腹茧症的临床症状有所不同,患者大多无症状,发现偶然且时间较晚。

本病例中,治疗方法是切除肠膜并游离肠环[7,13]。通常不需要肠切除。然而,在文献中很少有膜切除后症状复发的报道。如本报道病例所示,由于该病的炎症特点,短期类固醇治疗可能对复发病例有益。但是,在硬化性腹膜炎病例中使用类固醇尚需进一步证实。

结论

硬化性腹膜炎是机械性完全肠梗阻的罕见原因之一,在无其他明显肠梗阻病因的情况下应将其纳入鉴别诊断。迄今为止首选治疗方法是手术探查,通过手术切除肠上的致密硬化膜拉直大肠。术后短期使用类固醇也有益处。

参考文献(略)

注:省略图表

Exercise

1. Read the sample of "Case Report" and analyze its contents and structure. Recognize the signal markers and sentence patterns to realize its contents. Note the use of tenses for different contents in the writing.

2. Translate the following sentences in "Case Report" into English.

1)31 岁男性,是一名办公室职员,来急诊室就诊,主诉腹部正中疼痛(central abdominal pain)2 天,并伴有恶心(nausea),呼吸困难(dyspnea)但无呕吐(vomiting)。

2)在最近几年中,患者多次发作了轻度的类似疼痛,被诊断为肠易激综合症(irritable bowel syndrome),无手术史,慢性疾病和恶性肿瘤的家族史阴性。

3)腹部检查发现轻度腹胀(distended abdomen),主要在右下腹象限(right lower abdominal quadrant)有肌卫和压痛(guarding and tenderness)。触诊未发现明显的肿块或器官增大。肠鸣音(bowel sound)正常。

4)切除样本送组织病理学检查(histopathological examination),发现在肠粘膜和粘膜下层(mucosa and the submucosa)有许多大小不等的淋巴通道(lymphatic channels),有明显的炎性细胞浸润(inflammatory cell infiltration),样本中恶性细胞阴性。诊断为回肠淋巴管瘤(lymphangioma of the ileum)。

5)入院时,患者主诉持续干咳,恶心和呕吐 2 天,但无呼吸急促(shortness of breath)或胸痛。生命体征(vital signs)正常。体格检查发现患者粘膜干燥。其余部位检查基本正常。患者入院后行支持治疗(supportive care),包括 2 升生理盐水(normal saline)和治疗恶心的恩丹西酮(ondansetron)。

6)该病例报告强调了临床医生获取急症就诊患者近期旅行史或接触病患史的重要性,这样可以确保正确查明并迅速隔离(prompt isolation)具有 2019-nCoV 感染风险的病例,并有助于减少进一步传播(transmission)。

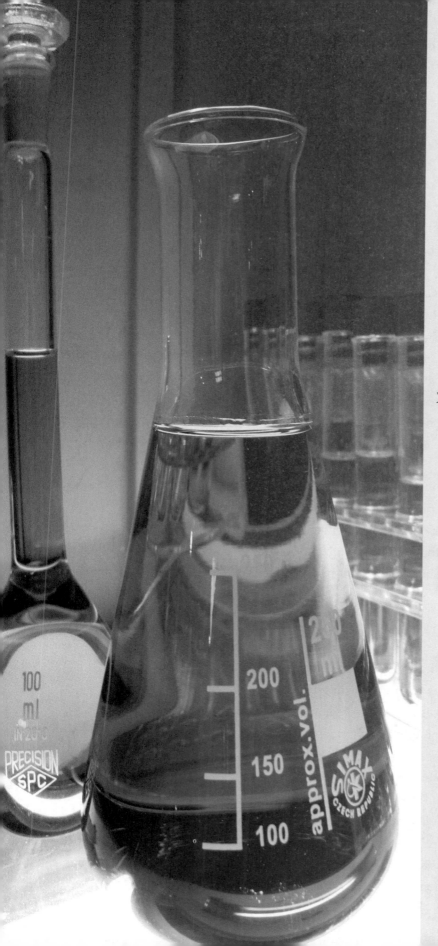

参考答案

第 2 章

1. Basic imaging features of CT in SARS were ground-glass opacities and pulmonary consolidation.

2. We randomly divided 54 healthy naive rats into three groups, with 18 in each group.

3. This study preliminarily demonstrated that using un-disinfected bottle is a major risk factor of diarrhea in infant-young children. If parents stop using bottle-feeding, the morbidity of diarrhea will be decreased by 73.7%.

4. These factors may have a significant impact on the occurrence, development and severity of pregnancy-induced hypertension and umbilical artery resistance index.

5. Acidosis is a common feature of ischemia and often leads to brain injury, however, its underlying mechanism remains ill-defined.

6. All these rabbits were separately euthanized 4, 8, and 12 weeks after the operation and then tracheal CT scanning, tracheal endoscopy, histopathological examination and scanning electron microscopic examination were performed.

7. The drug resistance of 3761 cases were monitored in this study. The primary drug resistance rate was 27.7% (958/3459) and the secondary drug resistance rate was 41.1% (124/302).

8. It is of benefit for the women with a history of recurrent miscarriage to receive progestogens for prevention and treatment of threatened abortion.

9. The characteristics of alcohol dependent patients include psychological dependence, physical dependence, withdrawal syndrome and tolerance.

10. We could not identify any predisposing factor for lactic acidosis other than renal impairment.

第 3 章

1. After treatment, the blood oxygen saturation increased.

2. Ethanol evaporates from the mixture rapidly.

3. Blood pH was measured with a radiometer capillary electrode.

4. There are still three main shortcomings: acute closure (50%), late restenosis (35%), and unsuitable treatment with PTCA (50%).

5. We performed an anterior lateral thoracotomy at the seventh intercostal space of the patient.

6. The patient was followed up after (her) discharge from the hospital.

7. Each of the 41 fecal specimens was treated as described in the text.

8. Ataxia telangiectasia may be associated with deficiency in DNA repair of the damage caused by ionizing radiation.

9. However, lipid peroxides may influence the genesis or the progress of atherosclerosis.

10. Pulse rate decreased by 40 beats/min, systolic blood pressure by 50 mmHg, and cardiac output by 18%.

11. The preparation of the cardioplegic solution should meet the following requirements: (1) a proper concentration of potassium ion must be maintained; (2) all principal electrolytes in the normal myocardium should be contained; (3) appropriate osmolarity should be sustained;and (4) the solution must be easy to prepare and stable.

12. Our approach aimed to pave the way toward a systematic unveiling of the chemical repertoire encoded by the human microbiome.

13. We recently observed bronchospastic reactions in an asthmatic patient after he ingested this drug.

14. None of the groups was found side effects.

15. Deaths within 30 days of operation were considered early mortalities, and deaths after 30 days, late mortalities.

第 4 章

1. 按主题句交代的顺序
2. 问题-答案模式
3. 按时间顺序
4. 使用连接语表明信息间关系
5. 保持一致的视角
6. 标记小主题+重复关键词

第 6 章

6.1

1. Effects of Environment in Vivo and in Vitro on the Differentiation of Mesenchymal Stem Cells of Bone into Neural Cells

2. Reno-protective Effect of Irebesartan, an Angiotensin—Receptor Antagonist, in Patients with Nephropathy Caused by Type 2 Diabetes

3. Use of Staphylococcus Aureus Conjugate Vaccine in Patients Undergoing Hemodialysis

4. Radioimmunoassay of Serum 17-OH-progesterone for Diagnosis and Treatment of Congenital Adrenal Hyperplasia

5. A Human Bi-specific Antibody Against Zika Virus with High Therapeutic Potential

6. Failure of Metronidazole to Prevent Preterm Delivery Among Pregnant Women with

Asymptomatic Trichomonas Vaginalis Infection

7. Increased Need for Thyroxine in Women with Hypothyroidism During Estrogen Therapy

8. Efficacy of Nitric Oxide, with or Without Continuing Antihypertensive Treatment, for Management of High Blood Pressure in Acute Stroke (ENOS): a Partial-factorial Randomised Controlled Trial

9. Once-weekly Dulaglutide Versus Bedtime Insulin Glargine, both in Combination with Prandial Insulin Lispro, in Patients with Type 2 Diabetes (AWARD-4): a Tandomised, Open-label, Phase 3, Non-inferiority Study

10. Targeting BCL2 with Venetoclax in Relapsed Chronic Lymphocytic Leukemia

11. Adjuvant Capecitabine for Breast Cancer after Preoperative Chemotherapy

12. Long-Term Renal Effects of Tenofovir Disoproxil Fumarate vs. Entecavir in Chronic HBV-Infected Patients

13. Predictive Value of the Urinary Dipstick Test in the Management of Patients with Urinary Tract infection-associated Symptoms in Primary Care in Indonesia: a Cross-sectional Study

14. High Intensity Focused Ultrasound Ablation Activates Anti-tumor Immunity

15. Interleukin-13 and Interleukin-18 for Regulating Expression of Nerve Growth Factor mRNA in Rats with Bronchial Asthma

6.2

1. 略

2.

1) Effects of prone positioning on survival of patients with acute respiratory failure

Background　Although placing patients with acute respiratory failure in a prone position improves their oxygenation by 60 to 70 percent of the time, its effect on survival is not known.

Methods　In a multicenter, randomized clinical trial, we compared conventional treatment (in the supine position) of patients with acute lung injury or acute respiratory distress syndrome with a predefined strategy of placing patients in prone position for six or more hours daily for 10 days. We enrolled 304 patients, 152 in each group.

Results　The mortality rate was 23.0 percent during the 10-day study period, 49.3 percent at the time of discharge from the intensive care unit, and 60.5 percent at 6 months. The relative risk of death in the prone group as compared with the supine group was 0.84 at the end of the study period (95 percent confidence interval, 0.56 to 1.27), 1.05 at the time of discharge from the intensive care unit (95 percent confidence interval, 0.84 to 1.32), and 1.06 at six months (95 percent confidence interval, 0.88 to 1.28). During the study period the mean increase in the ratio of the partial pressure of arterial oxygen to the fraction of inspired oxygen, measured each morning while patients were supine, was greater in the prone than that in the supine group (63.0±66.8 vs. 44.6±68.2, p=0.02). The incidence of complications related to positioning (such as pressure sores and accidental extubation) was similar in the two groups.

Conclusions   Although placing patients with acute respiratory failure in a prone position improves their oxygenation, it does not improve survival.

2) Effects of the combination of GLP-1 and chamomile oil on differentiation of mesenchymal stem cells into functional insulin-producing cells

Objective: To investigate the effects of the combination of GLP-1 and chamomile oil on differentiation of mesenchymal stem cells (MSCs) into functional insulin-producing cells (IPCs).

Materials and Methods: In this experimental study, adipose MSCs derived from the adult male New Zealand white rabbits were assigned into four groups: control (in which cells received no treatment); GLP-1 (in which cells were treated with 10 nM GLP-1 every other day for 5 days); chamomile oil (in which cells were treated with 100 ug/ml *Matricaria chamomilla* L. flower oil every other day for 5 days); and GLP-1+ chamomile oil (in which cells were treated with 10 nM GLP-1 and 100 μg/ml *M. chamomilla* flower oil every other day for 5 days). Characterization of isolated MSCs was performed using flow cytometry, Alizarin red S staining and Oil red O staining. The expressions of genes specific for IPCs were measured using reverse transcriptase-polymerase chain reaction (RT-PCR) assay. Insulin and the cleaved connecting peptide (C-peptide) in response to different concentrations of glucose were measured using ELISA kits.

Results: Our results demonstrated that isolated cells highly expressed MSC markers and were able to differentiate into osteocytes and adipocytes. Additionally, using GLP-1 in combination with chamomile oil exhibited higher levels of IPCs gene markers including NK homeobox gene 2.2 (*NKX*-2.2), paired box gene 4 (*PAX*4), insulin (*INS*) and pancreatic duodenal homeobox-1 (*PDX*1) as well as insulin and C-peptide secretion in response to different glucose concentrations compared to GLP-1 or chamomile oil alone (P<0.05).

Conclusion: Collectively, these findings establish a substantial foundation for using peptides in combination with natural products to obtain higher efficiency in regenerative medicine and peptide therapy.

6.3

1. 略

2.

1) The presence of a cardiovascular implantable electronic device has long been a contraindication for the performance of magnetic resonance imaging (MRI).

2) The human microbiome harbors thousands of bacterial species, varies in composition between different sites of the human body and between individuals, and has been correlated with several diseases

3) The increased risk of cardiovascular disease in people with metabolic syndrome has been well established by observational studies and meta-analyses, and considered to be partly attributable to the accompanying atherogenic dyslipidaemia, which is characterized by increased levels of triglyceride and small dense low density lipoprotein cholesterol.

4) Chemotherapy induced peripheral neuropathy remains one of the major limitations in oncology clinics due to the increasing number of cancer patients, the lack of effective treatment strategies and relapse of the disease.

5) In multicenter studies, tight glycemic control targeting a normal blood glucose level has not been shown to improve outcomes in critically ill adults or children after cardiac surgery. Studies involving critically ill children who have not undergone cardiac surgery are lacking.

6) The pathogenesis caused by these viruses in their respective host species is currently insufficiently understood, which is primarily due to the inability to obtain and keep these bat species under appropriate environmental and biosafety conditions.

7) The identification of a new therapeutic strategy to address the inflammatory and oxidative stress components of this metabolic disorder remains of great importance.

8) We hypothesized that this easily clinically identifiable cohort of patients would be the group most likely to have a favourable balance of treatment efficacy and safety and in whom tricagrelor could serve an unmet clinical need.

9) Therefore, in this study we explored the effects of TAT-Cx43 in neurons and astrocytes and compared them with those of other c-Src inhibitors currently being evaluated in clinical trials.

10) To evaluate the effect of amniotic suspension allograft in vivo, a well-established rat pain model of osteoarthritis was used to assess pain and other behavioral changes as well as cytokine levels in synovial fluid and serum.

6.4

1. 略

2.

1) In this multicenter, randomized, open-label trial, we adopted the same method and design to evaluate the same interventions, namely anticoagulant therapy with low-molecular-weight heparin. The research protocol (available online: NEJM.org) and trial design were approved by the Medical Ethics Committee of Leiden University Medical Center. The trial was funded by the Dutch Health Research Centre.

2) Participants in the study were recruited through advertisements in local newspapers and on-site recruitment. People were eligible if they were 18 to 60 years of age, working full-time and had no high-risk illnesses such as chronic cardiopulmonary disease, diabetes, or other serious conditions. Exclusion criteria were a history of immediate hypersensitivity reactions in eggs and thimerosal, or a history of influenza vaccination. Informed consent was obtained from all subjects in this study.

3) In this experimental study, 20 male New Zealand white rabbits with a mean weight of 2.5 kg, were obtained from Razi Institute, Iran. Rabbits were maintained in a chamber set at 25±1 ℃, with 12/12-hour light/dark cycles. They were placed in their cage with free access to food and water. All procedures and experimental tests were approved by the Animal Ethics Committee of Shahid Beheshti University of Medical Sciences.

4) Enrolled patients were randomly assigned, in a 1 : 1 ratio, to receive standard chemotherapy or placebo. The drugs were daunorubicin (60 mg/m² daily, administered intravenously on days 1, 2, and 3) and cytarabine (200 mg/m² daily, administered intravenously from day 1 to day 7). Mildotolin or placebo was administered in a double-blind manner (50 mg, orally twice daily) on day 8 to day 21.

5) Insulin levels in culture media were measured using rabbit insulin ELISA kit. First, cells were pre-incubated with Krebs-Ringer buffer at 37 ℃ for 2 hours. Then, cells were incubated with Krebs-Ringer buffer containing different doses of glucose (0, 15, and 30 mM) at 37 ℃ for 1 hour. Finally, culture media were collected and assessments were performed.

6) Male Wistar rats (240-300g, 8 weeks old) were randomly divided into two groups: a control (non-diabetic) group fed with a standard diet (n=6), and a diabetic group fed with a hypercaloric diet composed of 20 kcal% protein, 25 kcal% carbohydrates, and 45 kcal% fat (n=18). After 14 days, streptozotocin (STZ; Sigma-AldrichCo., StLouis, MO, USA) was injected into the caudal veins (35mg/kg body weight) of rats in diabetic group to induce T2DM. Non-diabetic rats received oral administration of the compound vehicle, which was a mixture of benzylalcohol, polysorbate80, disodium EDTA, hydroxyethyl

cellulose and water.

6.5

1. 略

2.

1) To confirm differentiation of cells treated with GLP and chamomile oil into insulin-producing cells, we measured mRNA levels of NKX-2.2, PAX4, INS and PDX1 using RT-PCR assay. Our results demonstrated that although cells treated with GLP or cells treated with chamomile oil significantly expressed NKX-2.2, PAX4, INS and PDX1, the expression of these markers was highest in cells treated with GLP+chamomile oil.

2) The catalase activity, superoxide dismutase activity and glutathione levels were significantly higher in allantoin-treated rats than in cisplatin-treated rats. The malonaldehyde levels and nitric oxide concentration of cisplatin-treated rats were higher than those of normal rats.

3) The tail withdrawal latency of cisplatin-treated (group 2) rats was significantly lower than that of normal rats (group 1), indicating development of hyperalgesia. Treatment with allantoin significantly increased the tail withdrawal latency compared to the cisplatin group.

4) CFA significantly increased the expression of NLRP3 in rat spinal cord tissues compared with the control group. However, the qRT-PCR analysis showed that after propofol treatment the expression of NLRP3 in the spinal cord tissues of CFA induced rats was significantly reduced.

5) To evaluate the function of cells, we measured C-peptide secretion by cells in response to different concentrations of glucose. As shown in Figure, no significant differences were found among different groups in the absence of glucose. Significant differences were observed in response to 15 and 30 mM concentrations of glucose.

6) The number of patients who died within 90 days was 231 in the hypothermia group vs. 247 in the normothermia group. The duration of mechanical ventilation or the length of stay in the ICU did not differ between the two groups among patients who survived or among those who died.

6.6

1. 略

2.

1) This trial demonstrates that long-term support with a left ventricular assist device resulted in substantial improvement in survival in patients with severe heart failure who were not candidates for cardiac transplantation. The patients in the medical-therapy group

received optimal medical care with digoxin, diuretics, angiotensin-converting-enzyme inhibitors, and beta-blockers from heart-failure specialists. The one-year mortality rate of 75 percent in this group exceeded the rates for the acquired immunodeficiency syndrome and breast, lung and colon cancer and was more than four times that in trials of beta-blockers.

2) We conducted a randomized trial examining the effect of coffee on insulin sensitivity using the gold-standard hyperinsulinemic euglycemic clamp in overweight Asian individuals. Consumption of 4 cups of coffee per day over 24 wk did not have a substantial effect on insulin sensitivity, measures of fasting glycemia, or other cardiometabolic biomarkers, but was associated with modest loss in FM.

3) Our study has shown that both approaches are valid treatment options, although an important clinical advantage of the endoscopic approach is the reduction in external pancreatic fistulas and hospital stay. In our view, patients with infected necrosis should be treated in tertiary referral centers by multidisciplinary teams where both the endoscopic and surgical step-up approach are available, because a combined approach might be required in some patients.

4) Our results are consistent with those from other multicenter trials involving other critically ill children. The SPECS (Safe Pediatric Euglycemia in Cardiac Surgery) trial and the CHiP (Control of Hyperglycaemia in Paediatric Intensive Care) trial showed no significant differences in ICU length of stay or mortality among children who had undergone cardiac surgery or in children who had not undergone cardiac surgery. The CHiP trial showed that among patients who had not undergone cardiac surgery, the mean 12-month health care costs were lower in the group that was assigned to a lower target blood glucose range than in the group that was assigned to conventional glycemic control, a finding that was most likely attributable to a shorter hospital stay for the index admission among those assigned to the lower target. Notably, the hospital length of stay in our trial did not differ significantly between treatment groups.

5) Previous studies have compared outcomes regarding transplants from cord-blood donors with those from other donor sources. Because of the previously reported profound effect of the presence of minimal disease before transplantation on outcomes in the context of non-cord-blood transplantation, this variable was examined closely. As with data in all retrospective analyses, our data may be subject to bias because which patients received which treatment was the result of nonrandomized selection (e.g., clinical priority).

6) A major strength of this study is its prospective design, enrolling a large cohort of children with the same generic risk from 4 countries with different infant feeding habits and following the same study protocol. Another strength is the dietary assessment method that allowed repeated measurements to capture changes in dietary habits in growing infants and young children over time prior to disease onset. The prospective design also reduced the

effect of changes in dietary habits because parents were unaware of their child's autoantibody status when the food records were collected.

7) Our study has certain limitations. First, informed consent was obtained only after hyperglycemia was confirmed, which created a delay between the onset and treatment of hyperglycemia. Second, it was not possible for the bedside team to be unaware of the study-group assignment. Concern for bias was mitigated by the explicitly defined intervention and primary outcome. Third, in order to compare two tight glucose-control targets within the range of usual care, we did not include a third group in which hyperglycemia was not treated. Thus, the two study groups had explicitly managed glucose and insulin adjustment.

8) In conclusion, the addition of an antiandrogen agent to salvage radiation therapy resulted in higher rates of overall, disease-specific, and metastasis-free survival than radiation therapy plus placebo among patients who were treated for biochemical (PSA) recurrence of prostate cancer after radical prostatectomy. The higher rate of overall survival with antiandrogen therapy than with placebo became evident in the second decade after therapy.

第 7 章

1. 略

2.

1) In this review, we explore what we have learned from systematic sequencing of cancer genomes. We discuss the current and potential future clinical applications of genome sequencing and reflect on both the promise and challenges around large-scale integration of genome sequencing into precision cancer medicine.

2) Resistance to therapy continues to be the biggest challenge in cancer today. There are as many underlying mechanisms of resistance as there are patients with cancer, because each tumour has its own defining set of characteristics that dictates tumour progression and that can eventually lead to death.

3) Outbreaks of mumps have very occasionally been seen in teenagers, despite a solid vaccination record. This highlights the need for surveillance of all age groups for disease outbreaks, and could be due to waning of protection induced by vaccines that are otherwise regarded as highly efficacious.

4) Although huge strides have been made in associating specific genes with particular disorders, establishing the causal role of individual variants within those genes remains problematic, and many patients with suspected rare genetic diseases are left without a definitive diagnosis.

5) However, neuroscientists and psychologists have begun to investigate techniques that may overcome these challenges. These new approaches are being used to address the prospect of purposefully editing human memories, with goals such as reducing the emotional consequences that stem from memories of traumatic events, diminishing cravings that are induced by drug cues in addicts or enhancing education.

第 8 章

1. 略

2.

1) A 31-year-old male, who is an office worker presented to emergency department complaining of central abdominal pain for 2 days, with nausea, dyspnea but no vomiting.

2) The patients had many attacks of similar pain but of milder intensity for the last years which was diagnosed as irritable bowel syndrome, the surgical histories were unremarkable and the family history was negative for chronic illnesses and malignancies.

3) The abdominal examination revealed a mildly distended abdomen, with guarding and tenderness mainly in the right lower abdominal quadrant. There were no any palpable masses or organ enlargement. The bowel sounds were normal.

4) The resected sample was sent for the histopathological examination which showed an evidence of numerous and variable sized lymphatic channels in the mucosa and the submucosa of the bowel, there was intense inflammatory cell infiltration and the sample was negative for malignant cells. The diagnosis was lymphangioma of the ileum.

5) On admission, the patient reported persistent dry cough and a 2-day history of nausea and vomiting; he reported that he had no shortness of breath or chest pain. Vital signs were within normal ranges. On physical examination, the patient was found to have dry mucous membranes. The remainder of the examination was generally unremarkable. After admission, the patient received supportive care, including 2 liters of normal saline and ondansetron for nausea.

6) This case report highlights the importance of clinicians eliciting a recent history of travel or exposure to sick contacts in any patient presenting for medical care with acute illness symptoms, in order to ensure appropriate identification and prompt isolation of patients who may be at risk for 2019-nCoV infection and to help reduce further transmission.